ENCYCLOPEDIA
OF WOMEN'S HEALTH
AND WELLNESS

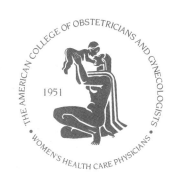

The American College of
Obstetricians and
Gynecologists

Women's Health Care Physicians

Encyclopedia of Women's Health and Wellness was developed under the direction of a panel of experts working in consultation with staff of the American College of Obstetricians and Gynecologists. Designed as an aid to patients, it sets forth current information and opinions on subjects related to women's health. The average readability level, based on the Fry formula, is grade 6–8. The information in this publication does not dictate an exclusive course of treatment or procedure to be followed and should not be construed as excluding other acceptable methods of practice. Variations taking into account the needs of the individual patient, resources, and limitations unique to the institution or type of practice may be appropriate.

Editorial Task Force
Jonathan S. Berek, MD
Sandra A. Carson, MD
Nancy Chescheir, MD
Susan Johnson, MD
Thomas Nolan, MD
Roger P. Smith, MD

Gerald B. Holzman, MD, ACOG Vice President, Education
Rebecca D. Rinehart, Director of Publications
Tatum Birdsall, Assistant Editor
Margo Harris, Senior Editor
Mary Clark, Design
Thomas P. Dineen, Manager of Production and Design

The assistance of the following ACOG staff is greatly appreciated:
Susannah Frazier, JD, Staff Attorney
Mary Hyde, MSLS, Public Services Librarian
Penny Rutledge, JD, General Counsel
Pamela Van Hine, MSLS, Director, ACOG Resource Center

Library of Congress Cataloging-in-Publication Data

Encyclopedia of women's health and wellness.
     p. cm.
    "Encyclopedia of women's health and wellness was developed by a panel of experts
working in consultation with staff of the American College of Obstetricians and Gynecologists."
    Includes index.
    ISBN 0-915473-60-7 (pbk. : alk. paper)
    1. Women—Health and hygiene—Encyclopedias. I. American College of Obstetricians
and Gynecologists.

RA778 .E583 2000
613'.04244—dc21

                                     00-029971

To order copies of this book, call 800-762-2264 ext 181 or visit the ACOG web site at <www.acog.org/books>.

CONTENTS

PREFACE

The American College of Obstetricians and Gynecologists (ACOG) celebrates its 50th year with the publication of the *Encyclopedia of Women's Health and Wellness*. This definitive guide to health care for women is itself a celebration of a field and organization that have fostered and promoted the quality of life of millions of women throughout the world.

The information in the *Encyclopedia of Women's Health and Wellness* is the result of a collaboration of experts in all areas of obstetrics and gynecology. It is much more than a compilation of material, however—it represents the collective voice of more than 40,000 obstetrician–gynecologists across the country. Each piece of information has been carefully weighed to ensure it meets certain standards: Is it accurate and based on good science? Is it appropriate to most women and practices? Can it improve the health care of women? The result is a solid base of information women can rely on to help them take an active role in their health.

The content of the *Encyclopedia of Women's Health and Wellness* evolved over time as the College's commitment to health education grew. It was originally part of the Patient Education Pamphlet series, designed to help doctors explain medical conditions and procedures to their patients. As preventive care and health maintenance became more important, topics covered health and wellness as well as disorders. The balance of these topics reflects the partnership between women and their doctors in promoting health, preventing disease, and providing good health care.

An educated woman can be more involved in her health care by partnering with her doctor to ensure her good health. The *Encyclopedia of Women's Health and Wellness* enables a woman to become familiar with her body and her physical and mental health, as well as a particular symptom or condition she may have. The first section of the book, "Women's Bodies," helps women understand how their bodies work at different periods of their lives. It sets the stage for the next section, "Women's Wellness," which focuses on a healthy lifestyle, routine care, and normal events in a woman's life. The section "Women's Health" covers specific disorders, tests, and procedures. Throughout there are references to special needs during pregnancy. Although much of the detail regarding pregnancy is covered in other ACOG publications, it was felt to be a factor key to many women and thus was included.

The information is designed for women of all ages, types, and backgrounds. It is intended for women who are healthy and want to stay that way as well as women who may have questions or concerns about their health. The *Encyclopedia of Women's Health and Wellness* can be a valuable reference to any woman as well as to her family and friends. Readers can rest assured that the information is sound, that it comes straight from the experts, and that its main goal is to improve the health of women.

INTRODUCTION

As America's leading authority on women's health care, the American College of Obstetricians and Gynecologists (ACOG) is committed to education of patients and the public. It is a serious commitment not taken lightly. For the 50 years of its existence, ACOG has been developing high-quality educational information for patients and the physicians who treat them. This book represents still another approach to meeting the goal of promoting women's health.

1

The *Encyclopedia of Women's Health and Wellness* is a consolidation of information developed to educate women about their health needs. Originally created as a part of ACOG's popular Patient Education Pamphlet series, much of the content is a distillation of material derived from hundreds of experts in the field of women's health. The information here has been reorganized to serve as a reference to women and their families who need vital, up-to-date health information.

Provide education for patients and the public

The book is organized into sections to help women find specific information that relates to them. The first section is about a woman's body—its structure and function. It creates a basis for the sections that follow. The next section, "Women's Wellness," promotes a healthy lifestyle. It is designed for women who want to know more about what they can do to maintain or improve their health. The section, "Women's Health" explains disorders and procedures. Throughout there are cross-references to related topics. The last section, "Resources," includes a complete list of resources, including websites, associations, and hotlines, for those who require more information. A glossary of terms used throughout the book also is included.

The content of the *Encyclopedia of Women's Health and Wellness* was assembled by a group of experts in various aspects of obstetrics and gynecology. It was carefully reviewed by physicians and other health professionals to ensure the information is current, accurate, and of value to women. Much of the content is based on guidelines produced by ACOG to help physicians in clinical practice. These guidelines are developed through a complex process of reviews by experts who assess the scientific evidence available to support the recommendations.

Develop and recommend practice guidelines

About ACOG

The American College of Obstetricians and Gynecologists is a nonprofit membership organization of more than 40,000 obstetrician–gynecologists. Founded in 1951, it is dedicated to the advancement of women's health through education, advocacy, practice, and research.

ACOG Fellows

All obstetrician–gynecologists (also known as ob-gyns) are doctors whose training equips them to give general care to women, as well as care related to pregnancy and the reproductive organs. Ob-gyns have graduated from college and medical school. They have completed an additional 4-year course of special training—a residency—in obstetrics and gynecology.

After residency, a doctor may be board certified by the American Board of Obstetrics and Gynecology, Inc. To become board certified, the doctor must pass two tests. The first is a written test to show that he or she has the knowledge and skills required to treat women. It covers both medical and surgical care. He or she also must show experience in treating women's health conditions for 2 years in practice after residency. At this point, he or she takes a second test—an oral exam given by a panel of national experts. This exam reviews the doctor's skills, knowledge, and ability to treat different conditions. It includes a review of cases treated during the past year. Doctors certified after 1986 must be recertified in 10 years.

There are four subspecialty areas in obstetrics and gynecology:

1. *Gynecologic oncology*— Care of women with cancers of the reproductive system

2. *Maternal–fetal medicine*—Care of a pregnant woman and the fetus before birth and for both a short period after birth.

3. *Reproductive endocrinology and infertility*—Care of women who have hormonal or infertility problems

4. *Urogynecology and pelvic reconstructive surgery*—Care of women with disorders of the genitourinary system

ACOG's Goals

The following goals have been set forth in ACOG's mission statement:

1. Define objectives for physician education in obstetrics and gynecology, determine needs, provide educational materials, and evaluate the process.

2. Develop and recommend practice guidelines for health care of women, including preventive and primary care.

3. Provide education for patients and the public in reproductive and general health care.

4. Serve as an advocate for women's health care, including access to services and to public and private sectors at all levels.

5. Evaluate, recommend, and provide services in regulatory and medical–legal aspects of women's health care.

6. Promote and support research and research training in women's health care.

7. Evaluate, recommend, and provide services in ethical and socioeconomic areas of women's health care.

8. Facilitate the evaluation of women's health care, including professional performance, through a range of peer-review activities.

9. Interrelate with other organizations and special interests within obstetrics and gynecology, other medical organizations, and health care in general.

All board-certified ob-gyns can treat patients with these disorders. Some doctors have special training that qualifies them to take a test to specialize in these areas. Such doctors often teach other doctors.

If the initials FACOG are behind your ob-gyn's name, it means that he or she is a Fellow (full member) of the American College of Obstetricians and Gynecologists (ACOG). All ACOG Fellows are board certified. Junior Fellows are currently in a training program or have recently finished training and are in practice preparing to pass the final oral exam.

Define objectives for physician education

Ob-gyns work with their patients as a partner in their health care. The health care team also may include other health professionals working with an ob-gyn:

▶ *Residents*—Provide care to patients at teaching hospitals after graduation from medical school.

▶ *Certified nurse-midwives*—Provide care focusing on pregnancy, childbirth, the postpartum period, care of the newborn, family planning, and gynecologic needs of women. They have an extra 12–18 months of education after graduating from an accredited nursing program and must pass a national certification exam.

▶ *Nurses*—Assist doctors in providing patient care and education. They have completed accredited nursing programs and passed tests.

▶ *Nurse practitioners*—Provide a wide range of services, including obtaining medical histories, performing physical examinations, and diagnosing and treating common illnesses and diseases. They are licensed registered nurses who have advanced education. In some states, they must pass a national certification exam.

▶ *Physician assistants*—Handle various medical duties. They have completed at least a 2-year educational program after college.

▶ *Dieticians*—Give advice and guidance on diet and nutrition.

▶ *Social workers*—Provide counseling and information on community services. They have studied in a special program and must be licensed.

▶ *Childbirth educators*—Teach parents-to-be about conception, pregnancy, birth, and parenting.

The advice of experts from many of these fields has been sought in compiling the information in the *Encyclopedia of Women's Health and Wellness*. It represents the full scope of today's practice of obstetrics and gynecology. As research continues and advances are made in the field, as new knowledge unfolds, ACOG will bring it to women.

Interrelate with ...
health care in general

The Future of Women's Health

The information in the *Encyclopedia of Women's Health and Wellness* reflects established medical practices developed over time that have proven to be accurate and effective. In many areas of medicine, however, mysteries remain to be explored through research. Increasingly, research efforts are being directed to women to allow scientists to learn more about how diseases affect women specifically.

Basic research leads to findings that help develop new products to detect disorders and treat them. Information is most useful and accurate when studies have certain features:

- Large number of people studied
- Controls in place to ensure objectivity
- Long length of time subjects are studied

The larger the numbers, the more controls, and the longer the time, the better the quality of information. Long-term studies can show patterns and trends that occur over time in certain groups. This helps to detect risk factors that can affect certain people. It also can help assess the effectiveness of tests to detect disorders, lifestyle changes, and treatments.

Promote and support research

Some major new research efforts are under way that show promise in providing new ways to prevent disease, detect disease in early stages, and treat patients. These programs will provide valuable information that can improve the quality of health care for women. Following are some long-term, large-scale studies that women will be hearing more about in the near future:

First and Second Trimester Evaluation of Risk (FASTER). This study is designed to show that screening for Down syndrome can be done earlier and better using a combination of ultrasound and testing of the blood of the mother (instead of blood testing alone). A total of 50,000 women will be studied over a 2-year period, and the results may affect more than 4 million women who have babies each year in the United States.

Heart and Estrogen/Progestin Replacement Study (HERS). This study of 2,763 postmenopausal women with coronary heart disease was done to assess the value of hormones (estrogen plus progestin) in preventing further heart disease. After 4 years of follow-up, researchers could not find a benefit for women who already had heart disease, although there could be some benefit for women who do not have heart disease.

Human Genome Project. This study is designed to map the genetic code of human chromosomes. There are 46 chromosomes in each cell in the human body, except for the egg and sperm, which each have 23. These chromosomes make up an estimated 80,000 genes in the human body. In all, there are 34 million chemical codes that make up the DNA that construct a person. By mapping this code, scientists can find genes that carry disease and thus identify those at risk.

The Nurses' Health Study. This study of more than 120,000 married female nurses ages 30–55 began in 1976. It was originally intended to study any link between oral contraceptive use, cigarette smoking, and risk of major illness in women. It has since been broadened to evaluate the health effects of lifestyle practices such as diet, exercise, and hormone therapy. The findings from this ongoing study have had a major impact in understanding the relationship of lifestyle factors to disease such as breast cancer, heart disease, colon cancer, fractures, and diabetes.

Postmenopausal Estrogen/Progestin Interventions (PEPI). This study was started in 1987 by the National Institutes of Health. It followed 875 postmenopausal women at seven medical centers for 3 years to assess the effect of hormone replacement therapy on risk factors for heart disease. The results are still being studied, but thus far show that hormone therapy can benefit the risk factors for heart disease.

Study of Tamoxifen and Raloxifene (STAR). One of the largest breast cancer prevention studies, STAR involves 22,000 post-menopausal women at risk for breast cancer to assess whether these treatments can help reduce the chance of developing it.

Women's Health Initiative. This long-term national health study evaluates the effect of hormone therapy, diet, and vitamin D and calcium supplements in preventing heart disease, breast and colorectal cancer, and osteoporosis in postmenopausal women. It is a 15-year project that involves more than 167,000 women ages 50–79.

Many other areas of research are still emerging. Following are some of those areas in which medical advances hold promise for the future of women's health:

▶ Vaccines to prevent infection, including sexually transmitted diseases

▶ Less invasive approaches to surgery, including alternatives to hysterectomy

▶ Health needs for aging women

▶ Screening and prevention of cancer of the cervix, ovary, and breast

▶ Using complementary and alternative medicine along with traditional treatments

▶ New approaches to treating infertility

▶ New drug therapy to treat diseases and disorders

Serve as an advocate for women's health care

As women assume a greater role in research efforts they also can become more aware and informed about their own health care. Working with their obstetrician–gynecologists, women can now truly become partners in their health care.

WOMEN'S BODIES

Women's bodies change throughout the course of their lives. These changes are natural events. Although the same changes take place in all women's bodies, each woman feels and copes with them differently.

This section is designed to acquaint women with the basic structure of the female body and how it functions. Knowing how the female body works can help women care for themselves. It also can help them be aware of what is normal—or abnormal. Although each woman is unique, all women share certain events, from puberty to menopause, that are part of life and birth.

THE FEMALE REPRODUCTIVE SYSTEM

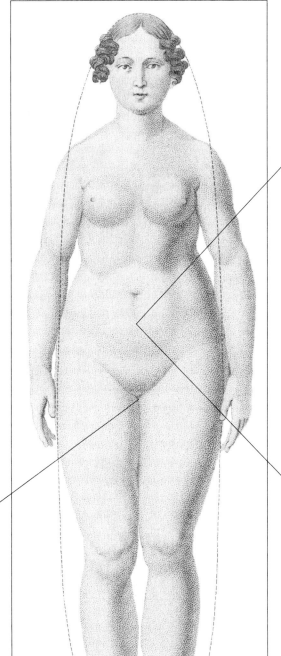

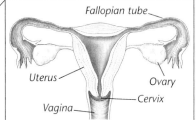

This is a frontal view of a woman's internal reproductive organs. The ovaries are glands, located on either side of the uterus, that contain the eggs released at ovulation. The fallopian tubes are a pair of ducts that connect the ovaries to the uterus.

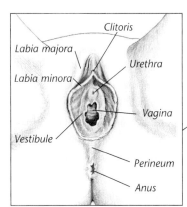

The outside of the female genital area is called the vulva. The outer lips of the vulva are called the labia majora. The inner lips are called the labia minora. The clitoris is at the top of the inner lips. For most women, the clitoris is a center of sexual pleasure. It is partly covered by a fold of tissue called the hood. The perineum is the area between the anus and vagina. The vestibule is found with the inner lips. The vagina and the urethra open into the vestibule.

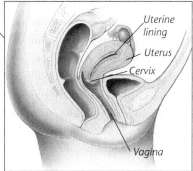

This is a cross-section of a woman's reproductive organs. The uterus is a muscular organ located in the female pelvis that contains and nourishes the developing fetus during pregnancy. The lower, narrow end of the uterus is called the cervix, which opens into the vagina. The vagina, also known as the birth canal, is a passageway surrounded by muscles leading from the uterus to the outside of the body.

THE MALE REPRODUCTIVE SYSTEM

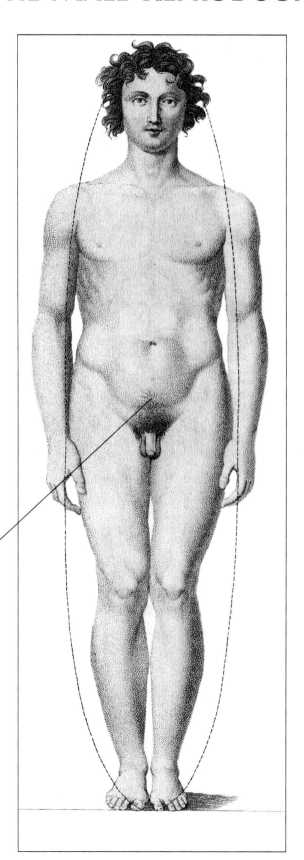

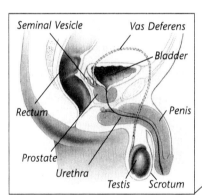

Seminal Vesicle *Vas Deferens*
Bladder
Rectum *Penis*
Prostate
Urethra *Testis* *Scrotum*

The penis is an external male sex organ that can become engorged with blood to increase its size and fullness. Sperm cells are made in a man's testes, in the scrotal sac below the penis. When the sperm cells mature, they leave the testes through small tubes called the vas deferens. As sperm move from the testes, they mix with fluid made by the seminal vesicles and prostate gland, small organs located near the bladder. The mixture of sperm and fluids is called semen. When the man ejaculates or climaxes during sex, semen moves through the urethra, a tube in the penis, into the woman's vagina.

Reprinted from J.P. Maygrier, *New Demonstrations of Childbirth*, 2nd ed. Paris: Bechet Je et Labe, 1840

▸ THE REPRODUCTIVE PROCESS

The reproductive process is controlled by hormones. During puberty, early adults have an increase in hormones that will trigger changes in them. One of these changes is the ability to reproduce. A woman begins to menstruate at this time and most women continue to do so until menopause. During the entire time a woman is having menstrual periods she can have children (unless there is a problem).

The Menstrual Cycle

Menstruation is the discharge of blood and tissue from the lining of your uterus each month. It is often called the menstrual period. Menstruation most often begins around age 12 or 13, but it may happen as early as age 8 or as late as age 16.

Menstruation is a key part of your reproductive cycle. An average menstrual cycle lasts 28–30 days, counting from the first day of one period to the first day of the next. Normal cycles can vary from 22 to 35 days.

Your brain controls your menstrual cycle. It uses messengers, called hormones, to trigger the events of your cycle.

Each month, after day 5 of your cycle, the lining of the uterus (endometrium) begins to grow and thicken to prepare for a possible pregnancy. Around day 14, an egg is released from one of your ovaries. This is called ovulation. The egg moves into one of the two fallopian tubes connected to the uterus, where it can be

Hormones

Hormones are chemicals that control when and how certain organs work. They are made by glands in the body. The menstrual cycle and pregnancy are controlled by key hormones that interact at various stages:

▸ *Estrogen and progesterone.* Produced by the ovaries, these hormones trigger changes in the lining of the uterus (endometrium), causing it to thicken during each menstrual cycle and to shed if pregnancy does not occur. Increases in these hormones when you are pregnant keep you from ovulating and having your period. During menopause, the ovaries stop making enough estrogen to thicken the lining of the uterus. This is when the menstrual periods stop.

▸ *Follicle-stimulating hormone (FSH) and luteinizing hormone (LH).* These hormones are made by the pituitary gland, a small organ located at the base of

the brain. One (FSH) causes eggs to mature, and the other (LH) causes them to be released by the ovaries.

▸ *Gonadotropin-releasing hormone.* This hormone, made by a part of the brain, tells the pituitary gland when to produce FSH and LH.

▸ *Human chorionic gonadotropin.* This hormone only occurs during pregnancy. It is made by cells that form the placenta, which nourishes the egg after it has been fertilized and becomes attached to the uterine wall. This hormone causes increases in estrogen and progesterone during pregnancy. It is the hormone that is detected in a pregnancy test.

The Menstrual Cycle

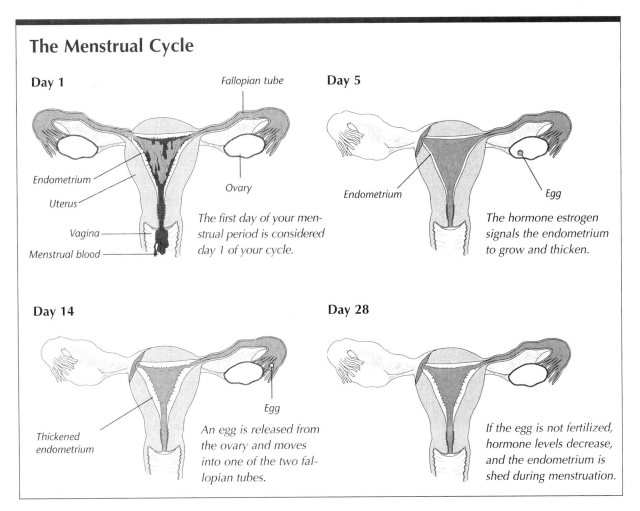

Day 1

Fallopian tube

Endometrium

Uterus

Vagina

Menstrual blood

Ovary

The first day of your menstrual period is considered day 1 of your cycle.

Day 5

Endometrium

Egg

The hormone estrogen signals the endometrium to grow and thicken.

Day 14

Thickened endometrium

Egg

An egg is released from the ovary and moves into one of the two fallopian tubes.

Day 28

If the egg is not fertilized, hormone levels decrease, and the endometrium is shed during menstruation.

fertilized by a man's sperm. If fertilized, the egg then moves into the uterus and begins to grow into a fetus.

On about day 28, if an egg is not fertilized, the endometrium is shed by bleeding. This bleeding is your menstrual period. Your period may last for 3–5 days. Some last as long as 7 days. The process of growth and thickening of the endometrium then starts again in the next cycle.

When Will It Start?

Most girls have their first period around age 12. In most cases the first period is very mild—only a few drops of blood. For some young women, menstrual periods occur monthly on a regular cycle. Others periods may not be regular. You may miss a period. Or, you may have two periods in one month. This can be normal, especially when you first start to menstruate. It takes a while for periods to get on a regular pattern.

How To Keep Track

It is a good idea to use a calendar to keep track of your periods. Mark the first day your period starts on your calendar with an "X." Count the first "X" as day 1. Keep counting the days until you have your next period. If you do this every month, you'll be able to tell how many days there are between your periods. It will help you know how many days your periods last and when your next period will start.

Ovulation

Signs that you may be ovulating include a twinge or cramp—called mittelschmerz, for "middle pain"—in your lower abdomen or back. You also may notice some breast tenderness, an increase in cervical mucus (vaginal discharge), or an increase in sexual desire around the time an egg is released.

To raise the odds of getting pregnant, sex must occur during a small window of time near ovulation. How do you know when you are ovulating? There's no foolproof method to make sure that an ovary has released an egg, but there are a number of methods that are useful. One method is to note changes in your body. Look out for telltale signs of ovulation: cramps, tender breasts, cervical mucus, or an increased desire to have sex. Other methods—especially when they are used in combination—can give you a pretty good idea:

▸ *Chart your cycle.* The simplest way to spot your fertile days is to check your menstrual calendar. First, figure out how long your cycles tend to last and pinpoint the day your next period is due to start. If your periods are regular, count back 14 days. If they are not regular, count back to the first day of your last period and divide the total. Chances are, the result will be the day you will ovulate.

▸ *Know when you are most fertile.* You also can detect ovulation by watching for changes in your cervical mucus. A few days after your period ends, rising estrogen levels trigger the production of cervical mucus. As your body prepares to release an egg, this mucus increases in volume and becomes thicker. (To get a good look at your cervical mucus, gently wipe your vaginal opening with a clean finger or a piece of toilet tissue before you urinate.) Just before ovulation, you produce more cervical mucus. It becomes clear, slippery, and stretchy—it looks and feels like a raw egg white. This

Ovulation

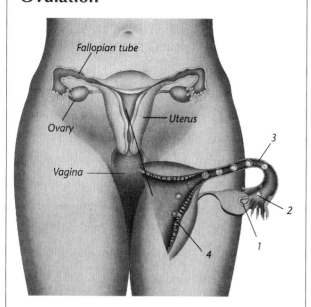

Each month during ovulation an egg is released (1) and moves into one of the fallopian tubes (2). If a woman has sex around this time, an egg may meet a sperm in the fallopian tube and the two will join (3). This is called fertilization. The fertilized egg then moves through the fallopian tube into the uterus and becomes attached there to grow during pregnancy (4).

Events That Occur at Ovulation

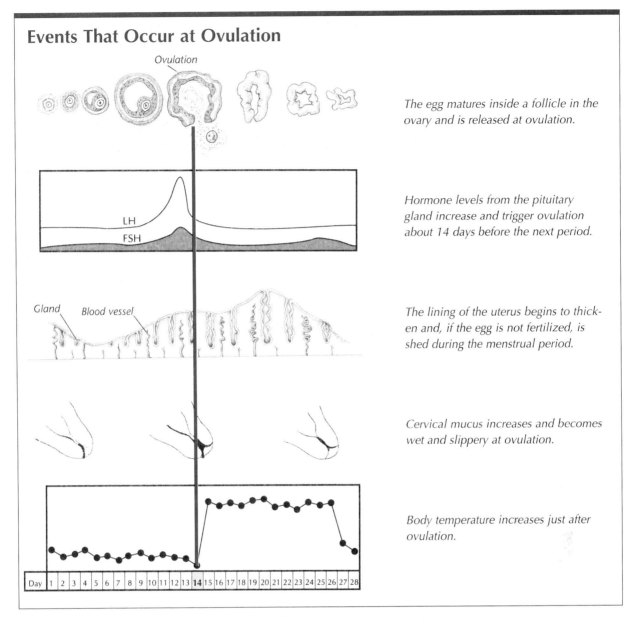

Ovulation

LH

FSH

Gland   *Blood vessel*

Day | 1 | 2 | 3 | 4 | 5 | 6 | 7 | 8 | 9 |10 |11 |12 |13 |**14**|15 |16 |17 |18 |19 |20 |21 |22 |23 |24 |25 |26 |27 |28

The egg matures inside a follicle in the ovary and is released at ovulation.

Hormone levels from the pituitary gland increase and trigger ovulation about 14 days before the next period.

The lining of the uterus begins to thicken and, if the egg is not fertilized, is shed during the menstrual period.

Cervical mucus increases and becomes wet and slippery at ovulation.

Body temperature increases just after ovulation.

kind of mucus smoothes the way for sperm to enter the uterus and swim up the fallopian tubes. Your fertile period begins with the first signs of slippery mucus and continues through the day you ovulate. After ovulation, an increase in progesterone makes cervical mucus sparse and dense. This makes it harder for sperm to swim through the cervix.

▶ *Track your temperature.* Most women's basal body temperature rises slightly—about half a degree—after they ovulate. To use this method, take your temperature at the same time every morning, before you get out of bed. Chart the temperature on a graph that also shows the days you menstruate. After you have done this for a few months, you'll begin to spot a pattern that will help you predict when you will ovulate. Your temperature will go up 24–48 hours after you ovulate.

> **Use ovulation-predictor kits.** Ovulation-predictor kits are home tests that you can buy without a prescription. They measure the level of luteinizing hormone (LH) in your urine. When LH levels rise, it means that one of your ovaries is about to release an egg.

Fertilization

The union of egg and sperm that results in pregnancy is called fertilization. Once an egg is released, it can be fertilized by a sperm.

Sperm cells are made in a man's testes, in the scrotal sac below the penis. When the sperm cells mature, they leave the testes through small tubes called the vas deferens. As sperm move from the testes, they mix with fluid made by the seminal vesicles and prostate gland, small organs located near the bladder. The mixture of sperm and fluids is called semen. When the man ejaculates or climaxes during sex, semen moves through the urethra, a tube in the penis, into the vagina. A woman does not have to climax to become pregnant.

When a man ejaculates into the vagina, sperm move up through the cervix, into the uterus, and out into the fallopian tubes. Sperm live 2–3 days or longer. If a sperm joins with an egg in one of the tubes, fertilization occurs.

Sperm cells are made all the time. Some couples worry that having sex too often—such as every day—will reduce the number of sperm and make it harder for the woman to become pregnant. Daily intercourse should not be a problem if the man has produced enough sperm. The sperm count is the number of active sperm in a milliliter (less than a half teaspoon) of semen. A normal sperm count is between 20 million and 250 million per milliliter.

Most couples are able to conceive within 6 months of having regular sex without birth control. Almost all (85 out of 100) are pregnant within a year.

▶ PUBERTY

As girls and boys mature, they go through puberty. During puberty, your body changes—inside and out. The changes don't come all at once, and they don't happen at the same time for everyone. It's normal for changes to start as early as age 8, or not until age 16. Even if nothing looks or feels different yet, the changes may have already begun inside your body.

Changes During Puberty

As you reach puberty, a part of your brain tells your sex glands—your ovaries—to start working. The sex glands then signal other parts of your body to start to grow. These signals are carried by hormones—special chemicals made by your body. Hormones cause your body to change and start being more like an adult:

▶ Your breasts grow.

▶ You will gain weight and grow taller.

▶ Your hips may get wider.

▶ You grow hair under your arms and around the genitals.

▶ Your body odor may change.

▶ You may get acne or pimples.

Boys also go through changes during puberty. They also grow hair in new places and go through other changes.

You might notice a change in your breasts first. They start to look as if the nipples are swelling. The breasts under the nipple also grow. One breast may even seem a little larger than the other, and they may feel sore at times. This is normal.

Hormones also cause changes that prepare a girl's body to be able to have a baby. The ovaries contain eggs, and one is released each month. This is called ovulation. The egg moves into one of the fallopian tubes. The lining of tissue builds up in the uterus. If the egg has not been fertilized, the lining of the uterus is shed as menstrual fluid during menstruation.

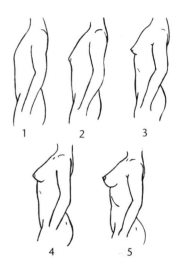

Your breasts grow in stages. Stage 1 shows breasts before puberty. Stage 5 shows breasts that are fully developed.

Your Menstrual Period

There is no way to tell when you will have your first period. The average age is 12–13, but it can happen earlier or later. The first period is usually very mild—only a few drops of blood. Periods usually last between 3 and 7 days and happen about once a month.

When you first start having periods, they may not be regular. There are times when you may miss a period. You may have two periods in 1 month. This is normal. It will take a while for your body to get on a regular pattern.

Looking and Feeling Your Best

The many changes your body goes through in puberty can sometimes make you feel awkward or ill at ease. While your body is changing, taking care of your body will help you feel and look your best.

Eating Right

Your body needs nutrients to grow. Eating a balanced diet will help keep you healthy. Eat plenty of bread, cereal, pasta, fruits, and vegetables and drink lots of milk. Eat less meat. Also, avoid eating too much fast food, which is loaded with fat.

One of the first signs of puberty is a growth spurt. This usually happens in girls about two years before boys.

Staying in Shape

To help keep your body in shape, you need to be active. Getting regular exercise can make your muscles stronger and give you more energy. It can also help decrease menstrual cramps.

Exercising can be fun if you find something that you like to do. Try a team sport such as soccer or basketball. Or try other activities, like riding a bike, rollerblading, dancing, walking, or jogging.

Dealing with Acne

People of all ages may get acne, but it is most common in adolescents. Almost 85% of women and men between the ages of 12 and 24 years develop some form of acne.

Acne is caused by glands under the skin that produce a natural oil called sebum. Puberty makes these glands produce extra sebum, which can clog the pores in your skin.

Washing your face often with water and mild soap usually helps get rid of the excess sebum in your pores. This will help reduce pimples and acne. If you have concerns about acne or pimples, there are medications that can help.

▶ THE REPRODUCTIVE YEARS

After a woman begins to ovulate and menstruate she is able to have a baby. Unless she is pregnant, her body will go through this process each month until she reaches menopause. At menopause a woman ceases having menstrual periods.

Starting at puberty, about age 8–16, and ending at menopause, about age 45–55, a woman is in her reproductive years. This is an important time when a woman can make choices that will affect the rest of her life.

During the reproductive years, women need to think about certain things:

▶ If and when they want to become pregnant

▶ Which method of birth control they would like to use to prevent pregnancy and sexually transmitted diseases

▶ How they can take care of themselves now—such as exercising, eating well, and getting routine health care from their doctor—to help prevent health problems in the future

▶ MENOPAUSE

Menopause is the time in a woman's life when she stops having menstrual periods. The years leading up to this point are called perimenopause, or "around menopause." Menopause marks the natural end of the reproductive years that began in puberty.

Your body changes at midlife, too. Around your mid-40s, you enter a transition phase called perimenopause. It is a time of gradual change leading up to and following menopause. In general, perimenopause extends from age 45 to 55, although the timing varies among women. During this time, the ovaries produce less of the hormone estrogen. Other changes occur in your body, as well. Because these changes happen slowly over time, you may not be aware of them.

The average age that women go through menopause is 51. Most women enjoy a healthy lifestyle for years afterward.

Menopause is a natural event. Today women can expect to live one third of their lives after menopause. The physical changes that occur around menopause should not prevent you from enjoying this time of your life.

Perimenopause

Some women compare perimenopause to puberty—another time when you have to adjust to big changes. These changes may make you feel unlike your usual self. Many changes of perimenopause are related to a drop in estrogen levels. Some are related to aging in general. The effects caused by the lack of estrogen can be treated. Hormone replacement therapy (HRT) can relieve symptoms as well as protect against certain diseases.

Menstruation

In your 40s, surging and falling hormones can cause changes in your menstrual cycle. These changes can be erratic. For instance, the number of days between periods may increase or decrease. Your periods may become shorter or longer. Flow may get heavier or lighter. You may begin to skip periods. Some months your ovaries may release an egg, some months they may not.

Although changes in bleeding are normal as you near menopause, they still should be reported to your doctor.

Hot Flushes

As you approach menopause, you may start having hot flushes (also known as hot flashes). About 75–85% of perimenopausal women get them. These flushes are the most common symptom of perimenopause.

A hot flush is a sudden feeling of heat that rushes to the upper body and face. The skin may redden like a blush. You may also break out in a sweat. A hot flush may last from a few seconds to several minutes or longer.

Hot flushes may come a few times a month or several times a day, depending on the woman. Some women will get hot flushes for a few months, some for a few years, and some not at all.

Hot flushes can happen anytime—day or night. Those occurring during sleep, called night sweats, may wake you up and leave you tired and sluggish the next day. Even though hot

Some women have found that alternative therapies may help relieve hot flashes. Roots from black cohosh, a tall North American forest plant, is one of the treatments most often used. Be sure to let your doctor know if you plan to use this treatment.

flushes are a nuisance, are sometimes embarrassing, and may interfere with daily life, they are not harmful.

Sleep Problems

Perimenopausal women may have to deal with sleep problems. Night sweats may disrupt your rest. You may have insomnia (trouble falling asleep), or you may be awake long before your usual time.

Perimenopausal women may not get enough REM (rapid eye movement) sleep. REM sleep is when dreams occur. A key role of REM sleep is to rest the brain. Without REM sleep, you will not feel rested. When normal sleep rhythms are broken, a woman's moods, health, and ability to cope may be affected. She may have trouble concentrating or become depressed.

Vaginal and Urinary Changes

As your estrogen levels fall, changes take place in the vagina. Over time, the vaginal lining gets thin, dryer, and less flexible. Some women have vaginal burning and itching. The vagina also takes longer to become moist during sex. This may cause pain during intercourse. Vaginal infections may also occur more often.

The drop in estrogen may thin the lining of the urinary tract and weaken supporting tissues. This can cause women to urinate more often. Also, the bladder may become more prone to infection. When the tissues get weak, some women may leak urine when they sneeze, cough, or laugh. This is known as stress incontinence. Some women get this problem even before perimenopause because their tissues have been stretched by childbirth. If you notice a loss of bladder control, tell your doctor. It often can be treated.

Bones

Once made, bone is always changing. Old bone is removed in a process called resorption, and new bone is formed in a process called formation. From childhood until age 30, bone is formed faster than it is broken down. The bones become large and denser. After age 30, the process begins to reverse: bone is broken down faster than it is made. This process continues for the rest of your life. A small amount of bone loss after age 35 is normal in all women and men. It usually does not cause any problems.

However, bone loss that happens too fast can result in osteoporosis. In osteoporosis, bones become too thin and weak, which can result in a break and disability. Some later symptoms of osteoporosis are back pain or tenderness, slight curving of the upper back, and loss of height.

Hormone replacement therapy (HRT) can slow or stop bone loss. For women who cannot take estrogen, there are other medications that may help. Calcitonin is one that slows

To prevent osteoporosis, the National Institutes of Health recommends 1,500 mg of calcium daily for women ages 50–65 who are not taking hormone replacement therapy, as well as for all women older than age 65.

bone loss. Another, called alendronate, has been shown to increase bone density and prevent fractures. Selective estrogen receptor modulators (SERMs) also help prevent bone loss by strengthening tissues of the bone.

To prevent osteoporosis, you should focus on building and keeping as much bone as you can before menopause. You can do that by getting plenty of calcium and exercise.

Just as muscles get stronger with regular exercise, so do bones. Active women have higher bone density than women who do not exercise. Regular weight-bearing exercise is best to strengthen bones and slow bone loss. Brisk walking is good. So are aerobic dancing, stair stepping, tennis, and jogging. Lifting weights also improves bone strength.

What Is Menopause?

Menstrual Changes
Even though periods tend to be irregular around the time of menopause, you should be aware of bleeding that is not normal for you. Call your doctor if you:

▶ Have a change in your monthly cycle

▶ Have very heavy bleeding with clots

▶ Have bleeding that lasts longer than normal

▶ Bleed more often than every 3 weeks

▶ Bleed after sex

At some point, the ovaries stop making enough estrogen to thicken the lining of the uterus. This is when the menstrual periods stop.

A small amount of estrogen is made by other glands and body fat after menopause. Women who are very overweight may not have symptoms of menopause because their extra body fat allows them to make estrogen even after the ovaries stop working.

Early Menopause
Early menopause can occur when a woman's ovaries suddenly stop working or are removed by surgery. With ovarian surgery, there is a sudden loss of estrogen. This may trigger severe symptoms. Women who have early menopause may need to take hormones to replace those made by the ovaries.

Although the removal of the uterus (a hysterectomy) ends menstrual periods, it will not cause early menopause unless the ovaries also are removed. If the ovaries remain after surgery, most women will go through menopause around the normal age.

A woman's ovaries are not always removed during a hysterectomy. Removal of the ovaries is called oophorectomy.

What To Expect

Menopause is a natural part of aging. The lower amounts of estrogen that come with menopause will cause changes in your body. These changes occur slowly, over time. Menopause, however, is different for everyone. Some women notice little difference in their bodies or moods. Others may find it difficult to cope with their symptoms.

Hormone Replacement Therapy

Your doctor may recommend hormone replacement therapy. Hormone replacement therapy helps relieve the symptoms of menopause. It replaces female hormones no longer made by the ovaries. Depending on your situation, you may begin hormone replacement therapy before menopause. If you are taking birth control pills, they will be stopped when you begin treatment.

Bone and Other Body Changes

Bone loss is a normal part of aging. At menopause, the rate of bone loss increases. Such bone thinning, called osteoporosis, increases the risk in older women of breaking bones. The bones of the hip, wrist, and spine are most often affected.

In the United States, 1 of every 3 adults aged 65 and older falls each year. Almost 3% of these falls cause fractures. Osteoporosis increases this risk.

The estrogen produced by women's ovaries before menopause protects them from heart attacks and stroke. When less estrogen is made after menopause, women lose much of this protection. The risk of heart attack and stroke then increases.

Emotional Changes

Menopause does not cause sudden mood swings or depression. However, the change in hormone levels may make you feel nervous, irritable, or very tired. These feelings may be linked to other symptoms of menopause, such as lack of sleep.

If you are under a lot of stress, the changes of menopause may be harder to manage. Many women in midlife are going through major life changes anyway. There may be stress in the family as time passes and roles change. There may be stress related to money or your job. Some women may be watching children leave home and are learning to deal with the "empty nest." Some are saddened that they can no longer have children. And more often, women find themselves part of the "sandwich generation," becoming caretakers for their children, grandchildren, and their aging parents. If you find it hard to cope, talk about your feelings with your partner, a close friend, a counselor, or your doctor.

Sexuality

Menopause does not have to affect your ability to enjoy sex. Although the lack of estrogen may make the vagina dry, estrogen replacement and vaginal lubricants can help moisten the vagina and make intercourse more comfortable. There are a number of lubricants available without a prescription. If you don't like one product, try another.

Regular sex may help the vagina keep its natural elasticity. If you have been having sex on a regular basis, you may not notice any major changes during menopause. If you have not been sexually active for a while, you may want to talk with your partner and perhaps your doctor, too, about ways to make sex more comfortable.

Some women find that they have less interest in sex around and after menopause. Lower hormone levels may decrease sex drive. It may affect your ability to have an orgasm, or it may take longer for you to reach orgasm.

Men, too, may find that their sex drive decreases as they age. It may take an older man longer to achieve an erection and ejaculate, or he may have problems with impotence. Impotence is usually caused by physical or medical problems, or it may be caused by medications. In many cases, impotence can be treated with success.

Talk with your partner about how you feel. Communication is key during this time of changes. This may a good time to experiment with your sex life. You and your partner may want to try different positions or engage in longer foreplay. There are many "how-to" books and videos available as guides.

Sex often becomes more enjoyable at this stage of life. Older couples may be more experienced and know how to please each other. They may have more privacy and time.

Despite the signs of menopause, you still may be able to get pregnant. You are not completely free of the risk of pregnancy until you have not had a menstrual period for one year.

▶ Health Care for Women 65 and Older

▶ See also *"Routine Care" in Women's Wellness*

Most women can expect to live about 80 years. With this life span, at least one-third of a woman's life is lived after menopause. Women can lead active and fulfilling lives well into their later years. They can become involved in their own health care by having routine screening tests and making healthy lifestyle choices. This may help prevent health problems in the years ahead.

Routine Health Care

All women age 65 and older should have a physical exam yearly. The exams should include certain routine tests. Your doctor may suggest other tests as well. It depends on your risk factors and health history.

Medications

Sometimes staying healthy includes taking medication. Many women in your age group take prescription drugs. Often they take more than one. When you visit your doctor, it's a good idea to bring a list of all the medications, vitamins, and natural remedies you may be taking. The list will help your doctor see if anything you are taking could be harmful.

When taking medications:

▶ Be sure to take them as they have been prescribed.

▶ Do not skip dosages.

▶ Create a system to remind yourself to take medications at the right time.

▶ Do not stop taking the drug without talking to your doctor, even if you are feeling better.

If you have concerns about your medication or its side effects, talk to your doctor right away. If you choose not to take the drug prescribed to you, let your doctor know.

Prescription drugs can be harmful if taken improperly. Taking the wrong dose or improperly mixing a prescription drug with alcohol or other prescription or over-the-counter drugs may cause serious problems. If you have questions, talk to your pharmacist or doctor.

Hormone Replacement Therapy

After menopause, many women take hormone replacement therapy. This replaces the estrogen their body is no longer making. Women who have a uterus also may take progesterone, another hormone that is no longer produced.

The major benefits of hormone replacement therapy are that it prevents osteoporosis and protects against heart disease—problems that can have long-term effects on your life and health. Other benefits include the reduced risk of urinary tract infections and cancer of the uterus. It also helps relieve hot flushes and improves memory in some women.

Like most treatments, hormone replacement therapy is not free of risks. If estrogen is used without progesterone, the risk of cancer of the uterus is increased. Also, there is a slight chance that use of hormone replacement therapy may increase the risk of breast cancer.

You should keep taking hormone replacement therapy if it has been prescribed to you. If you choose to stop taking it, tell your doctor.

There may be reasons why you should not take hormones, or you may choose not to. There are other options. Talk to your doctor about it.

Diet

A well-balanced diet is key to good health. It may be hard to eat a healthy diet all the time. You may not feel like eating, foods may not taste the same, or you may not be able or want to cook. However, try to keep a healthy weight. Poor nutrition increases your risk of vitamin deficiency and related problems. Extra weight increases your chances of having health problems. Avoid junk foods, sweets, and foods high in fat.

Include foods high in fiber in your diet. Drink eight glasses of water a day to prevent constipation. Make sure you drink more water in hot weather.

Your doctor may suggest you take vitamin and mineral supplements. For instance, women age 65 and older should have 1,500 mg of calcium per day to prevent osteoporosis (1,000 mg per day if you are taking hormone replacement therapy). You also need 10 micrograms of vitamin D per day.

It's hard for women to meet all of their calcium and vitamin D needs through diet. If you are not eating enough calcium, there are supplements you can take.

Exercise

Regular exercise is one of the best things you can do to promote better health. Exercise can help to:

▶ Lower your blood pressure and cholesterol level

▶ Lower your risk of heart disease, stroke, and type II diabetes

▶ Strengthen your heart, lungs, and bones

▶ Keep a healthy weight

▶ Keep your joints flexible and muscles strong

▶ Give you more energy

▶ Reduce stress, anxiety, and depression

Exercise may help relieve problems with sleeping. Mild exercise a few hours before bed or during the day can help you get a restful night's sleep.

It's never too late to begin to exercise. This is true even if you've never exercised or haven't done it for years.

Before you begin any exercise program, check with your doctor. There are plenty of low-impact programs to try. For instance, water aerobics is a good choice to ease movement and stress on joints.

A physical therapist can design an exercise program for you if you have been injured or ill, you are physically limited, or you have a problem with balance. Exercise is important for everyone. It is just as vital for someone who uses a wheelchair or walker.

Harmful Things

Just as starting to exercise at any time is good, quitting smoking and cutting back on drinking alcohol has benefits at any age. Alcohol use can be a problem in older women. If a woman age 65 or older lives alone, she may begin to drink too much and not be aware of it. Heavy drinking (more than two drinks a day) can:

▶ Cause health problems or make them worse

▶ Damage the liver over time

▶ Lead to vitamin and mineral deficiencies

▶ Increase risk of falls and accidents, including car crashes

▶ Increase risk of depression or cause it to worsen

Many women age 65 and older take prescription drugs. Alcohol can interact with a medication and cause problems.

Using tobacco increases a woman's risk of chronic health problems and premature death. Tobacco use in women increases the risk of:

▶ Cancer

▶ Heart disease and stroke

▶ Emphysema

▶ Bronchitis

▶ Pneumonia

Smoking is the single greatest preventable cause of illness and early death.

When older smokers quit, they increase their life expectancy, reduce their risk of heart disease, and improve lung function and circulation.

Mental Health

As people age, they go through life changes that can affect their mental health. Sometimes this can lead to depression.

Depression is a medical disorder, like diabetes, high blood pressure, or heart disease. It can be long lasting or related to a major life event. Many women age 65 and older face situations that can trigger depression:

▶ Retirement

▶ The deaths of spouse and friends

▶ Chronic illness

▶ Being alone

▶ Concerns about finances

One third of all older people live alone. Being with people daily often has a positive effect on attitude, general well-being, and eating habits.

A social network of friends and activities can promote good mental health. If you're feeling down most of the time, this may signal depression. Talk about it with your doctor. Treatment often can help.

Abuse

Sometimes women in your age group are victims of abuse or domestic violence. Abuse may come in the form of mental, physical, sexual, or financial abuse. Neglect also may occur. The source of abuse can be anyone but often is a spouse, caretaker, or other family members. Here are some questions to think about:

▶ Has anyone at home ever hurt you?

▶ Has anyone taken anything of yours without asking?

▶ Are you afraid of anyone?

If you think you are being abused, don't let the abuse go on. Seek help from someone you trust.

Sexuality

Changes brought about by aging or illness can affect sexual response in both men and women. Many of these problems can be treated. For instance, lubricants or hormone replacement therapy can help women with vaginal dryness. Medications can help men with impotence.

Women may enjoy sex more at this stage of life. Older couples may be more experienced and know how to please each other. They may have more privacy and time than when they were working or raising children. You may enjoy sex more at this time of your life because there is no risk of pregnancy.

A woman age 65 or older may have a healthy interest in sex, but she may lack a partner or her partner may not be able to have sex. Masturbation (stimulating your own genitals for sexual pleausure) or trying new ways of lovemaking can be good choices as people age. Keep trying. Being creative helps.

It also may be hard to find a place that is private. Many older people live in a care facility or with family members. Ask your family or caregivers for some private time.

Keep in mind the need for safe sex doesn't stop. You still need to prevent sexually transmitted diseases.

Injury Prevention

Falls and injuries can be pose a serious health risk for women age 65 or older. There are things you can do to prevent them:

▶ Is my home safe from falls?

  —Is there nonskid backing on throw rugs?

  —Are rooms well lit?

  —Are there handrails by stairs and in the bathroom?

  —Is there clutter?

▶ Should I use a walker or a cane to help my balance?

▶ Have I had my vision checked this year?

▶ Do I or others have concerns about my driving?

Almost 70% of women remain sexually active well into their older years.

▶ SEXUALITY

For most women, learning about sex is a lifelong process. Women—whether married or single, young or old—differ greatly in their sexual interest and response. A woman's sexual function is not limited to sexual intercourse. Also, her sexuality is more than just her sexual practices. It is the way she thinks and feels about herself as a woman. This includes her feelings about sex and how she relates to others.

As a parent you can help your children feel good about themselves and teach them how to relate to others. Part of being a parent is teaching your children about sex and sexuality.

Sexual identity is shaped and reshaped throughout life. A number of key factors affect your sexual development. These include early role models, religious teachings, and early sexual experiences—both good and bad.

Adult

A woman's sexual response peaks in her late 30s and early 40s in most cases. A woman can have a full physical and emotional response to sex through her whole life. Many women have an active sex life that gives them pleasure well into their late years.

Most couples follow a pattern when having sex. It starts with hugging and goes to kissing to body caressing to sex. Vaginal sex is the most common sexual activity. Couples also have oral sex—the second most common activity. Many women also enjoy masturbation, fantasizing, and watching their partner undress. How often a woman has sex varies greatly.

Most women are attracted to men. Some women are attracted to other women. The term "lesbian" refers to women who are mainly emotionally and sexually attracted to other women. Some women are sexually attracted to both men and women.

Many women have trouble with sex at some time in their lives. They may find it hard to talk about their sexual concerns—even with their partner, a trusted friend, or their doctor.

Children and Sexuality

Many parents feel uneasy talking about sexuality with their child. They wonder what type of information is right for the child's age. They may wonder how to

The Sexual Response Cycle

A woman's body follows a regular pattern during sex. There are four stages:

1. *Desire*—The feeling that you want to have sex

2. *Arousal*—Physical changes take place. Your vagina and vulva get moist and the muscles of the opening of the vagina relax. The clitoris swells and enlarges. The uterus lifts up, and the vagina gets deeper and wider.

3. *Orgasm*—The peak of the response. The muscles of the vagina and uterus contract and create a strong feeling of pleasure. The clitoris can feel orgasm, too.

4. *Resolution*—The vagina, clitoris, and uterus return to their normal state.

bring up the subject or answer all the child's questions. A good rule of thumb is to give children information about 2 years before you think they need it. If you talk about things you judge them to be ready for today, there's a good chance they've already passed that stage, or will pass it soon.

Most parents just need help getting started. Talking about sex for the first time may be the toughest part. After you've talked about sexual issues with your child once, you're likely to find the next time easier. There are no strict rules for teaching your child about sexuality. Each family and each child are different.

How Children Learn

Learning about sex is a lifelong process that begins at birth. When they are very young, children may learn from how they are held or touched. As they get older, children are exposed to many ways of thinking about sex. Family members, friends, the media, schools, and church all play a role. Sorting out what is right or wrong can be confusing. This is especially true if they see you, or others they admire, acting in ways that differ from what they've been taught. Early in life children start forming their attitudes about sex by watching their parents. If you never talk about sex at all, it suggests that sex is bad or shouldn't be talked about.

Your children will learn about sex whether you talk openly about it or say nothing at all. For very young children, parents are the center of their world. They watch you, admire you, and copy you.

Your child also learns about sex from TV, music, magazines, and the Internet where sex is often shown in a distorted way that does not match real life. The average teenager watches about 24 hours of TV a week where he or she sees many sexual references. A lot of that sex is casual. On afternoon and prime-time soap operas, which teenagers watch avidly, most of the sexual relationships are between unmarried partners. It is important for a parent to point out that sex is not as simple or easy as it is portrayed.

Many parents fear that talking about sex will increase sexual activity in their children, but it doesn't. Ignorance, not knowledge, creates problems. Lack of knowledge about sex and birth control adds to the high teenage pregnancy rate in this country.

As a parent, you can help your children learn about their sexuality in many ways. Educating your children promotes a better understanding of sex and a healthy attitude. You can give them a set of values, make sure they have correct information, and encourage open communication from early childhood into the adult years.

By the time the average person reaches age 70, he or she will have spent approximately 7 to 10 years watching TV. Talk to your child about making good choices of what to watch.

Communicating With Your Child

Children learn by watching how their parents:

▶ Dress

▶ Act around people of the same and the opposite sex

▶ Show affection

▶ Respond to nudity

Communication

If you find it hard to talk to your child about sex, it may help to talk with a third person. This person could be a doctor, member of the clergy, teacher, school counselor, relative, or family friend. There are also people specially trained to counsel teens.

Communication about sex should start early in your child's life. Teach your preschooler the proper names for body parts and explain where babies come from in simple terms. When your child asks a question, be prepared to answer it, if only briefly. For example, when your 5-year-old asks, "Where did I come from?" you might say, "You began in a special place inside Mommy called a uterus." Later your child may ask more about the uterus or another follow-up question. You can then build on the knowledge, bit by bit, as your child seems ready for it. If you begin when your child is young, it will be much easier to talk about sex when he or she is a teenager. Children who feel free to ask questions about sex will ask questions about other subjects, too.

Before you talk to your child about sex, first decide what your child should know at his or her age. Then plan how you will present the information:

▶ Discuss your attitudes about sex with your partner and what messages you want to convey to your child.

▶ Express your beliefs. If you think sex should wait until marriage, or should only take place in a loving, mature relationship, then say so.

▶ Make sure you have correct facts. There are many books on sexuality for children, teens, and adults. It's all right to say to your child, "I don't know the answer. Let's look it up."

Educating your child about sex should involve give and take, not an adult lecturing while the child listens. Key questions may not get asked or answered. Often it is the parent who should listen. Show you are listening by making eye contact and repeating key remarks your child makes.

Try always to be honest. Children soon learn whether they can trust their parents' answers. If they find they can't, they will stop asking questions. They will turn to friends, magazines, and television for answers—and may get wrong information.

Some people think that mothers should only talk to girls and fathers only to boys about sexuality. However, mothers can play a big role in shaping their sons' attitudes about sex, and fathers can do the same for daughters. Parents should be willing to discuss sex with all their children, whether they are boys or girls.

If your child is already a teenager, you may fear it's too late to start talking about sex. Although it's true that younger children respond more openly, it is never too late. Admit to your teenager if you are uncomfortable and say you'll do your best.

Young Children

Children first notice a difference between the bodies of boys and girls, adults and children, at the toddler stage. You can foster a good body image in your child by talking in positive terms. Your child may play with his or her own genitals and may express interest in the genitals of other children. This is normal. Do not respond with anger or scolding. Instead, talk to your child about what is correct behavior, such as controlling sexual actions in public. This is no different than teaching them not to hit others or talk loudly in school. Children should also learn that talk about sex is for private times at home, not in public.

Toilet training presents a good chance to convey positive attitudes about body parts and functions. Your reactions play a key role. For example, young children think that bowel movements are part of their bodies. If they are told that bowel movements are bad, they may feel that they are bad, too.

Young children should be taught that they are in charge of their bodies. They decide who can touch them, and where. Children need to learn about sexual abuse and should know to tell a parent or trusted adult if they have been touched in the wrong way.

Between the ages of 3 and 6, children are very curious about gender (boy versus girl) differences. This is when they make their first real effort to come to terms with being a girl or boy. Their interest in sex is open and honest, so it's an ideal time for parents

Before toilet training, think carefully about the words you will use to describe body parts, urine, and bowel movements. It may be best to use proper terms that will not confuse, offend, or embarrass your child.

What Your Child Should Know

By age 5, children should:

▶ Know correct terms for all sexual body parts

▶ Understand the concept of gender: "boy" and "girl"

▶ Know they have the right to say "no" to unwanted touch

▶ Know where babies come from

▶ Feel free to ask adults they trust about sexuality

By age 10, children should:

▶ Understand the facts about reproduction in humans and animals

▶ Know how male and female bodies grow and differ

▶ Know that different sexual orientations exist

▶ Understand basic facts about AIDS

By age 12, children should:

▶ Understand that human sexuality is a normal part of life

▶ Know that sexual feelings are normal

▶ Know what changes to expect in their bodies, including menstruation and "wet dreams"

▶ Understand that sex gives pleasure and also is the way to make a baby

▶ Know about methods of birth control and abortion

▶ Be aware of sexual abuse and other forms of sexual exploitation, and know how to respond to such dangers

▶ Know how sexually transmitted diseases are spread, prevented, and treated

to encourage children to ask questions. If this frankness can be nurtured at a young age, it may carry over to later stages when children are less open.

If children don't ask questions or seem curious about sex by age 5 or 6, parents should look for chances to bring up the subject. Most likely, the children are interested but may think sex is a subject parents won't discuss. Or, they may think it's bad to ask questions.

Primary School Years

During this time, a child's interest in sex continues. It is often less obvious, though, because many children feel their parents don't want to talk about sex. This is also the age when children tend to pick up sexual slang that offends the parents. Parents give mixed messages if they scold children for using such language, but then use it themselves. When children use bad language, parents should calmly explain what the words really mean and suggest other words that would be better.

Up to age 9 or so, children usually want brief and direct answers to their questions. Parents should respect a child's curiosity. Their questions are often about the body, how it functions, and why. Answer in simple but correct terms. If parents tell children more than they want to know, or explain concepts that are too advanced, children will get bored, stop listening, or change the subject. On the other hand, giving too little information isn't good either.

By about age 10, children should know about sexually transmitted diseases (STDs), especially AIDS (acquired immunodeficiency syndrome) and how it is transmitted. Your child may be hearing a lot about AIDS and may be worried about "catching it." Headlines and advertisements give ample chances to discuss AIDS, other diseases passed through sex, and use of condoms.

Early Adolescence

Most children start puberty between ages 11 and 13. Their interest in their personal sexuality usually increases a great deal. Their sexual organs mature, their sex glands start to produce hormones at an adult level, and they have spurts in height and weight.

Young people at this stage often compare themselves with their friends. Since bodies mature at different rates, children often wonder if they are normal. They may need to be assured that they are, even if they are developing a little sooner or later than their friends. Girls mature about 2 years ahead of boys—a fact that often disturbs both sexes.

Young adolescents are often shy about bringing up the subject of sex. Listen for hints that your child has questions, and be alert for words that will help you start to talk about sex. Girls

If you think your child is uncomfortable with his or her self-image, encourage him or her to eat healthy and exercise. You can help your child have a good body image by praising him or her on their appearance.

should be told of menstruation, and boys of erections and "wet dreams," long before they occur. These subjects should be discussed openly with both boys and girls.

Children should also be taught the benefits of abstaining from sex. In surveys, many adolescents say they wish they'd waited until they were older to start having sex.

Nonetheless, some children start experimenting with sex in their early teens. It is important to make sure they have accurate information about STDs, birth control, and "safer" sex. The practice of safer sex involves knowing one's partner, limiting sex to only one partner (who does the same), and always using a condom.

Almost 40% of all female teens did not use contraception the first time they had sex.

Your children may hear stories that make them feel "everybody is doing it but me." Remind them that their friends often exaggerate. Give them the facts: 4% of 12-year-olds have had sex. Although it's true that half of young people today have sex by age 17, the other half do not.

Help your children learn to say no to someone who tries to pressure them into sex. Explain that having sex before they are mature enough may make them feel bad about themselves and have a long-term impact. Discuss the "right" and "wrong" reasons to have sex. Sexual feelings are normal and natural, and children need to learn how to handle them.

Teenage Years

Young people reach their full physical growth during their teenage years. They become sexually mature and may have strong sexual urges. Many teenagers are having their first sexual experience at younger ages than their parents probably did.

The teenage years are when parents and children are most likely to have problems talking to each other. Teenagers become more independent and begin taking steps toward adulthood. Values that have been fostered in them since they were small are tested.

Parents often are afraid that talking about sex to their children may make it seem exciting and make them want to try it. However, studies have shown that teens whose parents have talked openly with them about sex are often more sexually responsible.

If you bring up sex and your teen claims to know it all already or shows a lack of interest in what you have to say, you might ask your child to tell you what he or she knows and then help correct any wrong information. Teens often think they know more than their parents. As hard as it may be to talk with your teen about sex, it is important to share your views, voice your concerns, and go over the facts.

Teenagers should be given a chance to talk openly about the risk of getting STDs, including HIV (human immunodeficiency virus). Teens should understand that having sex always carries a risk of disease or pregnancy, no matter what measures are taken. Let them know that it's okay to say no to sex. These days, abstaining from sex is more than a moral issue, it's a health and safety issue.

If your child—especially a daughter—dates someone older, it is likely she will face more pressure to have sex. Although less common in our culture, boys can feel pressure from women, too, and should feel free to say no. Emphasize that sex should be a loving act and that forcing sex is wrong.

Teenagers should also know about different forms of sexual behavior. They should understand terms such as heterosexual, homosexual, gay, lesbian, bisexual, and abstinence. Your children should be taught to respect a broad range of sexual expression so they can be sensitive to them.

Some parents will learn that their teenage son or daughter is homosexual. About 5–10% of adolescents are gay. Teens who are homosexual may feel very different and lonely. They may struggle with their sexual identity and keep the truth secret until they are older.

Homosexuality is not an illness. It is not something a person chooses. It just happens. If your child believes he or she is homosexual, learn as much about homosexuality as you can. Do not reject your child—continue to give love and support. He or she probably needs you now more than ever and has shown great trust by confiding in you. If you or your child have trouble coping with the child's homosexuality, you should consider counseling.

Additional Help

Your local bookstore and public library have books that may be helpful. Those aimed to adults—including books on child development and health—can help you brush up on the facts and learn ways to talk to your child and teach them about sexuality. There are also many good books for children and teens. Try to have at least one book that is written for your child's age level.

Parents, Families and Friends of Lesbians and Gays (PFLAG) offers support and understanding to parents of homosexuals. For more information contact:
PFLAG
1101 14th Street, NW, Suite 1030
Washington, DC 20005
(202) 638-4200

WOMEN'S WELLNESS

Making the right lifestyle choices is the best thing you can do to stay healthy. The choices you make now can make you feel better now and prevent health problems later.

You should see your doctor regularly for preventive health care. This can help you make choices that will prevent health problems. Preventive health care includes exams and screening tests, which look for problems even before you are sick. It also includes some immunizations to prevent disease.

There are some problems that are more likely to cause sickness, or even death, at certain times of your life. The goal of preventive care is to prevent or manage these problems early. Your obstetrician–gynecologist can serve as your primary care physician for this type of care.

Your obstetrician–gynecologist and staff are part of a health care team that can advise you on how you can have a healthy lifestyle, decrease risk factors, and prevent disease. This includes eating a well-balanced, low-fat diet, getting regular exercise, avoiding tobacco and other drugs, and using caffeine and alcohol only in moderation. Together, you can watch for signs of problems that are common in women your age. Problems found early are easier to treat and less likely to pose serious health risks.

▶ ACCIDENT PREVENTION

Many aspects of daily life can cause injuries, such as sports, recreation, or hazards on the job. If you use alcohol or drugs, your chances of having an accident are much higher.

Be sure you know how to handle work or recreation equipment correctly. Use safety equipment for sports, such as a helmet, kneepads, and protective eyewear.

Guns and other weapons cause many injuries and deaths each year. Many of these are accidental deaths. If you have a gun for hunting or protection, be careful. Store guns unloaded and locked away from children. It's best not to keep them in the house. Take a class on safe gun use.

Try to make the home as safe as possible. Older women especially are at risk of hip fractures due to falls. Install handrails along open staircases. Get rid of throw rugs that may slip.

Protect Yourself

Bike helmets have been shown to reduce the risk for head injury by almost 85% and the risk for brain injury by almost 90%.

▶ See also *Health Care Power of Attorney, Living Wills*

▶ ADVANCE DIRECTIVES

Medical advances have made it possible to keep people alive longer. This means many patients, families, and doctors have had to make some difficult life-and-death decisions. Advance directives help ensure that these decisions are made by you. The two most common types of advance directives are living wills and health care powers of attorney.

An advance directive is a legal document that tells others your wishes about your medical care when you are too sick to make your own decisions. If you have an illness or an injury that keeps you from being able to explain what you want, there is still a way to let others (including your doctor) know your wishes. The best way to do this is by writing directions in advance, when you are healthy and able to make decisions and express them.

Your Rights by Law

The federal Patient Self-Determination Act of 1990 is a law that requires hospitals and nursing homes to tell patients of their rights to make advance directives. They must put in the patient's medical record whether that person has an advance directive.

Also, states have their own laws about living wills and health care powers of attorney. The laws in your state will explain what your advance directive may contain and how and when it must be followed.

❱ ALCOHOL

Alcohol slows down your body. The more you drink, the more it slows your brain function. This affects talking, seeing, walking, and driving.

Light to moderate drinking rarely causes harm. Heavy drinking, though, can cause problems. It may damage the liver or cause cirrhosis, which can lead to liver failure and death. It may damage the heart muscle and other organs. It also may increase the risk of some cancers.

Alcohol use is linked with:

❱ About one half of fatal car crashes

❱ Two thirds of drownings

❱ One half of fires

❱ One half of severe falls

❱ Violence (including domestic violence)

❱ Suicide

Special Concerns for Women

Alcohol use has special risks for some women. Its use can lead to:

❱ Certain cancers (breast, for instance)

❱ Osteoporosis

❱ Early menopause

❱ Irregular periods

❱ Infertility

❱ Miscarriage in pregnant women

❱ Having a baby with fetal alcohol syndrome

What Is Problem Drinking?

Drinking becomes problem drinking when it harms your health, behavior, or relationships. The amount differs with each person. It depends on a person's weight, age, health, and family, medical, and emotional background.

Chronic alcohol abuse takes a heavier toll on women than on men. Female alcoholics have death rates 50–100% higher than male alcoholics. Related problems, such as brain and liver damage, progress faster in women.

How Much Is Too Much?

"Too much" means different amounts for different people. Here is one way to find out whether you are a light, moderate, or heavy drinker. Keep in mind that how often you drink is as important as how much you drink. You may not drink often, but if you drink too much at one time (binge), you still may have a problem.

Light: On average, less than one drink a day

Moderate: One or two drinks a day

Heavy: More than two drinks a day

You may not know if you have a drinking problem. Here are some signs:

> Drinking alone when you feel angry or sad

> Drinking in a pattern (every day or every week at the same time)

> Planning activities around drinking

> Drinking to relieve pain or stress

> Drinking more than you meant to or after you told yourself you wouldn't

> Drinking to get drunk

> Thinking a lot about drinking

> Showing a personality change when you drink

The box gives two tests that are used by experts to assess alcohol use versus abuse. If you are still unsure, check with your doctor.

A drink is defined as 12 grams of alcohol. That includes a:

> *12-ounce bottle of beer or wine cooler*

> *5-ounce glass of wine*

> *1½-ounce glass of liquor*

Do You Have a Drinking Problem?

Experts on alcohol abuse use many tests to find out whether a person has a drinking problem. The T-ACE questions and the CAGE test are two of the tests that your doctor may be to determine if you have a problem.

The T-ACE Questions*

Here's a test—called the T-ACE—used to assess problem drinking:

T   How many drinks does it take to make you feel high (**Tolerance**)?

A   Have people **Annoyed** you by criticizing your drinking?

C   Have you felt you ought to **Cut Down** on your drinking?

E   Have you ever had a drink first thing in the morning to steady your nerves or get rid of a hangover (**Eye Opener**)?

If your answer to the tolerance question is more than two drinks, give yourself a score of 2. Score 1 for each yes answer to any of the other questions. A total score of 2 or more may mean that you have a drinking problem. Talk to your doctor about your drinking habits. He or she can give you more information and refer you for counseling or treatment.

The CAGE Test†

Experts in treating alcohol abuse use the CAGE questions below to help them determine whether a person has a drinking problem. These questions can apply to other drugs, too.

C   Have you ever felt you ought to **Cut Down** on your drinking?

A   Have people **Annoyed** you by criticizing your drinking?

G   Have you ever felt bad or **Guilty** about your drinking?

E   Have you ever had a drink first thing in the morning (**Eye Opener**) to steady your nerves or get rid of a hangover?

If you answer yes to any of these questions, or if you notice an increased tolerance to alcohol or drugs, you may have a problem.

* Modified from Sokol RJ, Martier SS, Ager JW. The T-ACE Questions: practical prenatal detection of risk drinking. Am J Obstet Gynecol 1989;160:865.

† Source: Ewing JA. Detecting alcoholism: the CAGE questionnaire. JAMA 1984;252:1905–1907.

How Can I Get Help?

Problem drinkers can get help. If a woman has a drinking problem, she has some choices for treatment. Addiction to alcohol cannot be cured, but it can be treated with success. Treatment options include:

▶ Stopping drinking and safely getting alcohol out of your system with the help of a doctor

▶ Taking medication to help prevent relapse

▶ Counseling—including for friends and family members—to help cope with the stress of problem drinking

▶ BREAST SELF-EXAM

A breast self-exam is done to detect changes that could lead to breast cancer. To learn what is normal for your breasts and to find any problems, you should do a breast self-exam once a month. It is one of the best things you can do for your health. Finding and treating breast cancer early can save your life.

Most women who are diagnosed with breast cancer survive the disease. If it is detected early, breast cancer has a 5-year survival rate of over 95%.

Why Do Breast Self-Exams?

If breast cancer is found early, most women can be cured. That is why routine breast self-exams, mammography, and checkups by your doctor are vital (Table 1).

By doing a monthly breast self-exam, you learn how your breasts feel. This helps you detect any changes or signs of a problem.

All women should do the exam once a month. This includes women who:

▶ Have gone through menopause

▶ Are pregnant

▶ Are breastfeeding

▶ Have breast implants

Any changes or lumps should be discussed with your doctor.

How to Do a Breast Self-Exam

The best time to do the breast self-exam is a few days after your period ends each month. It's easier at this time because your breasts are less tender or swollen. If you are

Table 1. Screening Tests

Test	How Often
Mammography	Every 1–2 years for women aged 40–50
	Once a year for women aged 50 and older
	Once a year for a woman with a personal or family history of breast cancer
Doctor's exam of breasts	Once a year
Breast self-exams	Once a month

not having periods, try to do the exam on the same day each month. Some women choose the first day of each month to help them remember. There are two parts to a breast self-exam—looking and feeling.

Looking

In the first part of the exam, you are looking for any changes. This means you should make sure you have enough light when you are doing the exam.

Stand or sit in front of a mirror. Place your arms at your sides. Look at both breasts for:

▶ Dimpling, puckering, or redness of the breast skin

▶ Pulling in of the nipples

▶ Changes in breast size or shape

Look for the same signs with your hands pressed tightly on your hips. Then look with your arms raised above your head.

Feeling

In the second part of the exam, you are feeling for any changes. You can do this by lying flat on your back. Place a folded towel or pillow under your left shoulder and place your left hand over your head. You also can feel for changes when you are taking a shower or bath. It often is easier to examine your breasts when they are smooth and wet with soap and water. It's best to examine your breasts both ways—lying down and standing.

Examine one breast at a time. Feel with the pads (not tips) of your three middle fingers. With your right hand, keeping the fingers flat and together, gently feel your left breast without pressing too hard. The box lists three ways to do this.

With any pattern, be sure to examine the nipples also. Gently squeeze the nipple and check for any discharge. Examine the upper chest area and below the armpits—these places also have breast tissue. Then follow the same steps on the other breast.

You may find that one pattern works better for you than the others. Once you find the pattern that is easiest for you, use that pattern only.

Remember how your breasts feel each month. Mark any lumps or other changes on the diagram shown here. Show it to your doctor.

Signs of a Problem

If you notice any of these symptoms during your breast self-exam, call your doctor:

▶ Lump

▶ Swelling

▶ Skin irritation

▶ Dimpling

▶ Nipple pain

▶ Nipple retraction (nipple turns in)

▶ Redness of nipple or breast skin

▶ Scaly nipple or breast skin

▶ Nipple discharge

Any lump should be checked right away. Tests may be needed. In some cases, a biopsy may be done to look at the tissue.

Breast Self-Exam

Looking

The self-exam should always be done in good light. Stand or sit in front of a mirror. Place arms at your sides. Look for dimpling, puckering, or redness of the breast skin, discharge from the nipples, or changes in breast size or shape. Look for the same signs with your hands pressed tightly on your hips and then with your arms raised high.

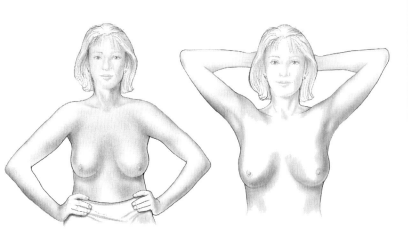

Feeling

Lie flat on your back. Place a folded towel or a pillow under your left shoulder. Place your left hand under or over your head. You also can feel for changes when you are standing.

With your right hand, keeping the fingers flat and together, gently feel your left breast without pressing too hard. Use one of the three methods shown here. Then lower your right arm and do the exam on the other breast.

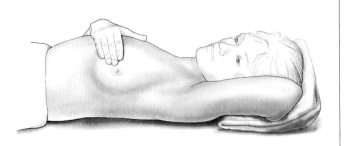

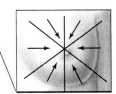

Don't Forget

- ▶ With any pattern, be sure to examine the nipples also. Gently squeeze the nipple and check for any discharge.
- ▶ Examine the upper chest area and below the armpits—these places also have breast tissue.
- ▶ Call your doctor if you notice any lumps or changes in your breasts.

Choose one of these methods

Circle. Begin at the top of your breast and move your fingers slowly around the outside in a large circle. When you return to the top, move your hand a little closer to the nipple and make a smaller circle. Do this in smaller and smaller circles until you have examined all of the breast tissue.

Lines. Begin in the underarm area. Slowly move your fingers down until they are below your breast. Move your fingers closer toward your nipple and go slowly back up, using the same motion. Use this up-and-down pattern all the way across your breast.

Wedge. Begin at the outside edge of your breast. Slowly work your way in toward the nipple, doing one wedge-shaped section at a time. Do this until the entire breast area has been examined.

▶ CAR SAFETY

Motor vehicle accidents are the leading cause of death in women under age 40. All women should drive safely and use safety belts. Buckle up every time you drive or ride. It takes only a few seconds.

When you are pregnant, you should take extra care to avoid things that might harm your baby. After birth, you still need to protect your baby. The best way to keep you and your baby safe in a car or truck is to use safety belts and child safety seats.

Safety Belts and Safety Seats Save Lives

Car crashes cripple and kill more people from birth to age 34 than anything else. Many of these deaths and injuries could have been prevented with safety seats and safety belts.

All states and the District of Columbia have child restraint laws. All states (except New Hampshire and the District of Columbia) have laws that require riders and drivers to buckle up. Most of the laws cover only people in the front seat. Some states also require that everyone in the car wear a seat belt.

In most cars the safety belt is one unit made up of the lap and shoulder belt. In some cars the lap and shoulder belts are separate. Always wear both. If a car only has a lap belt, wear it.

What Happens in a Crash

In a car crash, there are two collisions. The first is when the car hits something, or is hit, and comes to a sudden stop. The second crash happens a split second later when anyone not buckled in can fly forward, slamming into the steering wheel, windshield, dashboard, or front seat (from the back seat). The force of a 30-mph crash is like jumping headfirst off a three-story building.

In a crash or sudden stop, safety seats and belts hold everyone in their place. This helps keep them from smashing into the inside of the car or into each other. It also keeps them from being thrown through the windshield.

It takes only a second or two for an adult to buckle up. It takes only a couple of minutes to get a baby into the safety seat. Take the time to be safe—even when you are only going a short distance.

Buckling Up During Pregnancy

Your baby's first ride is in your belly. Although the baby is well-protected inside of your body, for the best protection in a vehicle,

For more information on car safety for you and your baby, contact:

National Highway Traffic Safety Administration 400 Seventh Street, SW Washington, DC 20590 Web site: www.nhtsa.dot.gov

wear a lap–shoulder belt while you're pregnant every time you travel. The safety belt will not hurt your baby. You and your baby are far more likely to survive a car crash if you are buckled in.

When wearing your safety belt:

▶ Always wear both the lap and shoulder belt.

▶ Buckle the lap belt low on your hipbones, below your belly.

▶ Never put the lap belt across your belly.

▶ Place the shoulder belt across the center of the chest (between your breasts)—never under your arm.

▶ Make sure the belts fit snugly.

The upper part of the belt should cross your shoulder without chafing your neck. Never slip the upper part of the belt off your shoulder. Safety belts worn too loosely or too high on the belly can cause broken ribs or injuries to your belly. But more damage is caused when they aren't used at all.

Safety Seats for Babies

You will need a safety seat for your baby's first ride home from the hospital. Plan to get a safety seat well before your due date. This will give you time to practice using the seat in your car before your baby's first car ride.

A car seat that has been in a crash may have been weakened and should not be used even if it looks fine. Call the manufacturer if you have questions about the safety of your car seat.

The safest place in the car for an infant is facing the rear of the car in the middle of the back seat. This helps support the baby's head and back. If the seat doesn't fit in the middle, place it in the back seat where it fits best. The back of the safety seat supports the baby's back, neck, and head in a crash.

If your baby's head flops forward, place a rolled towel under the front edge of the child safety seat. Also, place rolled towels or blankets on both sides of the baby's head and shoulders for support.

Two kinds of safety seats are made for babies—infant-only seats and convertible seats. Infant-only seats fit babies 17–22 pounds and always face the rear of the car. A convertible seat fits children from birth to about 40 pounds. It is used facing the back of the car for the first year, then can be turned to face the front when the baby is at least 1 year old and weighs at least 20 pounds.

Choosing the Best Seat

By September 2002, all new cars and trucks must have the same system to install child safety seats. This means every child safety seat will fit in a car or truck the same way. Special anchors—instead of seat belts—will hold the seat in place. All child safety seats will be redesigned to use the anchors. If you have an older model child safety seat, you can buy a special belt designed to fit the new anchors.

Until all new cars and seats have these anchors, some safety seats will fit in your car better than others. A seat that is easy to use will be the best for you and your child. When buying a seat, keep these tips in mind:

▶ Try locking and unlocking the buckle while you are in the store. Try changing the lengths of the straps.

▶ Try the seat in your car. If it doesn't fit, you'll need another model.

▶ Read the labels to check weight limits.

Using the Seat in Your Car

To protect your child, the safety seat must be secure in the car. First, place the seat in the middle of the back seat, facing the rear. Lock the seat into its base, if it has one. The base should not move more than 1 inch when pushed. The lap part of the seat belt should be tightly fastened to the seat frame. To make sure it's tight, push the safety seat down into the seat cushion while you tighten the belt around it. Check the car's owner's manual for instructions about using belts for safety seats.

The safety seat's harness should fit snugly around the baby. You should be able to slide one finger under the straps at your child's chest. The straps should be over your baby's shoulder. The chest clips should be placed at your baby's armpit.

If you want to cover your baby, first buckle the baby in without any covering. Then, place a blanket over the baby.

Air Bags

Many new cars have air bags to protect the driver and the passenger riding in the front seat. Air bags are inside the steering wheel and dashboard in front of the passenger seat.

In a crash, air bags inflate very fast. The force of an air bag can hurt people who are too close to it. To avoid injury to you and your child from an air bag, follow these steps:

▶ Never put a child age 12 and under in the front seat—children should always ride in back.

▶ Never put an infant seat that faces the rear of the car in the front seat.

▶ Buckle up with both the lap and shoulder belts on every trip.

▶ Keep driver and passenger seats as far back from the dashboard as you can.

If your car does not have a back seat or the back seat is not made for passengers, the air bag must have an on/off switch. To prevent injury, if a small child is in the car, the air bag should be turned off.

COMPLEMENTARY AND ALTERNATIVE MEDICINE

Complementary and alternative medicine (CAM) covers a broad range of healing philosophies, approaches, and therapies. It is defined as those treatments and healthcare practices not taught widely in medical schools and often not used in hospitals.

People use complementary and alternative medicine treatments in a mixture of ways. If the treatment is used along with standard medical therapy, it often is called complementary treatment. If the treatment is used in place of standard therapy, it is called an alternative treatment. CAM treatments often are not covered by health insurance plans.

In most cases, CAM treatments have not been studied as well as most standard medical treatments. Unlike prescription drugs, before they are sold, herbal products and dietary supplements do not have to be tested to prove they are safe and work well. As a result, consumers have no way of knowing if a product will do what the label claims. Also, you may not be able to find reliable information about a product, which makes it hard for doctors and patients to know if a certain CAM treatment is safe and helpful.

Most doses of standard medical therapy prescribed by doctors are standard. Accurate dosage information is not available for many CAM treatments and the ingredients can vary widely.

Some CAM treatments become part of standard medical practice after they have been shown to be safe and work well. Acupuncture is an example.

For more information on alternative medicine contact:

*National Center for Complementary and Alternative Medicine
NCCAM Clearinghouse
PO Box 8218
Silver Spring, MD 20907-8218
Phone: 888-644-6226
Web Address:
www.nccam.nih.gov*

Alternative Medicine Practices

▶ Alternative systems of medical practice include traditional Chinese medicine, homeopathy, ayurveda, naturopathy, chiropractic, acupuncture, and Native-American medicine.

▶ Bioelectromagnetic applications include the use of magnets for joint and nerve pain; low-frequency thermal waves; electromagnetic waves to treat bone fractures; and electrical nerve stimulation for pain relief.

▶ Diet and nutrition includes the use of vitamins, minerals, nutritional supplements, and diets to prevent cancer and heart disease. Treatments include intake of large amounts of certain foods or nutrients, vegetarian and macrobiotic diets, and diets named by their creator.

▶ Herbal medicine is the use of herbs or other plants that act as medicines in the body, such as St John's wort.

▶ Manual healing methods include massage, chiropractic and osteopathic manipulation, and biofield therapeutics, which includes Reiki, polarity, reflexology, and therapeutic touch.

▶ Mind-body interventions include yoga, relaxation methods, meditation, t'ai chi ch'uan, hypnotherapy, spirituality, support groups, and biofeedback.

▶ Pharmacologic and biologic treatments include folk medicine and medicinal plants.

Questions from Your Doctor

To learn more about a CAM treatment you may be using or thinking about using, your doctor may ask if you are:

▶ Using any herbal products, vitamins, or home remedies?

▶ Seeing any other health care providers?

▶ Pregnant or breastfeeding?

▶ Taking any prescription or nonprescription drugs?

▶ Allergic to any plant products?

If you are thinking about using a CAM treatment, it is a good idea to let your doctor know. Many alternative or complementary treatments can be used safely along with standard medical treatments. However, some may pose health risks. Even the safest methods can be harmful if they prevent you from getting an accurate diagnosis or from using a more effective proven treatment. Your doctor can help you sort out which treatments may be helpful and which could be health hazards.

▶ EXERCISE

Regular physical activity—exercise that is done on most days—has many health benefits. In spite of its advantages, however, more than 60% of American adults do not exercise on a regular basis. In fact, 25% of all adults are not active at all.

Benefits of Exercise

One of the most important benefits of regular physical activity is that it promotes cardiovascular fitness—that is, it strengthens your heart and circulatory system. Having a strong, healthy heart helps lower cholesterol and blood pressure levels—factors that can reduce your risk of heart disease. Regular physical activity also:

▶ Strengthens your muscles

▶ Increases your flexibility

▶ Gives you more energy

▶ Helps control weight

Physical activity helps build and maintain strong bones. Active women have stronger bones than women who do not exercise. This is important as women age and become prone to weakening of bones through osteoporosis. Regular physical activity may also reduce the risk of colon cancer.

Physical benefits are not all you get with regular exercise. Staying active promotes mental well-being, relieves stress, and reduces feelings of depression and anxiety. You feel good about your body when you exercise regularly, and therefore have a healthier body image.

You do not have to follow an intense exercise routine to benefit. In fact, even moderate daily physical activity totalling

Even 30 minutes a day of exercise has benefit, and the 30 minutes can be spread out through the day—a 10-minute walk, climbing stairs, cleaning, shopping, whatever gets you moving.

30 minutes, which may be spread throughout the day, can offer health benefits.

Types of Exercise

Two types of exercises—aerobic and resistance training—can help your body in a variety of ways. A combination of both is the most effective.

Aerobic exercise causes your heart and lungs to work harder and builds fitness. Improving the fitness of your heart and lungs increases your body's ability to use oxygen. It also burns more calories, which helps if you're trying to lose or maintain weight. Aerobic exercise includes, for example, walking, jogging, swimming, and dancing.

Resistance training builds muscle and slows bone loss. It strengthens muscles and bones by exerting force on them. As you build muscle, your body will become more toned. The more muscle you have, the better your body burns calories. Resistance training includes lifting weights and doing leg lifts or squats. Try to avoid exercising the same muscles 2 days in a row so they have time to recover. You can do resistance exercises for 30 minutes just 2–3 days a week to see results.

Stretching exercises also are good for your body. These exercises help to increase balance and flexibility.

Getting Started

Before starting an exercise program, you should be in good health. If you have a heart condition or are overweight, talk with your doctor first before beginning an exercise plan.

There are programs designed especially for certain women, such as older women or those with health problems. Some type of exercise is almost always of benefit. Rarely does a condition exclude you from all forms of exercise.

If it has been some time since you've exercised regularly, it's best to start slowly. Begin with as little as 5 minutes a day and add 5 more minutes a week until you can stay active for 30 minutes a day.

Many health clubs and gyms offer individual training services. You may want to consult a fitness instructor who can set a routine for you to follow under his or her supervision or on your own. A fitness instructor can show you how to perform certain movements to avoid strain or other injury. Instructors are often certified to ensure they are properly trained.

There are also many videos, books, and magazines available on exercise and fitness. They can provide tips on getting and staying in shape and can inspire you to stick with an exercise program. You may want to ask a fitness instructor to suggest a video that will match your level of fitness.

Stick With It!

Unless you have to stop your exercise program for a health reason, stick with it. Set short-term goals for yourself. If you get bored, try something different or exercise with a friend or family member. The health rewards of regular exercise are worth it!

Plan your exercise program to suit your interests and lifestyle. If you choose activities that you like, you're more likely to stick to it, which is most important. For example, gardening and dancing are great forms of exercise. Don't forget to count everyday chores and activities, such as climbing stairs, carrying bags, and washing the car. Table 2 lists activities that you can select to fit into your daily life. The harder you exercise, the more calories you burn.

Warming Up and Cooling Down

Make it a practice to start each exercise session with a warm-up period for 5–10 minutes. This is light activity, such as slow walking or stationary cycling at a low resistance, which prepares your muscles for more intense activity. You should also do warm-up stretches to help avoid muscle stiffness and soreness. Hold each stretch for 10–20 seconds—do not bounce. When you feel a pulling on the muscle, you will know that you are stretching enough.

After exercising, cool down by slowly reducing your activity. This allows your heart rate to return to near-normal levels. Cooling down for 5–10 minutes and stretching again will increase flexibility and prevent muscle soreness. Hold stretches for 20–30 seconds, and do not bounce.

Target Heart Rate

You should exercise so that your heart beats at the level that gives you the best workout. This is called your target heart rate. To check your heart rate, count the beats by feeling the pulse on the inside of your wrist. Count for the first 10 seconds. Multiply this count by 6 to get the number of beats per minute.

Table 3 gives guidelines for finding your target heart rate. It is about 60–80% of your maximum heart rate (the fastest your heart can beat). For example, if you are 40, your maximum heart rate is 220 minus 40, or 180. Your target heart rate is 60–80% of 180, or 108–144 beats per minute (180 × 0.6 = 108; 180 × 0.8 = 144). Exercise resulting in a heart rate above 80% of your maximum heart rate may be too much unless you're in top physical shape. Exercise resulting in a heart rate below 60% gives too little conditioning.

When you begin your exercise program, aim for the lower range of your target heart rate (60%). As you get into bet-

Table 2. Burning Calories

Keep track of the number of calories you burn while exercising or performing everyday activities:

Activity	Calories Burned Per 30 Minutes
Dancing	300
Jogging (5 mph)	230
Gardening	60–200
Shoveling snow	200
Climbing stairs	200
Low-impact aerobics	200
Mopping floors	100
Walking (3 mph)	100
Grocery shopping	100
Raking leaves	100

ter shape, gradually build up to the higher end of your target heart rate (80%). You should aim to exercise about 20–30 minutes while in your target heart rate.

How Often?

Physical activity should be a part of most, if not all, days of the week. A form of aerobic exercise should be done three times a week. You should maintain your routine throughout the year. If you stop for more than 2 weeks, you may need to work at a lower level when you start exercising again. Then increase the level of exercise as you feel able.

Things To Watch

If you are overdoing exercise, your body may give you some warnings. Be alert to injuries or any other changes in your body.

Injuries

Exercise and sports activities can increase your risk of injury to muscle, bones, and joints. It is important not to overdo it when you begin an exercise program. If your body is not used to exercise, it can suffer from muscle strains or other injuries. It is best to start slowly and warm up before you begin to exercise. In most cases, exercise-related injuries don't require extensive treatment. Your muscles may only need rest and time to heal.

Women who routinely exercise vigorously may get injuries as a result of repeated periods of excessive stress on their muscles and bones. These injuries include stress fractures, shin splints—which cause pain at the lower front part of the leg— and knee injuries. Exercises that can cause stress injuries include high-impact aerobics and running.

One way to avoid injury is to rest on some days or alternate between vigorous and lighter activity. Another way is to cross-train, which means doing different activities, such as tennis, swimming, and water aerobics to give variety to how you're using your muscles and joints. Also, pay attention to your body. If you don't feel well, take a break from exercise.

Menstrual Changes

Vigorous exercise over a long time span may cause changes in your menstrual cycle. Rarely, a woman's periods stop com-

Table 3. Target Heart Rate for Women

To find your target heart rate, look for the age category closest to your age and read the line across. For example, if you are 43, the closest age on the chart is 45; the target heart rate is 105–140 beats per minute. Your maximum heart rate is usually 220 minus your age. Your target heart rate is 60–80% of the maximum. These figures are averages to be used as general guidelines and do not apply to pregnant women.

Age	Target Heart Rate (beats per minute)	Average Maximum Heart Rate
20	120–160	200
25	117–156	195
30	114–152	190
35	111–148	185
40	108–144	180
45	105–140	175
50	102–136	170
55	99–132	165
60	96–128	160
65	93–124	155
70	90–120	150

National Heart, Lung, and Blood Institute. Exercise and your heart. NIH Publication No. 81-1677. Washington, DC: U.S. Government Printing Office, 1981

pletely. If you notice changes in your periods or if they stop altogether, see your doctor.

Never assume that menstrual changes are related to exercise. A thorough checkup is needed to find the cause.

▶ See also *Advance Directives, Living Wills*

▶ HEALTH CARE POWER OF ATTORNEY

In a health care power of attorney, you choose a person you trust to make your medical decisions for you when you cannot do so. They become your health care agent.

With a health care power of attorney, you may state your wishes about your medical care. Your agent is not required to follow them, though, because the power to make decisions becomes his or hers. In your health care power of attorney, you can list exactly which powers you are giving to your agent:

▶ Power to choose your doctors

▶ The right to decide whether you are hospitalized

▶ The right to accept or refuse treatment

The health care power of attorney is more flexible than a living will. If you use one, it is vital to choose your health care agent with care.

Do not expect a close friend or family member to know what your wishes will be for your care if you need life support. To make sure you get the kind of care you prefer, talk to your health care agent about what you want.

▶ HEALTH INSURANCE

Women often must choose health care insurance for themselves and their families. With the growth of different health care plans, it has become very important to choose the best one for your specific situation. Insurance may be offered through employers, and companies often change policies or coverage. Thus you need to be aware of all aspects of coverage.

What To Look For

Stay Informed

Read your health insurance policy and member handbook. Make sure you understand them, especially the information on benefits and coverage.

Evaluating a health plan can be challenging. What you need from a plan today may not be what you need 6 months from now. Your age, marital status, children, health, and income will affect which plan is best for you. You may also need to consider combining coverage from two companies if you and your spouse are both employed and have separate coverage.

Consider your own situation. Do you want coverage for your family, or just for yourself? Are preventive care and check-ups covered? How far must you travel to receive care? What kind of access would you have to your current doctor? These questions and others provided should be considered in making the choice that is right for you.

Choice of Care

Some plans require that you see a primary care provider—either a physician or nurse practitioner—before getting a referral to see other types of care providers, including obstetrician–gynecologists. Other plans do not limit access so tightly and allow you to go directly to your obstetrician–gynecologist.

Some health plans limit your choice of doctors. If the doctors you are currently using do not belong to the plan, you may have to switch doctors. Other plans offer direct access to the doctor of your choice. This means you can go to the doctor of your choice with first seeing another doctor for a referral. Your health plan may also affect which hospitals you can use and what treatment options are available.

If you already have health insurance, your choice of doctors may be limited to those in the plan. But, if you have a choice of plans, you may first want to think about which doctors you would like to use. Then you may be able to choose a plan that includes your choice.

Out-of-Pocket Costs

Another thing to consider before choosing your plan is the out-of-pocket costs—any money that you must pay for health care including monthly premiums (cost of an insurance policy). Some plans require you to pay a certain amount each time you visit a doctor or clinic (this is called a co-payment). There may also be a co-payment (or set price) for prescription medications—usually $2–10. You may also have to pay a deductible—an initial portion of your hospital bill—before your insurance company will begin to pay for your health care. A plan may have a lifetime maximum dollar limit (the maximum amount that a plan will pay for treatment of an individual or family) or an out-of-pocket maximum (the amount that you must pay before the insurance plan will fully cover the costs of treatment) on each person or family covered.

Completeness of Coverage

Some health plans may not pay for treatment of a medical problem or a condition that you had before you signed on with their company, such as pregnancy, high blood pressure, and cancer. This is called a preexisting condition. Some plans offer options for vision or dental care for an additional cost.

Types of Health Care Plans

Health care plans differ on how the health care provider is paid for his or her services. They can be either more traditional fee-for-service plans or managed care plans.

Fee-for-service plans pay the doctor of your choice, based on an established fee schedule. Managed care plans pay only for

Important Questions to Ask Your Health Care Insurer

Health Care

1. Does the plan provide and pay for:

    ▶ Immunizations?

    ▶ Preventive health exams and checkups, including Pap tests, mammography, cholesterol screening, and colon cancer screening?

    ▶ Preexisting conditions such as pregnancy, diabetes, and cancer?

    ▶ Infertility diagnosis and treatment?

    ▶ Elective sterilization such as tubal ligation or vasectomy?

    ▶ Contraception, including intrauterine devices, diaphragms, birth control pills, injections, and implants?

    ▶ Osteoporosis diagnosis and treatment?

    ▶ Hormone replacement therapy?

    ▶ Mental health services, including diagnosis and treatment of postpartum depression and eating disorders?

    ▶ Drug and alcohol abuse treatment?

    ▶ Comprehensive obstetric services?

    ▶ Obstetric anesthesia care?

    ▶ High-risk obstetric care and prenatal genetic screening?

    ▶ Well baby exam?

2. Are your doctors participants in the plan?

3. Does the plan allow you unlimited direct access to your obstetrician–gynecologist?

4. Will you be allowed to change your doctor if you're not happy with the one you have?

5. Can you use the hospital of your choice if you become sick or need treatment?

6. May you go to the emergency room or hospital without prior approval?

7. Is adequate coverage out of the geographic area provided?

8. Are prescription medications, including your current ones, paid for?

9. Is there an 800 phone number you can call with questions or problems?

10. Is there a good appeals process available if the plan refuses to pay for a treatment?

11. Does your doctor have a financial incentive to withhold care or referrals to specialists?

Expenses

12. What is the co-payment per doctor visit?

13. What is the co-payment for prescriptions?

14. What is the co-payment for inpatient hospital care?

15. What is the co-payment for emergency care or ambulance service?

16. What is the extra charge for seeing a doctor outside the plan?

17. What is the monthly premium?

18. What is the deductible?

19. What is the lifetime maximum dollar limit coverage per person/per family?

20. What is the out-of-pocket maximum per person/per family?

care provided by doctors enrolled in the plan. There are two types of managed care plans:

▶ Health Maintenance Organizations (HMOs) provide or arrange for health care services to members within a geographic area. The emphasis is on preventive health care. Most care may be provided by a primary care provider who may also be called a gatekeeper. Your primary care provider may refer you to another physician.

▶ Preferred Provider Organizations (PPOs) contract with independent providers (doctors, hospitals, and other health care providers) for discounted fees for services provided to plan members. Members usually have a wider choice of providers, but the cost of care by participating providers is lower.

Your Decision

To find out more about a given plan, ask other members about the health plan you are considering. Is the language of the policy clear? How are you treated by the plan's representatives? How easy is it to get your questions answered? These factors may all indicate how plan members are treated.

If you are given a choice of health plans, look at what each one has to offer. Do not hesitate to ask your health insurer specific questions that concern you. The questions provided can be used as a guide to help you choose the plan that offers the best value for yourself and your family.

Did You Know?

Women make 75% of the health care decisions for their families and are more likely to be the caregivers for a sick family member.

▶ INFORMED CONSENT

The more you know about your health care, the better equipped you are to make choices. During medical visits, your doctor will explain what's happening and why. Before you give your OK for a test or a treatment, be sure you know what it is and why it's needed. You also should be told about the risks, benefits, and options. This is called "informed consent."

You and your doctor are partners in your health care. You both have rights and responsibilities.

If you don't understand something you have heard, ask your doctor to explain it more clearly. The doctor will make a note in your chart that something has been explained to you. He or she also will note what you have chosen to do. In some cases, you may be asked to sign a form saying that you have been informed of something or that you have agreed to have a certain procedure done.

Partners in Health Care

Both you and your health care providers have rights and responsibilities. Your health care provider has the right to stop treating you as long as you have time to find other care. He or she has the responsibility to give you quality medical treatment while you are in his or her care.

You have the right to:

▶ Get quality care without discrimination

▶ Be given privacy

▶ Know the professional status of your health care providers and their fees

▶ Know your diagnosis, treatment options, and expected outcome

▶ Be involved in decisions about your care

▶ Refuse all or part of the treatment

▶ Agree or decline to be involved in research that affects your care

You have the responsibility to:

▶ Provide correct and complete health information

▶ Let your providers know that you understand what's being done to you and what you are expected to do

▶ Accept responsibility if you refuse treatment or don't follow the doctor's plan

▶ LESBIAN HEALTH

Roughly 4–10% of women in the United States identify themselves as lesbians. Lesbians are women who are mainly emotionally and sexually attracted to other women. Lesbians need the same health care as other women. However, they may be less likely to receive regular care because they may not trust the health care system or do not think they need the same kind of care as women who have sex with men.

Sexual Orientation

Sexuality is part of every human being. No one really knows why a person develops a certain sexual orientation—that is, whether a woman is a lesbian or homosexual (attracted only to women), bisexual (attracted to both men and women), or heterosexual (attracted only to men). Some experts think that sexual orientation is set before birth.

Every woman does not express her sexuality in the same way. Also, a woman may express her sexuality in different ways over her lifetime. Many lesbians have had sex with men at some time in their lives. Many factors affect sexual behavior.

Preventive Health Care

Obstetrician–gynecologists (ob-gyns) provide preventive health care and promote wellness for women. All women, including lesbians, should see their doctors regularly for preventive health care. Such care includes routine tests and exams that all women need, regardless of their sexual orientation. Preventive care can help detect health problems before they become serious. It provides a chance to learn ways to stay in better health.

You and Your Doctor

Talking about your sexual orientation with your doctor may be hard to do. You should be able to discuss with your doctor anything that affects your well-being. This includes your sexuality.

Many doctors don't ask about sexual orientation. It can be hard for you to reveal because you may be unsure about the doctor's response. The risk is worth it, though. Trust your doctor. If you don't, you may not tell your doctor things he or she needs to know about your health.

Sharing information about your sexual orientation with your doctor also helps him or her to be more aware of your health care needs. For instance, questions about your health may be phrased in a different way if your doctor knows you are a lesbian.

Women who have not told their families or coworkers they are lesbians may not want to discuss it with their doctor. They may worry that it will not be kept private. Doctors are required by law to keep your health information confidential (private).

The Well-Woman Exam

All women—whether they have sex with other women or men or do not have sex—should have a well-woman visit at least once a year. This visit includes a general check of your health and an exam of your breasts and pelvic (reproductive) organs. During the exam your doctor will:

▶ *Obtain a health history.* This includes asking questions about your past illnesses, family health history, your menstrual periods, use of medications, and whether you have ever been pregnant.

▶ *Do a physical exam.* This begins with a check of your weight and blood pressure. The doctor will also check your breasts for lumps and examine your pelvic organs.

▶ *Perform routine tests.* A Pap test and perhaps others, such as mammography or some blood tests, may be done. It depends on your age and other risk factors.

▶ *Provide counseling.* You will be given information to help you stay healthy. The doctor will answer any questions you may have.

If you do not want information about your sexuality in your medical record because you think it is likely to be seen by insurance companies or others, simply let your doctor know.

Gynecologic Health Concerns

Lesbians do have gynecologic problems. Because lesbians may avoid seeing a doctor, health conditions such as infections and cancers may not be noticed or treated.

Sexually Transmitted Diseases

You are at greater risk for STDs if you or your partner have had sex with other partners.

Sexually transmitted diseases (STDs), including HIV (human immunodeficiency virus), are less common in lesbians than in heterosexual women. These diseases can be passed from woman to woman, though. Sex can pose a risk.

There are steps you can take to protect yourself from STDs:

- Do not allow body fluids of another woman, including menstrual blood and vaginal fluids, to enter your body through cuts or other openings.

- During oral sex, make sure none of your partner's fluids get in your mouth. Cover her entire vagina with plastic food wrap, a dental dam (a square sheet of latex), or a cut-open condom or latex glove.

- Place a latex barrier or plastic wrap between your vaginas during vulva-to-vulva sex.

- Avoid sharing sex toys. If you do, always wash them in hot, soapy water or put a fresh condom on the toy before switching users.

- If you think you might have an STD, or have had sex with someone who has an STD, seek medical care. Do not have sex until both you and your partner have been tested and treated.

Cancer

Cancer of the cervix appears to be less common among lesbians than among heterosexual women. You still should be tested for it regularly. The risk of cancer of the cervix is higher in women who:

- Began having sex with men at a young age
- Have had more than one male sexual partner
- Have been infected with human papillomavirus (HPV)
- Smoke cigarettes
- Have been treated for an abnormal Pap test

Regular Pap tests can detect changes in the cervix that could be a sign of cancer or changes that could lead to cancer. When cancer of the cervix is caught early, there is a high cure rate.

Lesbians may be at an increased risk for certain other cancers. Women who have never given birth and have not used oral contraceptives (birth control pills) have a higher risk of cancer of the ovary and uterus. Exams for these two cancers are included in a gynecologic exam.

Women who have never had children and have never breast-fed are at a higher risk of breast cancer. Having routine breast exams and mammograms can help detect breast cancer early. Women older than 40 should have a mammogram every 1–2 years until age 50, and then annually after that. Mammograms may pick up tumors before they can be felt.

You also should examine your own breasts every month (known as a breast self-exam). See the Breast Self-Exam entry in this section to learn how to do this exam.

Emotional Health

An important health issue facing lesbians is emotional well-being. Revealing your homosexuality to family, friends, and coworkers is a hard to do. Some people have a hard time accepting that a person is homosexual. Because of this, you may worry about how your family and friends will react. You may fear or experience rejection. Lesbians who keep their sexual orientation to themselves, though, often become anxious, fear discovery, and may not get the support they need.

Your feelings and experiences can lead to isolation and depression. In a survey of nearly 2,000 lesbians, more than one third said they had suffered a long depression or sadness. This may make lesbians more open to alcohol and drug abuse.

The teen years can be a very hard time for many lesbians. Emotions change quickly. Sexual feelings awaken. There is intense pressure to "be like everyone else." For lesbian teens, adolescence can be trying and lonely.

Although there is no set time when a woman realizes she is lesbian, many women become aware of it during their adolescence. Lesbian teens may struggle with their sexual orientation and keep the truth secret until they are older. They may become depressed, do poorly in school, or even think about killing themselves. If you feel sad or depressed, get help as soon as you can. Your doctor or nurse can refer you to a counselor or support group.

Local gay or lesbian service centers provide information on support services; they are listed in the phone book.

Parenting

Many lesbians are parents. Lesbians may have children from previous relationships with men, they may adopt, become pregnant by artificial insemination or by having sex with a man, or serve as foster parents.

Laws about artificial insemination and adoption vary from state to state. If you are thinking about becoming a parent in this way, talk with your doctor about your plans. A preconceptional visit with your ob-gyn to plan for any pregnancy is a good idea.

▶ See also *Advance Directives, Health Care Power of Attorney*

▶ LIVING WILLS

A living will is a written statement. It tells your doctor and family what type of health care you will accept or refuse if you are not able to express your wishes. The laws about living wills vary from state to state, but most living wills:

▶ Tell doctors if you want them to do whatever they can to prolong your life.

▶ Tell doctors if you do not want to be kept alive with treatments that prolong your life:
  —Breathing machines (respirator)
  —Cardiopulmonary resuscitation (CPR)
  —Feeding tubes (inserted into your nose or abdomen and leading to your stomach)
  —Intravenous (IV) medication

A living will should be stated clearly in writing. That way, no one is confused about what you want. It deals only with medical care. It is different from a will that deals with your property.

You do not need a lawyer to prepare a living will, although you may wish to consult one. If you use a standard form, make sure the form is valid in your state. Be sure to follow the instructions, including those about witnesses.

The living will goes into effect only if you have a terminal condition (you are dying) and cannot make decisions for yourself. Until then, you can change your mind at any time about what you have written in your will. If you wish to make changes, you can complete new forms to replace the current ones.

Do I Need a Living Will?

There may be a time when you are too sick to make decisions for yourself. For instance:

▶ A car crash leaves you in a coma—how long do you want to be kept alive on life support?

▶ You had a stroke and become paralyzed—do you wish to be kept on life support?

Almost 3 out of 4 American adults have not filled out a living will of any kind, let alone talked with their family about how they want to die.

If you do not make a living will and are later not able to speak for yourself, your family and doctor may have a hard time deciding about your care. Living wills can spare your family from being forced to make tough decisions for you. It also allows you to express your wishes for your care.

When Should I Prepare a Living Will?

Only a small number of adults have prepared living wills. Most people don't want to think about becoming very ill and not being able to care for themselves. People are more likely to prepare a living will as they get older.

It's best to prepare a living will when you are healthy. No one knows when a serious accident or illness may happen. People of all ages can be injured in accidents.

A Gallup poll found that although 75% of Americans agree with living wills, only 20% had one.

How Do I Prepare a Living Will?

Forms for living wills are simple to fill out. You may be able to get them free from your hospital, insurance company, or doctor's office.

Before you fill out the forms, think about the choices you wish to make in your will. Discuss these issues with your family and your doctor.

Make a number of copies and give them to your doctors, family members, and friends. If you cancel or revise your living will, tell these people and give them copies of any new documents. You should keep the originals with your other important papers in a safe place.

What Are the Limits of Living Wills?

You also should be aware that states have different laws about living wills. Laws in some states are stricter than in others about when a living will can be used.

Most doctors want to honor the patient's wishes. If doctors don't agree with your will, though, they may not be required to honor it. In most cases, doctors do not have to follow a living will if they believe in good faith that it is not sound.

To protect the developing fetus, most states limit the rights of pregnant patients to refuse certain treatments. These limits may not be explained on the forms. To know

Your Living Will

Your living will should include your wishes for future medical care if there ever comes a time when you are terminally ill and cannot make decisions for yourself, including:

▶ Do you want life-sustaining treatments (including CPR) started?

▶ Do you want artifical nutrition and hydration started if it would be the main treatment keeping you alive?

▶ Do you want to be kept as comfortable and free of pain as possible, even if such care prolongs your dying or shortens your life?

▶ Do you want major surgery?

whether your state laws allow doctors to not regard your living will if you are pregnant, ask a lawyer.

▶ See also *Breast Cancer, Breast Problems, and Fibrocystic Breast Changes* in *"Women's Health"*

▶ MAMMOGRAPHY

Mammography is an X-ray technique used to study the breasts. It can help doctors find breast cancer at an early stage, when cancer treatment is more successful. About 1 in 9 women will develop breast cancer during her lifetime. The risk of breast cancer increases with age, and most cases occur after menopause. By age 50, yearly mammography should be a regular part of your health care.

What Is Mammography?

Mammography is a simple X-ray method. No dyes have to be injected or swallowed and no instruments will be put inside your body. The test involves passing low doses of X-rays through the breasts.

Because some growths are very small or are located deep within the breast tissue, they can be hard to detect. The test is a good way to detect growths before they are large enough to be felt during a physical exam. When growths are found in this early stage, they are easier to treat. Mammography is also useful for checking growths that have been detected during a physical exam. You should do a breast self-exam once a month.

Mammography can be done in a number of settings. These include a doctor's office or clinic or even a mobile screening van. You do not need to be admitted to a hospital for mammography. The test can be ordered by your doctor and performed by an X-ray technician specially trained in mammography. The results are read by a doctor specially trained in X-ray techniques. No matter where the test is done, you should get a report of the results from the radiologist or your doctor.

For more information about mammograms and breast cancer, call the National Cancer Institute's Cancer Information Service at 800-4-CANCER (800-422-6237).

Who Should Have Mammography?

Women ages 40–50 should have mammography done every 1–2 years. Women age 50 and older should have it done each year. If you have certain risk factors, your doctor may suggest you have this test done more often. If you have a mother, daughter, or sister with premenopausal breast cancer, your doctor may suggest that you start having mammography early—about age 35.

You also may need a mammogram if you have any of these signs:

▶ Unexplained lump or thickening in the breast or armpit

▶ Puckering or dimpling of the skin of the breast

▶ Discharge or bleeding from the nipple

▶ A recent change in the nipple, such as a retracted nipple (a nipple that has pulled inward)

▶ A change in the skin of the breast

> **Risk Factors**
>
> Most women who get breast cancer have no risk factors except age—as a woman gets older, her risk increases. But some women are at higher risk for developing breast cancer than others. These women:
>
> ▶ Have a sister, mother, or daughter who has had breast cancer
>
> ▶ Have had breast cancer before
>
> ▶ Began menstruating at an early stage
>
> ▶ Went through menopause at a late age

If any of these factors apply to you, talk to your doctor about having an exam and mammography done.

Mammography is vital for all women. The size of your breasts or whether you have breast implants does not matter. Women who have had breast cancer surgery also may need the test to examine the breast tissue that remains.

What To Expect During Mammography

The day you have mammography done, you may be asked not to wear any powders, lotions, or deodorants. Most brands contain substances that can show on the X-ray films and make them hard to read.

To get ready for the procedure, you'll need to put on a gown. When it's time for the test, you'll be asked to take off the gown and stand or sit in front of the X-ray machine. Two smooth, flat plastic plates will be placed around one of your breasts. The plates will flatten your breast so that the most tissue can be examined with the least radiation. After the first X-ray is taken, the plastic plates may be removed so that the breast can be X-rayed from one or more other positions. The procedure is then done again on the other breast.

The pressure of the plates may cause the breasts to ache. This discomfort will go away shortly. If you menstruate, you may want to arrange to have the test the week right after your period. The breasts often are less tender at this time.

If you have breast implants, tell your doctor. Mention your implants to the person who is giving you the test, too. There is some risk that the implant may burst during mammography. Therefore, extra care should be taken when the breast is compressed during the exam.

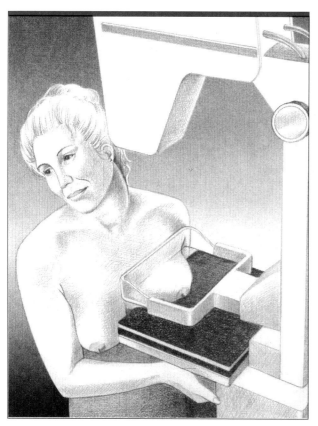

During mammography, your breast will be placed between two smooth, flat plastic plates so your doctor can take an x-ray and check for growths.

What Are the Benefits?

Mammography can detect some types of cancer long before a growth becomes large enough to be felt during an exam. If cancer is found early enough, there are more ways in which it can be treated with success, and the chance for cure is greater. Caught early enough, breast cancer often can be cured.

Are There Any Risks?

In most cases, mammography exposes a woman to a very low dose of X-rays—much lower than the level of radiation received naturally from the environment over the course of a year. In the past, there was some concern about the amount of radiation to which a patient was exposed during mammography. Improved equipment and techniques now result in very low exposure. Thus, risk is very low, even with repeated mammography.

Even when mammography is performed correctly at every step in the process, some cancers cannot be seen—even some that can be felt. The combination of self-exam, regular visits to your doctor, and mammography along with an exam will give the best results. That's why you shouldn't give up monthly breast self-exams just because you are having regular mammography. If you feel a lump, see your doctor.

What If the Test Result Is Positive?

About four of every five lumps found in the breast are benign—not cancer. To confirm the results of mammography, special mammography views or other tests, such as ultrasound, also may be helpful. You also may need to have mammography again if the results of the first test were not clear.

There are other tests that can tell your doctor more about the type of lump. They include:

▶ Needle aspiration, in which a needle is inserted into the lump to find out whether it is fluid filled or solid. A sample of fluid or tissue may be withdrawn for study under a microscope.

▶ Biopsy, a procedure in which the entire growth or a sample of breast tissue is removed for study under a microscope.

▶ MEDICATIONS

▶ See also
*Complementary and
Alternative Medicine*

Medications can help treat illness and infection and help you get well again. Drugs are useful for people of all ages, from infants to the elderly. Some drugs must be prescribed by your doctor. To prescribe a drug, your doctor will write an official order for the drug so your pharmacist can give it to you. Other medicines, known as over-the-counter (OTC) drugs, can be bought without a prescription. Most OTC drugs are for minor ailments.

Today there are many kinds of drugs available to treat many types of diseases. Research is being done every day to find new cures and treatments.

When taking any medicines, follow your doctor's advice. When using an OTC drug to treat a cold or other ailment, follow the package directions. Drugs may not work properly and can even cause harm if you take them the wrong way. You should never stop taking a drug before your doctor tells you to. Even if you feel better after a few days, take the medication as prescribed. Let your doctor know if you are taking any other drugs, including alternative medicine or over-the-counter medicine. And never take more or less than directed. Once a drug is past the expiration date stamped on the package, throw it away. Never take someone else's prescription drugs.

If a drug makes you feel worse or gives you a rash, call your doctor. Some people are allergic to certain drugs and some drugs do not mix well with other medications. Certain diseases, especially chronic ones like diabetes, call for taking two or more drugs at once. Most of the time this is safe, but sometimes bad reactions occur. If you are worried that your medicine is doing more harm than good, talk to your doctor. He or she may be able to prescribe another drug that may work better for you.

Women visit doctors more often than men, and they take more medications than men. You should always learn what your medicines are for and how to take them correctly. If you are pregnant or nursing, you need to be especially careful about the drugs you take. Your baby may also be affected. To help you take drugs safely, tell your doctor if you:

▶ Are taking any other drugs, even things like sleep aids, vitamins, or birth control pills

▶ Have any allergies or have ever had a bad reaction to a drug

▶ Are, or could be, pregnant

▶ Are nursing

▶ Foresee any problems taking the drug. For example, some people are unable to swallow pills

Generic Drugs

A generic drug is the drug's chemical name rather than the brand name. Though they contain the same active ingredients as brand-name drugs, generic drugs often are priced lower.

When you are well-informed, your medicine is more likely to work well and be safe. If you have questions, ask your doctor, nurse, or pharmacist. Be sure to learn:

▶ The drug's name and what it is supposed to do

▶ How much to take, when to take it, and for how long

▶ What side effects are possible, and what to do if they occur

▶ Whether you should avoid foods or drinks, such as cheese, milk, caffeine, or alcohol

▶ If you must avoid smoking while taking the drug

▶ If you should avoid sports or other activities, such as driving

The U.S. Food and Drug Administration (FDA) makes sure drugs work well and are safe. Most, but not all, drugs you can buy have been approved by the FDA. Be cautious if a treatment sounds too good to be true. You can call your local FDA office, listed in the blue pages of your phone book, to check whether or not a drug has been approved.

▶ See also *Nutrition During Pregnancy* in "Women's Health," *Weight Control*

▶ NUTRITION

Eating well is one of the best things you can do to stay healthy. A good diet increases your energy, improves your well-being, and lowers your risk of disease. What you eat is linked to your risk of serious health problems, such as heart disease, cancer, diabetes, and osteoporosis.

Too Much of a Good Thing

Vitamins A and D may have harmful effects if excessive amounts are taken regularly for a long period. Too much vitamin A may cause hair loss, liver damage, joint pains, and your skin may begin to peel. Overdosing on vitamin D may cause kidney damage and calcium deposits may form in your body tissues.

Nutrition and Your Health

A balanced diet is a basic part of good health. Every diet should include proteins, carbohydrates (sugars and starches), fats, vitamins, and minerals. Your body needs a regular supply of these nutrients to grow, to replace worn-out tissue, and to provide energy.

The amount of nutrients you need each day is called the Recommended Daily Allowance (RDA). To be sure that your diet gives you the RDA of nutrients, you need to know which ones are in the foods you eat. On foods that have labels, you will see a column labeled "% Daily Value." This column helps you see how the food fits into your diet by showing the amount of the RDA a serving supplies. The box shows you how to read a food label. Your daily goal is to reach 100% of each nutrient.

Reading Food Labels

All packaged foods must be clearly labeled with nutrition information. Reading all food labels can help you make smart food choices. The label will tell you how many grams of fat and how many calories are in each serving.

You may see the terms "enriched" or "fortified" on a food label. Both terms mean that vitamins or minerals have been added to the food. The difference is that enriched foods have vitamins or minerals added back to them, and fortified foods have vitamins or minerals added that weren't there from the start. Both make it simple for you to get the vitmins and minerals you need.

Serving Size: The amount served and eaten. The numbers on the label refer to this amount of food.

Total Fat: The amount of fat in one serving

Nutrients: A list of the nutrients the product contains. Nutrients often listed here are total fat, cholesterol, sodium, total carbohydrates, and protein.

Calories: Amount of energy the food supplies

Percent Daily Values: The percentage of nutrients this product provides based on the RDA. It is based on a diet of 2,000 calories.

Nutrition Facts

Serving Size 1 Package (46.8g)
Servings Per container 1

Amount Per Serving

Calories 180   Calories from Fat 18

	% Daily Value
Total Fat 2g	**3%**
Saturated Fat 0g	**0%**
Cholesterol 0mg	**0%**
Sodium 1100mg	**46%**
Total Carbohydrate 36g	**12%**
Dietary Fiber less than 1g	**1%**
Sugars 2g	
Protein 5g	

Vitamin A 0%	•	Vitamin C	0%
Calcium 0%	•	Iron	3%

*Percent Daily Values are based on a 2,000 calorie diet. Your daily values may be higher or lower depending on your calorie needs:

	Calorie	2,000	2,500
Total Fat	Less than	65g	80g
Sat. Fat	Less than	20g	25g
Cholesterol	Less than	300mg	300mg
Sodium	Less than	2,400mg	2,400mg
Total Carbohydrate		300g	375g
Dietary Fiber		25g	30g

Calories per gram:
Fat 9   •   Carbohydrate 4   •   Protein 4

Daily Food Choices

The first step toward healthy eating is to look at the foods in your daily diet. Eating a variety of foods each day helps ensure a balanced diet.

The Food Guide Pyramid can help you choose the foods to plan a balanced diet. It shows the number of servings you should have each day from each of these six food groups:

1. Bread, cereal, rice, and pasta

2. Fruit

3. Vegetable

4. Meat, poultry, fish, dry beans, eggs, and nuts

5. Milk, yogurt, and cheese

6. Fats, oils, and sweets

The Food Guide Pyramid

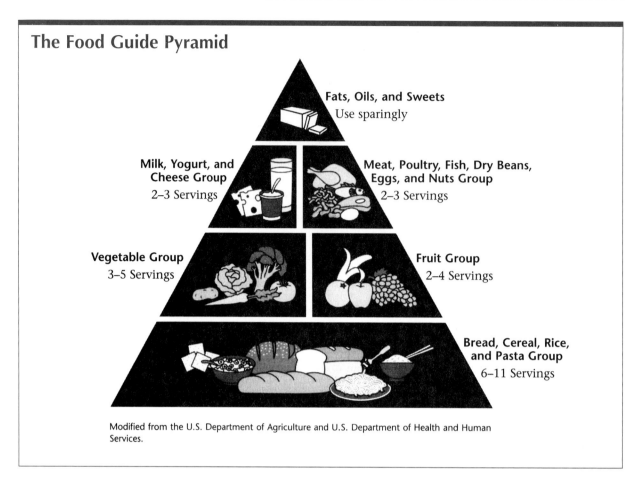

Fats, Oils, and Sweets
Use sparingly

Milk, Yogurt, and Cheese Group
2–3 Servings

Meat, Poultry, Fish, Dry Beans, Eggs, and Nuts Group
2–3 Servings

Vegetable Group
3–5 Servings

Fruit Group
2–4 Servings

Bread, Cereal, Rice, and Pasta Group
6–11 Servings

Modified from the U.S. Department of Agriculture and U.S. Department of Health and Human Services.

Make it a point to choose most of your foods from the bread, cereal, rice, and pasta group. This group has the largest number (6–11) of recommended servings. Although this may seem like a lot, it really isn't. For instance, one slice of bread is equal to one serving, and so is ½ cup of rice or pasta or 1 ounce of cereal. So, if you eat a bowl of cereal for breakfast, two slices of bread for lunch, and 1 cup of rice or pasta and a roll for dinner, you will get all you need of that food group.

Calories and Fat

When our body digests food, it breaks the food down into carbohydrates, proteins, and fats. It then converts these into energy. Different types of foods have different amounts of calories.

What Are Calories?

A calorie is a measure of the energy we get from food. The number of calories we need each day differs from person to person. It depends on your age, how active you are, and your body size. Most people should have an intake of around 2,000 calories per day.

One pound is equal to 3,500 calories. In order to lose 1 pound, you must eat less or be more active so you will burn more calories.

Try to eat the least amount of calories your body needs. The more calories you eat, the more you need to burn to keep from gaining weight. You can burn calories with exercise. Calories from food that are not used are stored in the body as fat.

Foods in the carbohydrate group have 4 calories/g, fats have 9 calories/g, and proteins have 4 calories/g. That is, for each gram of carbohydrate you eat, your body gets 4 calories of energy.

What Is Fat?

Fat is found in food. Your body only makes fat from the food you eat. Your body needs some fat to function. Too much fat in your diet, though, can raise the cholesterol in your bloodstream. This may increase your chance of getting high blood pressure and heart disease. Too much fat also can add to your weight.

There are two kinds of fat found in food—saturated and unsaturated. Saturated fat is solid at room temperature. Unsaturated fat is liquid at room temperature. Unsaturated fats are better choices than saturated fats—they don't raise your cholesterol as much. The best choice, though, is to limit all fats.

Fat should make up less than 30% of the total calories in your daily diet. Use the formula in the box to add up the amount of fat in your diet.

It is easy to reduce the amount of fat in your diet. Start by eating more fruits, vegetables, and whole grains. Switch from foods high in fat to foods low in fat. For instance, choose skim milk instead of whole milk. Be aware that most "fast food" and prepared foods like snacks and microwave meals have high amounts of fat in them.

You also can reduce the fat in your diet by changing the way you prepare foods:

- Broil or bake instead of frying
- Skim liquid fat from soups
- Trim all fat from meats
- Remove skin from poultry
- Cut back on butter, margarine, cream, oil, and mayonnaise

Do You Need Vitamin Supplements?

It may be hard to get all the nutrients you need from your diet. Some women, espe-

Finding Fats

Saturated fats are found in:

- *Fatty meats, especially prepared meats*
- *Whole-milk dairy products (butter, cheese, ice cream)*
- *Snacks and other foods that contain coconut and palm oils*

Unsaturated fats are found in:

- *Olive, peanut, and canola oils*
- *Liquid margarine*

Fat: How Much Is Too Much?

Fats should make up less than 30% of the total calories in your daily diet. Based on a 2,000-calorie-a-day diet, this is about 60 grams of fat each day. If you eat fewer than 2,000 calories a day, you should eat fewer than 60 grams of fat.

Each gram of fat has 9 calories. To find the total calories from fat, multiply the number of grams of fat in a serving shown on the label by 9. For instance, 1 ounce of potato chips has 10 grams of fat. This means that 90 of its calories comes from fat (10 × 9 = 90). If the potato chips have a total of 150 calories, 60% of the calories come from fat (divide 90 by 150 = .60 or 60%). If more than 30% of the calories are from fat, that food is high in fat.

An ounce of pretzels has 110 calories and 1 gram of fat. This means that 9 calories (1 × 9) come from fat. Those calories are only 8% of the total (9 divided by 110).

cially those who are pregnant or in menopause, may need to take extra vitamins or minerals. Talk with your doctor before taking any vitamin other than a multivitamin. Do not take more vitamins than your doctor suggests. Iron, calcium, and folic acid are key supplements women should think about taking.

Iron

Iron is needed to make new blood cells. If you are not getting enough iron, anemia (low blood count) may occur. Women may become anemic because of loss of blood during menstruation or childbirth. Anemia may make you feel tired. If anemia becomes severe, it can make you feel weak and look pale.

The RDA for iron for nonpregnant women is 15 mg a day. Pregnant women need 30 mg. To increase your iron intake, eat iron-rich foods, such as liver, meat, dried beans and peas, prunes, and prune juice. It also helps to eat foods rich in vitamin C, like oranges and tomatoes, at the same meal with an iron-rich food. Vitamin C helps your body use iron better.

Calcium

Bone is made up of calcium and protein. Bones can become thin and brittle if your diet is low in calcium. Calcium helps keep bones strong. See Table 4 to find out how much calcium you need each day.

Dairy foods are rich in calcium, but you should choose low-fat products such as yogurt or cottage cheese. See Table 5 for other foods that contain calcium.

It may be hard to get enough calcium by diet alone, so you may wish to take calcium supplements. You can buy calcium supplements in a number of forms, such as calcium citrate or carbonate.

Vitamin D is needed for your body to use calcium. Your skin makes it when it is exposed to sunlight. Women who don't get out in the sunlight very often may need a supplement.

Some women have symptoms such as nausea, diarrhea, and indigestion after eating milk products. This is known as lactose intolerance. If you have lactose intolerance, your doctor may prescribe calcium supplements.

Folic Acid

Folic acid is needed for healthy growth of a baby during pregnancy, especially during the first months. Not getting enough folic acid in your diet increases the risk of hav-

Almost 4,000 babies born in the United States each year have serious birth defects of the spine (spina bifida) or brain (anencephaly). Between 50% to 75% of these cases could be prevented if the mother took enough folic acid before and during the early weeks of pregnancy.

Table 4. Calcium Counts

The amount of calcium you need each day depends on your age. If you are pregnant, you need the same amount of calcium as suggested for your age group. See the table below to find out how much calcium you should be getting.

Age	Allowance (in mg) Recommended Daily
15–18	1,200
19–24	1,200
25-50	800
50+	800*

* To prevent osteoporosis, the National Institutes of Health recommends 1,500 mg daily for women ages 50-65 who are not taking hormone replacement therapy, as well as for all women older than age 65.

Source: National Academy of Sciences

ing a baby with certain birth defects of the spine and skull. Women should take folic acid before they become pregnant and during their pregnancy.

Folic acid is needed in the first weeks of pregnancy—before a woman may even know she's pregnant. After this time, it is too late for folic acid to help prevent birth defects. Also, many pregnancies are unplanned. For these reasons, any woman who can become pregnant should take folic acid every day.

Good sources of folic acid in foods are dark leafy greens (like spinach and collard greens) and citrus fruit (like oranges and lemons). It also can be found in enriched bread, pasta, flour, crackers, cereal, and rice.

It is hard to get all the folic acid you need just from your diet, so women should take vitamin supplements. Women who might get pregnant should have 0.4 mg of folic acid daily. Pregnant women should have at least 0.4 mg each day. Women who have had a child with a spine or skull defect are more likely to have another child with this problem. These women need higher doses of folic acid— 4 mg daily.

A Healthy Weight

To stay healthy, you should keep your weight at the level best for your height. You may have seen height and weight tables that suggest weights for men and women based on body frame size—small, medium, and large. Today, many doctors use the body mass index (BMI) table shown here to see if your weight is healthy.

The BMI compares a person's height to their weight to see if they are over-weight. Having a BMI of 20–24 is normal, and 25–29.9 is overweight. A woman with a score of 30 and higher is obese.

If your weight is not in the normal range, try to lose the extra pounds. You can lose weight by eating healthy foods and exercising. Talk to your doctor about a weight loss plan that is right for you.

Table 5. Foods Containing Calcium

Food	Amount	Calcium (mg)	Fat (g)
Milk and Dairy Products			
American cheese	1 oz	195	8.4
Cheddar cheese	1 oz	211	9.1
Swiss cheese	1 oz	219	7.1
Ice cream—hard	1 cup	176	14.1
Low-fat milk	1 cup	298	4.7
Skim milk	1 cup	303	0.4
Low-fat plain yogurt	1 cup	415	3.4
Nuts			
Almonds	1 oz	66	16.2
Sesame seeds, dried, hulled	31/2 oz	100	53.4
Seafood			
Scallops, steamed	31/2 oz	115	1.4
Shrimp	31/2 oz	63	0.8
Green leafy vegetables			
Broccoli, cooked	2/3 cup	88	0.3
Kale, cooked, without stem	3/4 cup	187	0.7
Spinach, cooked	1/2 cup	83	0.3
Turnip greens, cooked	2/3 cup	184	0.2
Other foods			
Chili con carne with beans	5 oz	61	9.9
Cream of celery soup made with milk	1 serving	135	33.0
Figs, dried	5 medium	126	1.3
Slice from 12-inch cheese pizza	1 piece	144	4.4
Pudding, chocolate	1/2 cup	147	6.6
Raisins, dried, seedless	5/8 cup	62	0.2

Body Mass Index

To calculate your body mass index (BMI), find your height in inches in the left column. Then look across the line to find your weight in pounds. The number at the top of that column is your BMI.

Height (inches)	19	20	21	22	23	24	25	26	27	28	29	30	31	32
							Weight (pounds)							
58	91	96	100	105	110	115	119	124	129	134	138	143	148	153
59	94	99	104	109	114	119	124	128	133	138	143	148	153	158
60	97	102	107	112	118	123	128	133	138	143	148	153	158	163
61	100	106	111	116	122	127	132	137	143	148	153	158	164	169
62	104	109	115	120	126	131	136	142	147	153	158	164	169	175
63	107	113	118	124	130	135	141	146	152	158	163	169	175	180
64	110	116	122	128	134	140	145	151	157	163	169	174	180	186
65	114	120	126	132	138	144	150	156	162	168	174	180	186	192
66	118	124	130	136	142	148	155	161	167	173	179	186	192	198
67	121	127	134	140	146	153	159	166	172	178	185	191	198	204
68	125	131	138	144	151	158	164	171	177	184	190	197	203	210
69	128	135	142	149	155	162	169	176	182	189	196	203	209	216
70	132	139	146	153	160	167	174	181	188	195	202	209	216	222
71	136	143	150	157	165	172	179	186	193	200	208	215	222	229
72	140	147	154	162	169	177	184	191	199	206	213	221	228	235
73	144	151	159	166	174	182	189	197	204	212	219	227	235	242
74	148	155	163	171	179	186	194	202	210	218	225	233	241	249

National Heart, Lung, and Blood Institute. Clinical guidelines on the identification, evaluation, and treatment of overweight and obesity. Washington, DC: U.S. Department of Health and Human Services, 1998.

▶ See also *Biopsy, Cervical Cancer, Cervical Disorders, and Colposcopy* in *"Women's Health"*

▶ PAP TEST

Since it first came into use 50 years ago, the Pap test has lowered the number of deaths from cancer of the cervix by 70% in the United States. The Pap test detects changes in the cells of the cervix (the opening of a woman's uterus). These changes could lead to cancer. The Pap test helps find these changes early so they can be treated before they become serious. By having a Pap test, a woman can help prevent cancer of the cervix.

The Cervix

The cervix is the lower, narrow end of the uterus. It opens into the vagina. The cervix is covered by a thin layer of tissue (like the skin inside your mouth). As with all cells, the cells that make up this tissue grow all the time. During this growth, the cells at the bottom layer slowly move to the surface of the cervix. When these cells reach the surface, they are shed. During this process, some cells can become abnormal.

For the Pap test, a sample of cells is taken from the surface of the cervix. The test can find abnormal cells that could lead to cancer of the cervix and the vagina. It is not used to detect cancer in other parts of the body.

A Regular Part of Your Health Care

Having a regular Pap test is an important part of your overall health care. When you start having the test and how often you have it depends on your history. You should have your first Pap test by age 18 or when you start having sex with men—whichever comes first.

Since women began getting Pap tests in 1943, deaths from cervical cancer have decreased by about 70%. Forty years ago almost 20,000 women died each year from cancer of the cervix. Today that number is down to almost 5,000.

Pap tests should continue past menopause. If your tests show abnormal results or if you have had cancer, your doctor may advise you to have a Pap test more often. If you have had a hysterectomy for benign (not cancer) disease, you should still have the Pap test if you have any of the risk factors listed.

Some women have a higher risk of developing cervical changes. Your risk may be higher if you:

▶ Have had more than one sexual partner or a male sexual partner who has had more than one partner

▶ Had intercourse for the first time at an early age

▶ Have had certain sexually transmitted diseases (STDs), such as genital warts (human papillomavirus) or herpes

▶ Are infected with human immunodeficiency virus (HIV) or have a weakened immune system (such as a transplant patient)

▶ Smoke cigarettes

If you have any of these risk factors, it is important for you to have a Pap test each year. If you have no risk factors and have had three normal tests in a row, your doctor may suggest you have the test done less often. You should still see your doctor each year for a pelvic exam.

Pap Test

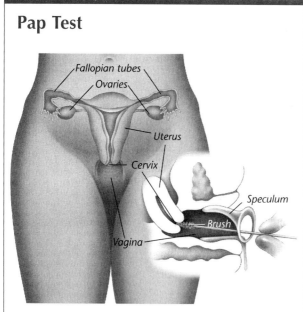

For the Pap test, a speculum is inserted into the vagina. A small sample of cells is collected from the cervical canal with a small brush or swab and a scraper.

Abnormal cells may go through several stages of change before cervical cancer appears. This usually happens over a number of years. If cancer does occur, symptoms may include bleeding, pelvic pain, or discharge. In most cases there are no symptoms, though.

The Test

The Pap test can be done during a pelvic exam. Do not douche or use vaginal medication, spermicides, or lubrication for 2–3 days before the test. These products may wash away or hide any changed cells. It is best to schedule the Pap test for a time when you're not having your menstrual period.

A speculum will be inserted into your vagina. This device gently opens the vagina so the cervix can be seen. A small brush and scraper are used to remove cells from the inside and outside of the cervix. You will not feel any pain.

The cell sample is then placed on a glass slide to be sent to the lab for testing. A technician or doctor uses a microscope to look for cells that do not appear normal. The results are classified based on how the cells look. Your health insurance often will pay for this Pap test.

There are several new methods designed to improve the accuracy of test results. Your doctor may suggest you use one of them. One method sends the cells to the lab in a bottle of liquid. The cells then are transferred to a slide and read in the standard way. Other methods use the help of a computer to find abnormal cells.

It is not clear that these methods detect cervical cancer better than the standard Pap test. Your insurance company may not pay for these newer types of tests.

The Results

The results of your Pap test are most often classified by a system developed by the National Cancer Institute (the Bethesda System). The classification of the cells helps doctors plan treatment:

▶ *Normal:* Only normal cells were seen on your Pap test

▶ *Atypical squamous cells of undetermined significance (ASCUS):* Mildly abnormal changes were seen in cells lining the outer cervix

▶ *Atypical glandular cells of undetermined significance (AGUS):* Mildly abnormal changes were seen in the cells lining the inner cervix

- *Squamous intraepithelial lesion (SIL):* The cells that were tested show certain abnormalities. SIL can be low-grade or high-grade.
  —Low-grade SIL includes mild changes and changes linked to human papillomavirus (HPV). Some types of these viruses have been linked to cancer of the cervix.
  —High-grade SIL includes moderate and severe changes and very early "precancer"

- *Cervical intraepithelial neoplasia (CIN):* Changes were seen on the cells on the surface of the cervix. Normal cells are replaced by a layer of abnormal cells. This is called dysplasia. CIN can be one of three grades:
  —CIN 1 includes mild dysplasia
  —CIN 2 includes moderate dysplasia
  —CIN 3 includes severe dysplasia and carcinoma in situ (CIS). CIS is not a true form of cancer. It is most likely to develop into cancer if not treated, though.

- *Cancer:* The cells have spread into other tissues

These terms may be confusing. Table 6 helps explain how they relate to each other.

Is the Pap Test Always Accurate?

Like any test, the Pap test is not always accurate. It may report abnormal cells are present when they aren't. This is known as a false-positive result. A Pap test may also miss abnormal cells— known as a false-negative.

False-negative results can occur for a number of reasons:

- The sample contains too few or too many cells

- An infection or blood covered up abnormal cells

- Douching or vaginal medicines have washed away abnormal cells

Because Pap test results are based on how cells on a slide look, even experts may not agree. Sometimes the reason for false-negative results is not known. Your doctor may suggest a test be repeated.

Follow-Up

If the lab reports any abnormal finding, the doctor may arrange for further tests. This may be as simple as a repeat Pap test in a few weeks or a few months.

Table 6. Pap Test Terms

Term	CIN	SIL
Human papillomavirus (HPV)	1	Low-grade
Mild dysplasia	1	Low-grade
Moderate dysplasia	2	High-grade
Severe dysplasia	3	High-grade
Carcinoma in situ (CIS)	3	High-grade

Sometimes your doctor will do an exam called a colposcopy to decide if you need treatment. A magnifying device called a colposcope is used to look at the cervix. With this device, your doctor may be able to see changes that suggest abnormal cells.

Colposcopy may help the doctor decide whether a cervical biopsy needs to be done. For a biopsy, the doctor removes some of the cells to be studied under a microscope. You may feel a little pain during the biopsy.

Treatment depends on the findings. In many cases, all that is required is to remove a thin layer of cells from the surface of the cervix. New cells often are normal and no further treatment is needed.

▶ See also *Pap Test*

▶ PELVIC EXAM

If you are sexually active or are 18 or older, you should have a pelvic exam every year. As a part of this exam, the doctor will check your abdomen, pelvis, vagina, and rectum by feeling them. A Pap test also may be part of the exam.

You will be asked to lie on a table with your legs raised and your knees bent and spread apart. The doctor first examines the outside genitals (vulva). He or she then will insert a slender device called a speculum into the vagina to view the vagina and cervix and take a sample of cells for testing. After the speculum is removed, the doctor inserts one or two gloved fingers into the vagina and reaches up to the cervix. The uterus and ovaries can be felt from the inside with this hand while the other hand presses on the abdomen from the outside. This allows the size, position, and shape of these organs to be checked.

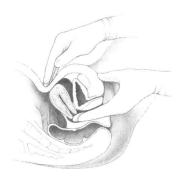

The doctor checks the pelvic organs for any changes during a pelvic exam.

During the exam, your doctor also may insert a gloved finger into your rectum. The exam can help your doctor detect any tumors or lumps or other problems that may be present in the pelvis or the rectum. Your doctor may also test a sample of your stool for hidden blood that may indicate colon or rectal cancer. This is called a fecal occult blood test.

▶ ROUTINE CARE

Women of all ages can help stay healthy by getting routine care from their doctor. Keeping track of certain tests and immunizations (vaccines) you need—as well as the results of those tests—will help you prevent health problems and keep track of special needs you may have.

Immunizations can protect you from infections. There are some tests and immunizations that all women in certain age groups should have. Some women may have risk factors that require further care. Be aware of things that cause illness or problems in your age group—if you know what poses a risk to your health, you can play an active role in trying to prevent it.

Routine Needs

Some health problems are more likely to occur at certain ages. Visiting your doctor for routine care will help you learn what are common problems for women your age. Your doctor also can show you ways to help prevent or treat them.

At routine visits, your doctor will do a physical exam. He or she will measure your height and weight, examine your breasts, and take your blood pressure.

If you are sexually active or are age 18 or older, you should have a pelvic exam every year. As a part of this exam, your doctor will check your abdomen, pelvis, vagina, and rectum by feeling them. Along with the pelvic exam, your doctor may do a

Leading Causes of Death in Women

Ages 13–18

1. Motor vehicle accidents
2. Murder
3. Suicide
4. Cancer
5. All other accidents
6. Diseases of the heart
7. Congenital anomalies (problems from birth)
8. Chronic obstructive pulmonary diseases (such as bronchitis or asthma)

Ages 19–39

1. Accidents
2. Cancer
3. Human immunodeficiency virus infection
4. Diseases of the heart
5. Murder
6. Suicide
7. Cerebrovascular diseases (such as stroke)
8. Chronic liver disease and cirrhosis

Ages 40–64

1. Cancer
2. Diseases of the heart
3. Cerebrovascular diseases (such as stroke)
4. Accidents
5. Chronic obstructive pulmonary diseases
6. Diabetes
7. Chronic liver disease and cirrhosis
8. Pneumonia and flu

Ages 65 and Older

1. Diseases of the heart
2. Cancer
3. Cerebrovascular diseases
4. Chronic obstructive pulmonary diseases
5. Pneumonia and flu
6. Diabetes
7. Accidents
8. Alzheimer's disease

Pap test. This test checks for changes in the cervix that could lead to cancer. You also may receive needed immunizations.

Starting at age 45, all women should have their cholesterol level checked once every 5 years. A woman age 45 and older also should have a fasting glucose test every 3 years to check for diabetes.

Starting at age 50, all women should have mammography once a year. Also at age 50, a woman should have a fecal occult blood test once a year and a sigmoidoscopy every 3–5 years.

Special Needs

Many women have special risk factors that may require further care (Table 7). For instance, members of some ethnic groups are more likely than other people to have certain health problems. Also, where you live, your lifestyle, and your personal and family medical history play a role in the type of health care you may need.

Table 7. Tests and Immunizations for High-Risk Women

You should have this test or immunization	If you
Test	
Blood count (anemia)	Are of Caribbean, Latin American, Asian, Mediterranean, or African descent; have a history of heavy menstrual flow
Bacteriuria testing	Have diabetes mellitus
Cholesterol testing	Have lipid disorders in your family; have a family history of coronary heart disease before age 55; have a history of coronary heart disease
Colonoscopy	Have a history of inflammatory bowel disease or polyps on the colon; have a family history of polyps, cancer of the rectum and colon, or cancer family syndrome
Fasting glucose testing	Have a first-degree relative with diabetes (get tested every 3 years); had gestational diabetes; are obese; have hypertension; are a member of a high-risk ethnic group (African American, Hispanic, or Native American)
Genetic testing or counseling	Have been exposed to agents known to harm a fetus; are planning a pregnancy and are age 35 or older; have someone in your family (including you) who has a history of a genetic disorder or birth defect; have a partner with a history of a genetic disorder or birth defect; are of African, Acadian, Eastern European Jewish, Mediterranean, or Southeast Asian descent
Hepatitis C virus (HCV) testing	Have injected illegal drugs; received treatment (clotting factor concentrate) for a blood disorder before 1987; are on long-term hemodialysis; received blood from a donor who later tested positive for HCV infection; received a blood transfusion or organ transplant before July 1992; are exposed to HCV-positive blood at work
Human immunodeficiency virus (HIV) testing	Are seeking treatment for other STDs; inject drugs; have a history of prostitution; have a past or present sexual partner who is HIV-positive or bisexual or injects drugs; have lived for a long time or were born in an area with a high number of HIV-infection cases; had a blood transfusion between 1978 and 1985; have invasive cervical cancer; are pregnant

(continued)

Table 7. Tests and Immunizations for High-Risk Women *(continued)*

You should have this test or immunization	If you
Test	
Lipid profile assessment	Have high cholesterol; have a parent or sibling with blood cholesterol of 240 mg/dL or higher; have a first-degree relative with coronary artery disease before age 55; have diabetes; smoke
Mammography	Have had breast cancer; have a first-degree relative (mother, sister, or daughter) or multiple other relatives who have a history of premenopausal breast or breast and ovarian cancer
Rubella titer assessment	Are childbearing age and no proof of immunity
Sexually transmitted disease (STD) testing	Have had more than one sexual partner or a partner who has had more than one sexual partner; have had sexual contact with someone with an STD; have a history or repeated episodes of STD; have attended a clinic for STDs
Skin exam	Work or play in the sunlight often; have a family or personal history of skin cancer; have precancerous lesions
Thyroid stimulating hormone testing	Have a strong family history of thyroid disease; have an autoimmune disease
Tuberculosis skin testing	Have HIV infection; have close contact with persons known or thought to have tuberculosis; have medical risk factors known to increase risk of disease if infected; were born in a country with high rates of tuberculosis; abuse alcohol; inject drugs; live in a long-term care facility (including a nursing home, prison or jail, or mental health institution); are a health professional working in a high-risk care facility
Immunizations	
Chickenpox (varicella) vaccine	Have no evidence of having had chickenpox; have household contact with people who are immunocompromised; are a teacher or daycare worker; live in a long-term care facility or institution (including college, the military, or prison); travel overseas; are a nonpregnant woman of childbearing age
Flu vaccine	Want to reduce the chance of catching the flu; live in a long-term care facility; have chronic cardiopulmonary disorders; have a metabolic disease (such as diabetes or renal problems); are a health care or daycare worker; are in your second or third trimester of pregnancy during flu season; are planning to become pregnant
Hepatitis A vaccine	Travel overseas; use illegal drugs; work with nonhuman primates; have chronic liver disease; have a blood disorder; have had sex with a man who has had sex with other men; are not immune to measles, mumps, or rubella; work in food service, health care, or daycare
Hepatitis B vaccine	Use IV drugs or have sex with someone who uses IV drugs; receive clotting factor concentrates; are exposed to blood or blood products at work; are a patient or employee in a dialysis unit; have chronic renal or hepatic disease; have household or sexual contact with a carrier of hepatitis B virus; have had sex with more than one person; have had sex with a sexually active bisexual or homosexual man; are an international traveler; live or work in an institution for the developmentally disabled or in a prison or jail
Measles–mumps–rubella vaccine	Were born in 1957 or later and have no proof of being immune or being vaccinated; were vaccinated in 1963–1967; are a health care worker; are starting college; travel overseas
Pneumococcal vaccine	Have a chronic illness; are exposed to pneumonia outbreaks; are immunocompromised; are pregnant and have a chronic illness

Immunizations

Immunizations are injections (shots) that help prevent infections. They are a routine part of preventive care. Your doctor will tell you which ones you need. Check Table 8 to see which are standard for your age group. If you have certain risk factors, you may need other vaccines.

Find out which tests and immunizations you need and how often. If you don't remember when you were last tested or immunized, your doctor may be able to test you to see if you are immune to the disease.

Table 8. Tests and Immunizations for Women

Test/Immunization	What and Why	When
Ages 13–39		
Pap test	A sample of cells is taken from the cervix during a pelvic exam to look for changes that could lead to cancer	Yearly when sexually active or by age 18 (doctor and patient decision to have less often if three normal test results in a row)
Tetanus–diphtheria booster	A shot to immunize against the diseases tetanus and diphtheria	Once between ages 11 and 16, then every 10 years
Hepatitis B vaccine	A shot to immunize against the disease Hepatitis B	One series for those not previously immunized
Ages 40–64		
Tests and immunizations for ages 13–39 plus:		
Mammography	An X-ray of the breast to look for breast cancer	Every 1–2 years until age 50; yearly beginning at age 50
Cholesterol testing	A blood test that checks levels of cholesterol (a substance that helps carry fat through the blood vessels) because levels that are too high can lead to hardening of the arteries	Every 5 years beginning at age 45
Fecal occult blood testing	A test of a stool sample for blood, which could be a sign of cancer of the colon or rectum	Yearly beginning at age 50
Sigmoidoscopy	A scope placed into the rectum or colon to look for colon cancer	Every 3–5 years after age 50
Fasting glucose testing	A test to measure the level of glucose because it if is too high it could signal diabetes	Every 3 years after age 45
Age 65 and Older		
Tests and immunizations for all ages plus:		
Urinalysis	A test to measure the levels of substances, such as glucose, in your urine	Yearly
Flu vaccine	A shot to help prevent influenza	Once a year
Pneumococcal vaccine	A shot to help prevent pneumonia	Once

▶ SMOKING

Smoking is a leading cause of death. In fact, a woman who smokes cigarettes shortens her life by 5–8 years. Smoking increases a woman's risk of cancer, heart disease, and reproductive problems. If you quit smoking, over time you can reverse some of the negative effects on your body.

About Cigarettes and Smoking

With each puff of a cigarette, a smoker's body is exposed to more than 2,500 chemicals. Many of these chemicals are known to cause cancer. For instance, cigarettes contain:

▶ *Nicotine*—a highly addictive drug

▶ *Carbon monoxide*—the poisonous gas in car exhaust fumes

▶ *Tar*—a gummy substance used to pave roads

Smoking is the most preventable cause of illness and death. It doubles the risk of heart disease and cancer of the cervix in women. Women who smoke are 12 times more likely to get lung cancer than women who have never smoked. Smoking increases the risk of many other cancers as well.

Smoking also is linked with reproductive problems such as infertility and early menopause. Even people, especially children, around smokers suffer health problems from being exposed to secondhand smoke.

How Can I Quit?

More than 3 million Americans quit smoking each year. You can do it, too. No matter how long you have been smoking, quitting has benefits.

Getting Started

Follow these steps to help you get started:

▶ Decide that you want to quit. Try to avoid thinking about how hard it might be. Instead, imagine your life smoke free.

▶ Focus on your reasons for quitting—to improve your health, protect your family, or save money. These reasons will help keep you going.

▶ Tell your family and friends that you plan to stop smoking. Get their support. If they smoke, you may want to ask them to quit too. It may help to have a friend quit with you.

▶ Know what to expect when you quit. Learn how to handle urges to smoke and the stress that comes along with quitting.

When You Smoke, Your Family Smokes

Children whose parents smoke are at increased risk for respiratory infections, including pneumonia and bronchitis. Children who are exposed to secondhand smoke are also at increased risk for developing asthma, a chronic disorder in which a person has trouble breathing and may cough a lot.

▶ Set a target date for quitting. This may make it easier to keep your promise. Your target date can be your birthday, your anniversary, or any other day. Mark the date on your calendar. This also will help you keep track of the exact day you became a nonsmoker—a date you can celebrate each year.

Nicotine Replacement Products

To help you quit, you may want to try nicotine replacement products. Using one of these products almost doubles your chances of quitting.

Nicotine replacement products release nicotine into your body. This can provide relief of cravings and withdrawal symptoms while you get used to life without smoking. They are available in a special chewing gum, skin patch, nasal spray, inhaler, or tablet.

You can buy some of these products over-the-counter. Others may require a prescription. Certain health insurance plans cover nicotine replacement products. Your doctor can help you decide which product is right for you.

You should never smoke when using these products. It could cause a stroke or heart problems.

If you smoke and are pregnant or breastfeeding, ask your doctor to help you quit smoking. You should not use nicotine

Nicotine Replacement Products

One of the nicotine replacement options listed here may help you quit smoking.
Discuss your dosage level with your doctor.

Patch

The patch can be used for up to 8 weeks. As soon as you wake up each morning, place a new patch on a smooth, flat place on your body between your waist and your neck. Each day, place the patch on a new spot on this area of your body. This will help prevent a rash.

Inhaler

The inhaler is shaped like a cigarette holder. When you inhale, nicotine is absorbed through the tissues of your mouth. It can be used up to 16 times each day for 3 months. Then, dosage should be decreased. It should not be used longer than 6 months. Side effects of the inhaler include mouth and throat irritation and cough.

Nasal Spray

Nicotine nasal spray must be prescribed by a doctor. The inhaled spray sends nicotine through the nasal passages into the bloodstream. The nasal spray should be used no longer than 6 months. Side effects of nasal spray include nasal and sinus irritation.

Gum

Chew at least one piece of gum every 1–2 hours for at least 1–3 months for the best results. Following a schedule will help you get the most benefit out of nicotine gum.

The gum must be chewed slowly, until a "peppery" taste comes out. Then, you should "park" it between your cheek and gum. You should chew and "park" off and on for about 30 minutes. Side effects of the gum include hiccups, upset stomach, or sore jaw. In most cases, these side effects go away if the gum is used the right way.

replacement products unless your doctor says they are safe for you and your baby.

Another product your doctor may suggest to help you quit smoking are bupropion hydrochloride tablets. These tablets are antidepressants and must be prescribed by your doctor. This medication helps reduce withdrawal symptoms and the urge to smoke. The treatment begins 2 weeks before your quit date. Treatment lasts about 7–12 weeks. Side effects of this medication include dry mouth, trouble sleeping, feeling shaky, and skin rash. If you are taking another antidepressant, you should not use these tablets to help you quit smoking.

Quitting Day

When the target date comes, throw away all your cigarettes. Clean your clothes to get rid of the cigarette smell.

Try to keep busy on your quitting day—exercise, go to the movies, or take long walks. It may help to spend most of your free time in places where smoking is not allowed, such as libraries, stores, and museums. Remind your family and friends that this is your quitting day. Ask them to help you through the first week or so—it is the hardest.

On the third Thursday of November, the American Cancer Society sponsors the Great American Smokeout. This yearly event is designed to help smokers quit cigarettes for at least 1 day—in hopes they will quit forever. More people quit smoking on this day than any other day of the year.

After You Quit Smoking

Once you stop smoking, there will be times when you feel you must have a cigarette. When you feel these urges, take steps to control them. Intense cravings only last a short time. By thinking about something else, you can keep your mind away from the cravings. Try using substitutes to keep the cravings down.

If you have a cigarette, don't be too hard on yourself. One slip doesn't mean you've failed. It takes time and patience to quit a habit. Many people have to try more than once—and try more than one method—before they become ex-smokers. Find out what set you back, and try again.

If you feel you need extra help, ask for it. Your doctor can offer support and medical advice. Many people who can't stop smoking on their own get help by joining special programs. You can contact the local chapter of the American Lung Association, the American Cancer Society, or other local groups to help you quit. The groups are listed in the phone book.

Rewards of Quitting

When you quit smoking, the benefits start right away. Quitting reverses much of the damage caused by smoking. The odor of stale cigarette smoke will begin to fade from your clothes, car, and home. The smoke stains on your fingernails will go away. A

The Rewards of Quitting

As soon as you stop smoking you will notice a change in your health:

Within 12 hours of quitting

▶ Levels of carbon monoxide and nicotine in your system decrease quickly.

▶ Your heart and lungs begin to repair the damage caused by cigarette smoke.

Within a few days of quitting

▶ Your sense of smell and taste may improve.

Within 3 months of quitting

▶ Your circulation improves.

▶ You breathe easier.

▶ Your voice sounds less hoarse.

Within 1 year of quitting

▶ Your risk of having a heart attack decreases by 50%.

Within a few years of quitting

▶ Your risk of getting life-threatening diseases (for instance, lung cancer, cancer of the mouth, and heart disease) is reduced to nearly that of a nonsmoker.

person who stops smoking can reduce the risk of heart disease to the same level as someone who has never smoked at all. Plus, you'll have the bonus of not spending your money on cigarettes. Reward yourself by buying something special with your savings.

Effects of Quitting

The first week after quitting is the hardest time. You may feel irritable, anxious, and hungry. You may have trouble sleeping. You may feel dizzy or drowsy and have headaches.

These feelings are known as withdrawal symptoms. Withdrawal symptoms may begin within a few hours, peak in 2–3 days, and last up to a month.

Your doctor can suggest ways to help you get through the withdrawal stage. Nicotine replacement products may help.

What About Weight Gain?

Many people who are thinking about quitting worry about gaining weight. Keep in mind that the benefits of quitting far outweigh the drawbacks of gaining a few pounds.

If you're concerned about gaining weight after you quit, make sure you eat right. It is also good to start a regular exercise program. Exercise helps you feel better, keeps your weight down, and may help ease any withdrawal symptoms. Using nicotine gum also may help delay or prevent weight gain.

Some ways to keep your weight down when you quit include:

▶ Follow a regular exercise program.

▶ Make sure you have a well-balanced diet with the right amounts of protein, carbohydrates, and fat.

▶ Drink a glass of water before each meal.

▶ Have low-calorie foods for snacks—fruits and vegetables, fruit juices, or air-popped popcorn without butter.

▶ Plan menus with care and count calories.

▶ WEIGHT CONTROL

▶   See also *Nutrition*

Keeping a healthy weight is good for your physical and mental well-being. Proper eating habits and moderate exercise are crucial to keeping your weight healthy and your body fit.

Being overweight is a problem for many people in the United States. People who are overweight eat more calories than they use. They are more likely to have medical conditions and some cancers. Extreme weight loss and being very underweight also can be bad for your health.

What Is a Healthy Weight?

To stay healthy, you should keep your weight at the level best for your height. Different tables have been used to show ideal weights. You may have seen tables that suggest different weights for men and women based on age, height, or body frame sizes. Today many doctors use the body mass index (BMI) chart (see page 68) to check if your weight is healthy.

The BMI compares a person's height to their weight to see if they are overweight. Having a BMI of 20–24 is normal, and 25–29.9 is overweight. A woman with a score of 30 or higher is obese.

The shape of your body is also a factor in keeping a healthy weight. Excess fat in the abdomen (an "apple" shape) is believed to be a greater health risk than fat in the hips and thighs (a "pear" shape). To check your body shape:

▶   Measure around your waist near your navel while you stand relaxed. Do not pull in your stomach.

▶   Measure around your hips, over the buttocks, where they are largest.

Research in adults suggests that you may be at greater risk for a number of diseases, such as diabetes and heart disease, if your waist is the same size or larger than your hips.

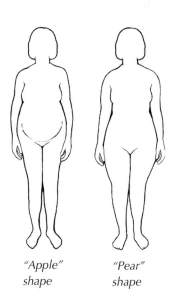

"Apple"
shape

"Pear"
shape

About Fat

Everyone must have some body fat. Fat provides a form of energy. Energy not used is stored in the fat cells.

If you are overweight, you likely have too much fat stored. Fat normally makes up about 20–25% of a woman's body weight. In most cases, men have less body fat—about 15–20% of their body weight.

A certain amount of body fat helps women to maintain their estrogen levels. Estrogen is a female hormone that controls a

More than 50% of American adults are overweight. If you are overweight, your risk of premature death is higher than a person who is not, even if you are otherwise healthy. Overweight people are at an increased risk for heart disease, stroke, and diabetes.

woman's menstrual cycle. The shape of a woman's body is partly the result of estrogen. Having too little body fat may cause estrogen levels to decrease. If these levels are too low, a woman's menstrual periods might become irregular or even stop.

Factors That Affect Weight

People who are overweight often eat too much and exercise too little. Every function of the body—from building cells to moving muscles—requires energy. Energy is measured in calories. Calories measure how much fuel is in a certain food. When this fuel is burned, calories are used. The body uses only as much of its daily intake of food as it needs for energy. The energy that remains is stored as fat in the body.

An average woman needs about 2,200 calories a day. If you eat 3,500 calories more than you burn off, you will gain one pound. A number of factors effect weight gain:

If you are extremely overweight, your doctor may prescribe medication to help you lose weight. There are two types of medication available. To get the best results with these medications, you must reduce the amount of calories you eat and exercise regularly.

▶ People tend to weigh more as they age. It is normal for people to be a little heavier as they grow older. Doctors think this does not pose a risk to a person's health.

▶ A woman might not lose all of the weight she gained during pregnancy. If this happens with each pregnancy, the weight can add up.

▶ A woman may have a hard time losing weight because of her metabolism—how your body uses the energy found in the foods you eat. People burn food at different rates. Even if you do not overeat, you might find it hard to lose weight or keep a healthy weight if you don't exercise.

▶ People gain extra weight when fat cells fill and grow. In most people, fat cells increase with growth spurts, such as in infancy and childhood. If you have children, their doctor can help you plan a healthy diet for them. It should include some fat—it is needed for growth. Too much fat in their diet, though, can result in adding fat to their bodies that will be hard to lose later.

Health Hazards of Being Overweight

Many health concerns directly relate to being obese or overweight. The more you weigh over the suggested range, the higher your risk of heart disease. Heart failure occurs almost three times more often in obese women than in women of normal weight. High blood pressure and a lifestyle that is not active raise the risk of heart disease. These risk factors are often found in overweight people.

Many overweight people have high cholesterol. High cholesterol can lead to coronary artery disease. This disease is a clogging of the arteries by cholesterol or fat deposits. With excess weight, the heart has to work harder. The risk of coronary artery disease increases and less blood gets to the heart. In time, arteries in the neck may clog. At some point, blood clots may move through the arteries and increase the risk of heart attacks or stroke. In fact, the risk of stroke among overweight people is four times greater than for people of healthy weight.

Diabetes is one more hazard of being overweight. People with diabetes have levels of sugar in their blood that are too high. Doctors estimate that 85% of people with diabetes have the type related to being overweight. These people have enough insulin in their bodies, but the insulin cannot do its work of keeping sugar levels in the blood under control. As a result, sugar needed to nourish your body cannot get into the cells. A healthy diet and regular exercise can go a long way toward helping people with diabetes control the disease.

Gallbladder disease is found most often in obese women. Gallstones have been linked to high-calorie diets.

Overweight women are more likely to have certain kinds of cancer. Cancer of the endometrium is five times more common in overweight women than in women with healthy weights. Breast, colon, and rectal cancers also are more common in overweight women. These types of cancer may be linked to diet. Some of these risks can be reduced by eating a healthy, low-fat diet and exercising.

Problems During Pregnancy and Childbirth

Both overweight and underweight women may have problems getting pregnant. The more overweight or underweight they are, the less likely pregnancy will occur.

If overweight women become pregnant, they may face certain problems during pregnancy. They are more prone to diabetes or high blood pressure during pregnancy, which are linked to being overweight. Obese women also are more likely to have a cesarean birth because their babies are too large to fit safely through the birth canal. There is an increased risk of complication during any surgery—including a cesarean birth—for any obese person.

Excess weight gained during pregnancy might be hard to lose after the birth of a child. If a woman is 20% overweight before she becomes pregnant, she needs to gain less than mothers of normal weight. A doctor will be able to tell a woman how much weight she should gain based on her weight before getting pregnant. A woman should never try to lose weight while she is pregnant.

A woman with a body mass index (BMI) of more than 30 is thought to be obese. Women who are overweight or obese may have problems during pregnancy. A woman with a normal BMI (20–24) is advised to gain about 25–35 pounds during pregnancy. An overweight or obese woman should gain less (about 15–25 pounds).

Health Through Weight Control

There is no magic answer to taking off weight and keeping it off. The best way to lose weight is to exercise and eat fewer calories. Losing weight requires a long-term commitment to good eating habits and regular exercise. "Yo-yo" or on-and-off dieting is not healthy. Healthy habits help to reduce or reverse health hazards of being overweight. A person who loses weight will feel better and find it easier to be more active.

Losing weight is hard. A doctor or nurse, sometimes working with a nutritionist, can help you plan a healthy weight-loss program. You may need some emotional support as well. Ask your doctor about support groups or counseling options.

Take a good look at your eating habits. You may wish to keep a food diary. It can help you find patterns of what you eat and why, when, and how. Avoid extremes of diet (fewer than 1,000 calories a day) unless your doctor is guiding your diet. Do not use over-the-counter weight loss aids without talking to your doctor—they may be harmful and cause problems.

Look at how active you are, too. You may have to find ways to get more exercise.

If you are a smoker, you may be afraid to quit because you might gain more weight. Trying to break more than one habit at the same time can be hard, but it's worth it for your health. Ask your doctor for advice.

Your new healthy eating and exercise habits could improve your family's and friends' health as well. This may help you to stay on track.

Calculate Your BMR

The number of calories your body needs to maintain its basic functions, such as breathing and keeping your heart beating, is called your basal metabolic rate (BMR). You can compute your BMR using the following method: 665 + [4.36 × body weight in pounds] + [4.32 × height in inches] − [4.7 × age in years] You will need to consume more than your BMR to provide energy for daily activities, such as walking, exercising, working, and shopping.

Nutrition

The United States Department of Agriculture guidelines for health suggest that you eat a variety of foods and maintain a healthy weight. You should choose a diet of healthy foods from the four food groups (Table 9) to make sure you get all the nutrients you need. These include:

- Carbohydrates
- Fiber
- Protein
- Vitamins
- Minerals
- Water

If you are trying to lose weight, you still need all these nutrients. Choose foods that are low in fat from the four food groups in the table. Also, learning to read a food's label will help you make healthy food choices.

Table 9. A Low-Fat Diet

For a balanced diet, choose foods from each of the four food groups each day.
For a diet low in fat and high in fiber, check the following lists for examples
of foods to select and avoid.

Food Group	Choose More Often	Choose Less Often
Fruits and Vegetables	Citrus fruits (oranges, grapefruit); dark-green, leafy vegetables (spinach, collard greens, endive); yellow-orange vegetables (carrots, sweet potatoes,squash); apples, berries, pears; cabbage, broccoli, cauliflower, brussels sprouts	Avocados, olives
Whole-Grain and Enriched Bread	Whole-wheat, rye, oatmeal, and pumpernickel breads; whole-grain and bran cereals; bagels and English muffins; brown, wild, or white rice; pasta with low-fat sauce; pretzels	Refined-flour breads and cakes; biscuits, croissants, crackers, chips; packaged rice and pasta mixes; pasta with cheese or meat sauces; cookies, pastries; granola
Milk and Milk Products	Low-fat or skim milk; low-fat or nonfat yogurt and cheeses (ricotta, farmer, cottage, mozzarella); sherbet; frozen, low-fat yogurt; ice milk	Whole milk; butter; yogurt made from whole milk; sweet, sour, or whipped cream; creamy toppings; coffee creamers; cream cheese; cheese spreads; Brie, Camembert, hard cheese (Swiss, cheddar)
Meat, Poultry, Fish, Eggs, Nuts, and Beans	Low-fat poultry (chicken, turkey) without skin; fresh or frozen fish and shellfish; water-packed canned tuna; lean meat trimmed of all fat; cooked dry beans and peas	Beef, veal, lamb, and pork cuts with marbling, untrimmed of fat; luncheon meats; sausage, hot dogs; peanut butter nuts, seeds; trail mix; tuna packed in oil; duck, goose

Exercise

There are many benefits to a regular exercise program. Exercise
speeds up the metabolism, which helps you lose pounds. It also
strengthens and tones muscles and conditions the heart.
Exercise may give you more energy and improve your mood
and self-image.

It is best to begin an exercise program slowly. If you have a
question about your health, consult your doctor. For the best
results, you should exercise at least 3 times a week for 30 minutes at a time. Once you become more fit, you can exercise
longer—up to 45–60 minutes at a time every day. The best type
of exercise for weight loss is steady, aerobic exercise that works
the heart and lungs. Although pregnant women should not try
to lose weight, moderate exercise usually is safe in pregnancy.

When you exercise, you increase muscle mass (which weighs
more than fat) and decrease your fat. This means you may lose
weight slowly, even though you are losing fat. It often takes
weeks before you notice results in your exercise program. But
don't be discouraged: your clothes may feel looser before your
scale reflects the loss.

About two thirds of the people who try to lose weight by cutting calories without exercising gain the weight back within a year. Dieting slows your metabolism. This makes your body burn fat more slowly and makes it harder to lose weight.

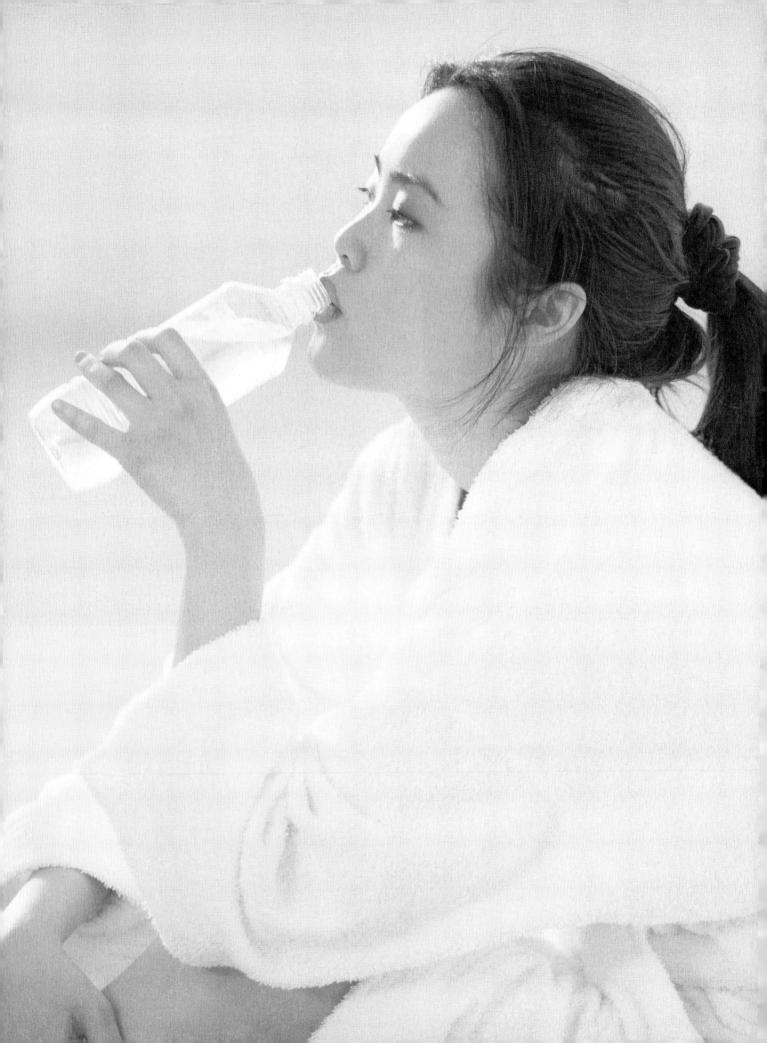

WOMEN'S HEALTH

A woman's health is a responsibility she shares with her doctor. The doctor is responsible for taking care of the basic health needs and for treating problems. This includes giving women information about a healthy lifestyle, as well as doing tests and exams to look for disease.

It is up to women to follow a healthy lifestyle and to be aware of any changes in their bodies that may signal a problem. Even if a woman is not having any problems, it is important for her to see her doctor regularly for routine checkups.

This section is designed to explain certain conditions and diseases that may affect a woman's health and the kind of care a woman can expect to receive when diagnosed with these conditions.

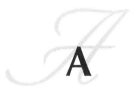

A

▶ ABLATION

The lining of the uterus—the endometrium—is shed each month during a woman's menstrual period. Sometimes the bleeding is too heavy or goes on too long and treatment is needed. If bleeding does not respond to medication, your doctor may suggest endometrial ablation. This procedure treats the lining of the uterus to control or stop bleeding. It does not remove the uterus.

Heavy Bleeding

If you soak through one sanitary pad or tampon an hour for several days in a row or have periods that last longer than 7 straight days, you may have heavy uterine bleeding. This also is called menorrhagia. Women with such menstrual cycles should be checked by a doctor.

Most women lose about ¼ cup of blood during their menstrual period, although it may seem like more. Some women have longer periods or heavier bleeding. One in five women has heavy bleeding at some point during her childbearing years. Heavy bleeding is most common for women between ages 40 and 50, as they approach menopause. It also can be caused by hormonal changes or certain medical conditions, such as problems with blood clotting. Although there are other causes of heavy bleeding, such as growths, ablation is not used to treat these problems.

Losing too much blood can lead to anemia (lack of iron in the blood). It also can lead to problems with your daily function. In most cases, the doctor first tries to treat the bleeding with medication. If the bleeding can't be controlled, ablation may be used.

About Ablation

Ablation destroys a thin layer of the lining of the uterus. This stops menstrual flow in many women. Some women still have light bleeding or spotting. A few women may have regular periods. This is because the ovaries and uterus were not removed.

Most women are not able to get pregnant after ablation. Thus, if you may want to become pregnant, you should not have endometrial ablation. Although pregnancy is not likely after ablation, you should keep using some form of birth control until menopause. You also may want to think about sterilization as an option.

Women who have had ablation still have all their reproductive organs in place. Because of this, you still need to have routine Pap tests and pelvic exams after ablation.

You will talk with your doctor and have a number of tests before the procedure is done. The tests may include:

- Hysteroscopy

- Ultrasound

- Endometrial biopsy

Before the Procedure

A few weeks or months before the procedure, your doctor may prescribe medication that will help thin the lining of your uterus. This will help expose the cell layer that needs to be removed.

Side effects of the medication include vaginal dryness, hot flushes, and night sweats. The effects will go away.

The Procedure

Ablation is a short procedure. It is done as outpatient surgery in most cases. This means you can go home the same day. You most likely will be given some form of pain relief or sedative to help you relax before the procedure. The type of pain relief used depends on the type of ablation procedure, where it is done, and your wishes. You should discuss this with your doctor.

There are no incisions (cuts) involved in ablation. Recovery takes about 2 hours, depending on the type of pain relief used.

Your doctor will use one of a number of types of energy to burn away the lining. These may include electrical, laser, or thermal ablation. As new techniques emerge, your doctor can explain them.

Electrical

A loop or rollerball tool can be used to destroy the thin inner lining of the uterus. For the procedure, the walls of the cervix are widened to allow passage of a device called a hysteroscope. The doctor looks through it to see the inside of your uterus on a monitor. Your uterus is filled with fluid to expand it. Then, the ball or loop is pulled across the endometrial surface. The rollerball or loop applies an electric current to the surface as it is pulled across the lining. This current destroys the lining.

Ablation often is used as an alternative to hysterectomy (removal of the uterus). After either of these procedures, a woman likely will no longer have periods or be able to get pregnant. Before you decide on treatment, think about all your options.

Laser

A laser device burns the lining using a high-intensity light beam. Like the rollerball and loop, the laser reaches the lining of the uterus through the hysteroscope. The laser then destroys the lining of the uterus.

Thermal

With thermal ablation, a balloon device filled with fluid is inserted into your uterus. Heat and energy are applied to increase the temperature and destroy the lining.

Risks

There is some risk involved with any procedure. Most problems result from:

▶ Pain relief

▶ Blood loss

▶ Infection

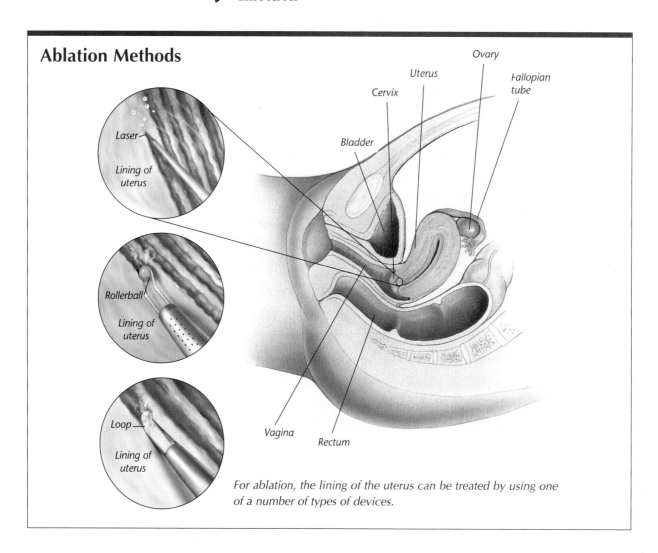

Ablation Methods

For ablation, the lining of the uterus can be treated by using one of a number of types of devices.

The ablation procedure has certain risks. The device used may pass through the uterine wall or bowel. Rarely, the fluid used to expand your uterus may be absorbed into your bloodstream. This may cause too much fluid in your body and can be serious.

After the Procedure

Some minor side effects are common after endometrial ablation:

▶ Cramping, like menstrual cramps, for a day or two

▶ Small amount of thin, watery discharge mixed with blood, which can last a few weeks

▶ Frequent urination for 24 hours

▶ Nausea

Ask your doctor about when you can exercise, have sex, or use tampons. In most cases, you can expect to go back to work or to your normal activities within a day or two.

Your doctor will arrange follow-up visits to check your progress. It may take a few months to achieve results.

▶ ABORTION, INDUCED

▶ See also *Birth Control*

Each year, about 1.37 million women in the United States have an induced abortion. It is a procedure that is low-risk when done in the proper setting.

The decision whether to have an abortion may be hard to make. If you decide to have an abortion, the earlier you have it, the safer and easier it will be for you. If you decide to continue the pregnancy, you will need to begin prenatal care as soon as you can.

Before having an abortion, explore your feelings and beliefs to be sure it's the right step for you. Talking with someone may ease any emotional stress and help you decide. Many people can help you, such as your partner, a relative, or a close friend. You can talk it over with your doctor or a counselor as well.

Common Questions About Abortion

What Is Induced Abortion?

Abortion means expelling or removing the developing fetus from a woman's uterus before the fetus is viable (can live outside the uterus on its own). The medical procedure used to do this is induced abortion. About 90% of abortions are done in the first 12 weeks of pregnancy. Some are done later, often for medical reasons. The woman may be extremely ill, for example, or something may be wrong with the fetus.

The length of a pregnancy is measured in weeks from the first day of your last normal period. Thus, if you missed your period, on the day that it was due you would be about 4 weeks pregnant.

Do I Need Anyone's Permission or Consent?

Abortion has been legal in the United States since 1973. No doctor, however, is required to perform an abortion.

In some states there are special legal requirements. For instance, some states require that minors get parental consent, notify their parent(s), or gain court approval before they can have an abortion.

Who Performs the Abortion?

Abortions are done by a doctor or other health professional who has been trained to do the procedure. Your own doctor may perform abortions. If not, he or she can refer you to someone who does. You can also find out about abortion services through your state's medical society, the local health department, or a family planning clinic.

Where Is the Abortion Performed?

An abortion is done in a doctor's office, a clinic, or a hospital. Where it is done depends on several factors, such as the procedure planned, your health, and the length of your pregnancy. For instance, early abortions can be performed safely in a doctor's office or clinic. Later abortions often are performed in hospitals or in special clinics. It may depend on what facilities are available in your region. It also may depend on the state law.

Wherever the abortion is done, you should also be able to get counseling, as well as recovery care. Family planning services should also be provided. Be sure to check that a full range of services is available and all the options and details are discussed. Your doctor can refer you to a good facility.

The National Abortion Federation has a hotline that can provide information and guide you to providers in your area. The hotline number is 800-772-9100.

How Is Abortion Performed?

The two most common kinds of abortion are suction curettage and labor-inducing abortion. Suction curettage is a surgical procedure that removes the contents of the uterus by a suction instrument that is inserted into the uterus. Labor-inducing abortion involves giving a woman drugs to start labor. Ask your doctor which type will be done. You need to know what to expect.

The same methods of dilation (widening the cervix) can be used for suction curettage or labor-inducing abortion. The doctor may dilate the cervix with instruments right before the abortion. Sometimes, doctors use laminaria to widen the cervix. Laminaria are thin rods that are inserted into the cervix. They absorb moisture and swell. This slowly stretches the cervix. It takes several hours, or even overnight.

Suction Curettage

The most common type of abortion in the United States is suction curettage. It is a type of surgery that may also be called vacuum curettage. Later in pregnancy, this procedure may be called dilation and evacuation (D&E).

For the procedure, you are positioned as for a pelvic exam. A speculum is inserted into the vagina to hold it open. Then, the cervix is dilated. The doctor uses local anesthesia by injecting it around the cervix to numb it. Sedatives may be used to help you relax. Sometimes the doctor uses general anesthesia, which puts you to sleep. A small, flexible, plastic tube is inserted into the uterus. It is attached to a suction or vacuum pump, which removes the pregnancy.

This procedure takes about 10 minutes or less. You may be able to go home as soon as an hour later. The later your pregnancy, the longer the procedure will take.

Labor-Inducing Abortion

For later abortions, labor may be induced with drugs. They can be put in the vagina, injected into the uterus, or given through an intravenous (IV) line. Labor-inducing abortions are nearly always done in a hospital.

Prostaglandins are the most widely used drugs for labor-inducing abortions. They cause the uterus to contract. Other agents, such as saline, urea, or oxytocin, are used less often. Sometimes more than one drug is used to induce labor.

These drugs usually cause labor within 12 hours. The abortion usually occurs within 12–24 hours. If the placenta is not expelled by about 2 hours later, the doctor may use forceps and curettage to remove it. Labor-inducing drugs may cause side effects such as nausea, fever, vomiting, and diarrhea.

Other Methods

Another type of procedure to induce abortion is called menstrual aspiration. With this method (done within 1–3 weeks after a missed period), a syringe is used to remove a pregnancy from the uterine lining.

The Rh Factor

When you are pregnant, your blood will be tested to see if it is has the Rh antigen—a protein on the surface of red blood cells. If it does, you are Rh-positive. If it doesn't, you are Rh-negative. An Rh-negative woman may develop antibodies to an Rh-positive fetus. This causes it to fight the Rh factor as if it were a harmful substance. To prevent this problem, after an Rh-negative woman gives birth or has an abortion, miscarriage, or ectopic pregnancy, she is given a medication called Rh immune globulin (RhIg). This drug tricks the immune system into thinking it has already made antibodies and blocks it from making any more. This prevents any chance of the woman developing antibodies that would attack a future Rh-positive fetus.

Mifepristone is a type of medication used to induce abortion. It causes an abortion by making it difficult for a fertilized egg to attach to the uterus. It is used in Europe, but the Food and Drug Administration (FDA) has not approved it for use in the United States.

Risks

Abortion is a low-risk procedure. An early abortion has less risk than a later one. Both are lower risk than carrying a pregnancy to term. Fewer than 1 in 100 women has complications from an early abortion. For later abortions, up to 2 in 100 women have complications. Although an abortion is low-risk, some problems may arise.

▶ *Incomplete abortion*—Rarely, the pregnancy is not removed completely. Bleeding and infection may occur. If the abortion is incomplete, your doctor may need to perform follow-up suction curettage or scrape the lining of the uterus (the endometrium).

▶ *Infection*—An infection can occur when bacteria from the vagina or the cervix get into the uterus. Your doctor may give you antibiotics to prevent this or to treat the infection if it happens.

▶ *Hemorrhage*—Some light bleeding after an abortion is normal. Some bleeding problems need to be treated. Bleeding is rarely heavy enough to require a blood transfusion.

▶ *Damage to the uterus*—During the abortion, the tip of an instrument may pass through the wall of the uterus (perforation) or tear the cervix. If this happens, your doctor may need to operate to repair the injury. Other organs, such as the bowel and bladder, also can be injured if there is perforation. In these cases, surgery will be needed to repair the organ. The risk of perforation or cervical tear is about 1 in 1,000 abortions. The risk increases with the age of the pregnancy.

▶ *Ectopic pregnancy*—When a pregnancy is not in the uterus, it is called an ectopic pregnancy. It is usually in the fallopian tube. Sometimes an ectopic pregnancy cannot be found until an abortion is tried. If you have an ectopic pregnancy, it will not be ended by an abortion and will need another treatment.

▶ *Death*—The risk of death from abortion is lower than 1 in 100,000 women who have suction curettage. It is slightly higher for other procedures. The risk of a woman dying from giving birth is at least 10 times greater than the risk from an early abortion.

Afterward

Normal physical effects after abortion vary. You may have soreness or cramps for a day or two. You may have light bleeding for up to 2 weeks. However, you may generally perform any activities you feel up to doing. Ask the doctor who did the abortion if there are any limitations.

Normal menstruation usually starts again 4–6 weeks after an abortion. You can get pregnant soon after the abortion, so use birth control right away.

Signs of a Problem

▶ Cramps that last longer than 2 days

▶ Severe abdominal or back pain

▶ Bleeding that is heavier than a normal menstrual period

▶ Foul-smelling discharge

▶ A fever (above 100.4° F)

Even if you do not have these symptoms, you should have a follow-up exam to make sure that you are healing properly.

Psychologic Effects

You may have a wide range of feelings about having an abortion. It is a stressful time, and you have made an important decision. You may feel happy and sad at the same time. Many women who decide to continue the pregnancy feel the same. Some of your feelings may be due not just to the abortion but to having an unintended pregnancy. If unhappy feelings don't go away in a few weeks, seek counseling.

Future Pregnancies

Most doctors agree that an abortion does not affect your ability to get pregnant or how a future pregnancy will turn out. Doctors do not know much about the risk for women having more than one abortion. It is possible that more than one abortion might increase the risk for low-birth-weight or for preterm birth.

▶ ABUSE

▶ See also *Alcohol* in *"Women's Wellness"*

Abuse is forceful, controlling behavior that makes a woman do what the abuser wants without regard for her rights, body, or health. A woman is defined as abused if she has had intentional, usually repeated, physical or emotional harm done to her by a man with whom she is or has been in an intimate relationship.

What Is Abuse?

Abuse can take any of several forms. In most violent relationships, though, mental abuse and "bullying" go along with physical force:

▶ *Battering and physical assault*—Throwing objects at the victim, pushing, hitting, slapping, kicking, choking, beating, or attacking with a weapon.

▶ *Sexual assault*—Abuse of the vaginal area or forced intercourse, whether vaginal, oral, or anal.

▶ *Emotional and psychologic abuse*—Forcing the victim to perform degrading or humiliating acts, threatening to harm a partner or her children, attacking or destroying valued possessions and pets, or exerting inappropriate control over a woman's life.

Exerting inappropriate control includes depriving the woman of money, food, sleep, clothing, or transportation; isolating her from her family and friends; and controlling her reproductive choices by forbidding sterilization or sabotaging the use of birth control.

Abuse During Pregnancy

Pregnancy can be a time of added emotional stress for both parents, and abuse often begins or increases during pregnancy. Many pregnant women are abused by their male partners.

Abuse during pregnancy puts both the mother and the fetus at risk. At this time, the abuser is more likely to direct his blows at the woman's breasts and abdomen. Harm to the fetus may include low birth weight, direct injury from blows to the mother's abdomen, and miscarriage. The fear of harm to her unborn baby often will motivate a woman to change an abusive relationship.

In other cases, abuse may decrease during pregnancy. In fact, some women feel safe only when they are carrying a child. They know from experience that "he never hits me when I'm pregnant." This may lead to repeated pregnancies as a way of escaping abuse.

Relationship to Child Abuse

More than half of men who abuse their female partners also abuse their children. Others threaten to abuse their children.

Children who witness family violence or who are abused themselves can be deeply upset by what they see or experience. The fear, helplessness, and anger children feel in an abusive home often take a serious toll. Children may have chronic headaches, stomachaches, diarrhea, bed-wetting, or problems with nightmares and sleeping. Often they have difficulty in school. Sometimes they withdraw from their studies and their friends. Other times they lash out in anger and get into frequent fights.

Children may come to believe that physical violence is a way of dealing with problems. Children who are abused are more likely to get into an abusive relationship when they grow up.

Get Help!

If you or someone you know is in an abusive relationship, help is available. Call the Domestic Violence Hotline at 800-799-SAFE.

The Abusive Relationship

Because women in abusive relationships are at risk for repeated physical and emotional injury, it is important to understand some of the traits that often characterize the men and women in these relationships. Partners in abusive relationships come from all economic and ethnic groups—from all walks of life.

A male abuser often has a family background of violence and may have low self-esteem and low self-confidence. He may be excessively jealous of his partner's relationships with others and refuse to take responsibility for his behavior, blaming his partner for his violent acts. Often he has a problem with alcohol or drugs. This may seem like the cause of the problem, but it is really just an excuse. In reality, the abuse seldom stops when alcohol or drug use does.

An abused woman also has low self-esteem and low self-confidence. Many women believe they somehow cause the abuse and that they can control the abuser by trying to please him or avoid getting him angry.

Women stay in abusive relationships for a number of reasons. They often have conflicting feelings—love and loyalty, guilt, fear of retaliation, or fear of being alone. Whatever her reasons for staying, the daily life of an abused woman is often frightening and chaotic.

The Cycle of Abuse

Many abused women find themselves caught up in a cycle of abuse that follows a common pattern in many relationships. Unless the woman takes some sort of action to break the cycle, the violence usually becomes more frequent and more severe over time:

▶ *Phase 1*—Tension mounts as the abusive partner increases his threats of violence, often calling the woman names or shoving her. During this phase, the abused woman often will try to please the abuser or calm him down. Usually, though, her efforts only delay the violence.

▶ *Phase 2*—The abuser becomes violent and throws objects at his partner; hits, slaps, kicks, or chokes her; abuses her sexually; or uses weapons, such as belts, knives, or guns.

Is Your Relationship Safe?

Women with a history of family violence, sexual assault or incest, or physical abuse from a male partner are at increased risk of being in an abusive relationship.

Disagreements and arguments, even heated ones, are part of a normal relationship. Physical violence or other abusive behavior is not. Everyone has a right to get angry. But no one has the right to express anger violently, to hurt you. Does your partner ever:

▶ Frighten you with threats of violence or by throwing things when he is angry?

▶ Say it's your fault if he hits you?

▶ Promise it won't happen again, but it does?

If you answered "yes," you may be involved in an unhealthy relationship. Remember, no woman deserves to be abused.

▶ *Phase 3*—The abuser apologizes and expresses guilt and shame. He promises the violent behavior will not happen again. He often buys his partner gifts. Sometimes the abuser will blame the violence on the woman, saying it wouldn't have happened if she hadn't said or done something to make him angry.

Over time, the man tends to put less time and effort into making up. He has learned that his violence is controlling his partner, and he will work less hard at being forgiven or at explaining away his behavior.

If You Are Abused

Get Help

The first step in breaking a violent pattern in a relationship is to tell someone. Let someone know about your situation so you can contact that person in case you need to leave a dangerous situation. The person you tell may be a nurse or doctor, counselor or social worker, a close friend or family member, or a clergy member.

At first, you may find it hard to talk about the abuse. But many abused women feel a great sense of relief—and some sense of safety—once they have told someone outside the home.

Feelings of shame are common at this point. Keep in mind that *no one deserves to be abused*. Violent behavior is the fault of the one who is violent, not the victim.

Most areas have many resources that can help in a crisis. These resources include the police department, crisis hotlines, rape crisis centers, domestic violence programs, legal aid services, hospital emergency rooms, and shelters for battered women and children. Many counselors and health professionals are specially trained to deal with domestic violence. Check your local phone directory for listings.

Plan a Quick Exit

Having an exit plan can help you and your children get out of a violent situation quickly. You can take these steps ahead of time:

▶ *Pack a suitcase*—Keep a change of clothing for you and your children, toilet articles, and an extra set of keys to the house and car with a friend or neighbor.

▶ *Keep special items in a safe place*—Have important items handy so you can take them with you on short notice. These may include prescription medi-

---

Elder Abuse

Sometimes women older than age 65 are victims of abuse or domestic violence. Abuse may come in the form of mental, physical, sexual, or financial abuse. Neglect also may occur. The source of abuse can be anyone but often is a spouse, caretaker, or other family member. Here are some questions to think about:

▶ Has anyone at home ever hurt you?

▶ Has anyone taken anything of yours without asking?

▶ Are you afraid of anyone?

If you think you are being abused, don't let the abuse continue. Seek help from someone you trust.

cines, identification, extra cash, checkbook, and credit cards. Also include medical and financial records, such as mortgage or rent receipts. Be sure to take a special toy or book for each child.

▶ *Know exactly where you will go*—Regardless of the time of day or night, know a friend, relative's home, or a shelter for battered women where you can go.

▶ *Know where you'll go if you cannot escape the violence*—Call your doctor or go to the emergency room if you are hurt. Give your doctor complete information about how you were injured. Ask for a copy of the medical record so you can file charges if you wish.

▶ *Call the police*—Physical abuse is a crime. Give the police complete information about the incident. Be sure to get the officer's badge number and a copy of the report in case you want to file charges later.

Make Changes

At some point you will have to think about the long-term situation. You will be faced with some tough decisions. No matter what choices you make, counseling can be of great help. Counseling can help you improve your self-image. It can also help you with the practical matters that will arise as you begin to make changes in your life, such as finding a job or dealing with money concerns or children's problems.

Sometimes a woman who has been abused eventually decides to break away from her partner for good. If this is the case and you are married to the abuser, it is important to get a lawyer who is experienced in dealing with abuse cases. If money is a concern, check out the resources in your area—many communities have legal aid services on an affordable basis. Ask your doctor, counselor, or the staff of a hotline to recommend one.

There are hard decisions to be made if you are changing an abusive relationship. It will take time to sort things out. You may feel pressure from family or friends or have conflicts over your religious beliefs. Allow yourself the time you'll need to decide what to do.

If you want to try to improve the relationship between you and your partner, he should also get counseling. Counseling for the man in an abusive relationship is important in order to change it. Some men do find it possible, through counseling, to change their violent behavior.

▶ See also *Pelvic Pain*

▶ ADENOMYOSIS

Adenomyosis occurs when the endometrium buries itself in the muscle wall of the uterus. This can cause menstrual cramps. It also can cause pressure and bloating in the lower abdomen before periods and more bleeding during periods. A hysterectomy may be needed to treat this condition if the pain or bleeding becomes severe.

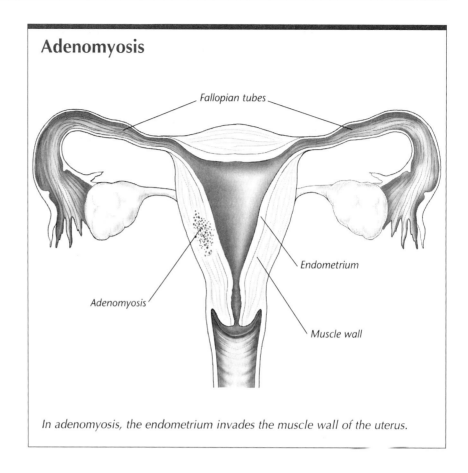

Adenomyosis

Fallopian tubes

Endometrium

Adenomyosis

Muscle wall

In adenomyosis, the endometrium invades the muscle wall of the uterus.

▶ See also *Endometriosis, Pelvic Inflammatory Disease*

▶ ADHESIONS

Adhesions are the result of scarring that binds together the surfaces of organs and structures inside the abdomen or uterus. This can happen because of endometriosis, surgery, or a severe infection such as pelvic inflammatory disease. Adhesions can involve the uterus, fallopian tubes, ovaries, and bowels. They can attach any of these structures to each other or to the sides of the pelvic area. Adhesions may cause pain. They often can be separated during laparoscopy.

▶ See also *Pregnancy Choices*

▶ ADOPTION

You may be anxious or worried about taking care of or raising a child. Choosing to have and care for a baby is a very important decision. It needs careful thought. If you cannot raise a child but do not want to have an abortion, adoption may be a good option. In an adoption, a child legally gets new parents. The baby will get a new birth certificate with the new parents' names on it.

If you choose adoption, prenatal care is as important as if you were going to raise the child yourself. Be sure to start care early and see your doctor regularly.

Not all babies are readily adoptable. Babies of color may be harder to place with adoptive parents. Some adoption agencies specialize in finding families for children of color. Babies with disabilities may also be harder to place. An agency may need to place a child in a foster home until a family can be found.

You may have a variety of feelings when the baby is adopted—anger, grief, a sense of loss, or relief—that may continue for a long time. These feelings could return to you on the child's birthday, even years after the baby has been adopted. Counseling can help you come to terms with this decision. It may be available from the agency providing the adoption service or from a local family services agency.

Women who adopt a child may be able to breastfeed. Talk to your doctor for information.

The Process

Shortly after the baby is born, the birth mother (the woman who gives birth to the baby) signs papers that end her rights to the child and gives her consent to the adoption. If the father's identity is known and he admits to being the father, he must also sign consent forms. He may sign the papers before the baby is born. After the adopting parents agree to accept the baby and have taken him or her home, they file legal papers asking to adopt the baby. A judge approves the adoption, and after a waiting period (usually 1–6 months, but sometimes longer), the adoption is final. Each state has its own laws about permission and consent and about the waiting period before the adoption is final.

Types of Adoption

There are two kinds of adoptions—open and closed. In open adoption, the birth mother and the adoptive parents know something about each other. They may meet and exchange names and addresses. The birth father may also be included. In a closed adoption, the birth mother and adoptive parents do not meet or know each others' names. Sometimes in a closed adoption, the files can be opened later. The laws in each state differ. Some protect the privacy of all involved more than others.

An adoption can be handled by an agency or, in some states, independently. Both agency and independent adoptions may handle open and closed adoptions. Check your state laws.

In an agency adoption, most agencies choose the adoptive parents after careful screening and study. Some agencies let birth mothers help choose. Sometimes babies go directly to their adopting parents from the hospital, but sometimes babies first may be placed in foster care.

In independent adoptions, which are legal in most states, babies are placed in the adoptive parents' home without an agency. They may be done through lawyers, doctors, counselors, or independent organizations. The birth mother may know who the new parents are. The new parents and the home setting must be approved by the state agency responsible for adoptions and by the court before the adoption is final.

In an independent adoption, one lawyer is available to represent both the birth mother and the adopting parents. It is in the best interest of the birth mother, however, to hire her own lawyer. The adopting parents are often asked to pay for this. State bar associations can provide names of lawyers who handle adoptions.

One advantage of agency adoption is that the agency often provides counseling, support services, and follow-up after the adoption. There also may be fewer legal problems with agency adoptions. However, agencies may not allow adoption by single parents or parents over a certain age. Independent adoptions are often more flexible and may have shorter waiting periods.

Financial Help

If you arrange an adoption through an agency, ask the agency what kind of financial help— both medical and legal—it offers. If you cannot afford a private lawyer, you may be able to find legal aid. This is available in most areas. Sometimes it is located at a university law school.

Most, if not all, states allow the adopting parents to pay the birth mother's legal and medical fees. Although these and certain other fees, such as counseling, often can be paid for the birth mother, it is illegal for anyone to profit from an adoption.

▶ See also *Alcohol* in *"Women's Wellness"*

▶ ALCOHOL USE IN PREGNANCY

Drinking alcohol during pregnancy can be harmful to you and your growing baby. Thus, the best course is not to drink at all during pregnancy. This will give your baby the best start in life.

Protect Your Baby

Pregnancy is an exciting time. A new life is growing inside you. Now is the time to take special care of your body. If you eat the right foods and avoid things that are harmful, you give your baby the best chance to be healthy.

Some things—such as alcohol—can harm your baby's health. The degree of harm depends on the amount of alcohol you drink, how often you drink, and when in pregnancy you drank alcohol. Early pregnancy, when many of the baby's organs are forming, is a time to be extra careful. If you have questions or concerns about any alcohol you may have had before you knew you were pregnant, talk to your doctor.

When you are pregnant, the baby inside you is exposed to what is in your bloodstream. A little bit of alcohol may not affect you, but it may hurt your baby.

Alcohol quickly reaches the fetus through your bloodstream. It crosses the placenta to the baby.

In adults, the liver breaks down alcohol. Your baby's liver is not yet able to break down the alcohol. Thus, its effects are more harmful to the baby.

Harmful Effects

Alcohol may affect the baby in many ways. The more you drink, the greater the risk.

Growth and Development

Drinking alcohol may cause a baby to be too small. This condition is called intrauterine growth restriction (IUGR). Alcohol use also increases the chance of having a miscarriage or preterm baby.

Alcohol use can cause heart defects. It also may affect the brain. This can lead to problems with memory, learning, speech, and behavior. You may not be able to see these problems until later in life.

Fetal Alcohol Syndrome

Fetal alcohol syndrome is a mixture of physical, mental, and behavioral problems. Fetal alcohol syndrome is the most severe effect of drinking during pregnancy. It most often results from heavy drinking (two or more drinks a day) or binge drinking (more than three drinks on one occasion). Even a few drinks once in a while can put your baby at risk for fetal alcohol syndrome.

A baby with fetal alcohol syndrome may have:

- Short height or low weight
- Small head
- Problems with joints and limbs (such as clubfoot)
- Abnormal facial features
- Heart defect

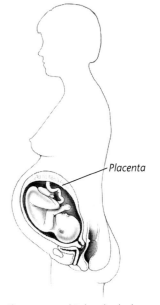

Placenta

If a woman drinks alcohol when she is pregnant, the alcohol reaches the baby through the placenta.

Some babies are born with all of these problems. Others show signs of only some of them. Severe ear infections and vision and dental problems may appear later in life.

There is no cure for fetal alcohol syndrome. The problems will be with these children all of their lives.

Getting Help

It may be hard to stop drinking. If this happens, you may need help.

You may not know if you have a drinking problem. Here are some signs:

- Drinking alone when you feel angry or sad
- Drinking in a pattern (every day or every week at the same time)
- Planning activities around drinking
- Drinking to relieve pain or stress
- Drinking more than you meant to or after you told yourself you wouldn't
- Drinking to get drunk
- Thinking a lot about drinking
- Showing a personality change when you drink

Talk to your doctor about your drinking habits. He or she can give you more information and refer you for counseling or treatment, if needed.

See also *Hormone Replacement Therapy*

ALZHEIMER'S DISEASE

Alzheimer's disease is a condition that leads to the gradual loss of mental functions: thinking, memory, and language. The disease can occur in people in their 30s, 40s and 50s, but most people diagnosed with Alzheimer's are older than 65. Women are twice as likely as men to get it. Alzheimer's disease affects about 4 million people in the United States.

Symptoms and Diagnosis

The most common symptom of Alzheimer's disease is forgetfulness. At first, this symptom usually is mild (forgetting names of people you know, having trouble solving simple math problems) and only seems to be a minor bother. Then forgetfulness becomes more serious (forgetting your name or address, getting lost). These symptoms may cause someone to see a doctor.

To diagnose Alzheimer's disease, the doctor may want to take a complete medical history of the patient and run a series of tests. The medical history will help the doctor explore specific problems the patient has been having. The tests may include basic blood and urine tests to assess memory and language functions and studies of the brain to help the doctor rule out other causes of the symptoms.

Management

There are some drugs that can relieve symptoms in the early stages of the disease, but there is no cure for Alzheimer's disease. Planning for the future and paying for care may become difficult.

This disease may progress quickly once it is diagnosed. It varies from person to person. Over time, family members or other caregivers will need to provide more care for the patient. Eventually the person with Alzheimer's disease will need care 24 hours a day. Living with Alzheimer's disease is different for each patient and caregiver.

For more information on Alzheimer's disease, call the Alzheimer's Association at 800-272-3900

▶ AMENORRHEA

▶ See also *Reproductive Process* in *"Women's Bodies"*

Some women never start menstruating during their teenaged years, while some women who have been having regular periods suddenly stop menstruating. This condition is called amenorrhea, or the absence of menstrual periods

The most common reason for a missed period is pregnancy. A woman who has been having sex and misses a period should consult her doctor. But there are many other possible causes—an abrupt weight change, severe stress, or heavy exercise. At other times, problems with the pituitary gland (a gland located near the brain that controls growth and other changes in the body), the thyroid gland (a gland in the lower neck that helps regulate metabolism), the adrenal glands (located above the kidneys), or the reproductive organs are the cause of amenorrhea.

A girl should see her doctor if she has not started having periods by age 16, or if her breasts have not begun to develop by age 13–14. Although many women sometimes miss a period, any woman who misses periods often should see her doctor.

See also *Birth Defects, Chorionic Villus Sampling, Genetic Disorders*

AMNIOCENTESIS

Amniocentesis is the most common procedure used to test for birth defects. It is done at 16–18 weeks of pregnancy in most cases. It is done in a hospital or in the doctor's office. You don't need to stay overnight.

Who Should Be Tested?

Your doctor can tell you about your genetic risks and the tests you can have. Only you and your partner can decide whether to have a test. You should learn about the tests and any risks involved. How far along your pregnancy is and whether the tests can be done in your area are two points to think about.

Testing should be offered to:

▶ Pregnant women who will be 35 or older on their due date (the risk of having an infant with a chromosomal problem such as Down syndrome increases with the age of the woman).

▶ Couples who already have had a child with a birth defect or have a family history of certain birth defects.

▶ Pregnant women with other abnormal genetic test results.

A normal test result on the fetus cannot ensure that the baby will be normal. This is for a number of reasons. First, each test performed on the fetus looks for a certain problem. There may be a problem that the test was not designed or able to find. Second, some problems cannot be detected by testing. Finally, no test is 100% foolproof.

The Procedure

With amniocentesis, a sample of amniotic fluid is withdrawn through a needle from the sac that surrounds the fetus. Amniotic fluid contains cells from the fetus that can be tested. These cells have the same genetic makeup as the fetus.

For the procedure, the patient lies down with her abdomen exposed. First, ultrasound is used to show the doctor where to insert the needle to try to avoid touching the fetus. The needle then is guided through the abdomen and the uterus into the amniotic sac. A small sample (about 1 ounce) of fluid is withdrawn. If you are carrying twins, the doctor will need to take a sample from each sac. The fetus will produce more amniotic fluid to replace the fluid that is withdrawn.

The amniotic fluid is sent to a lab. The cells are grown in a special fluid for several days. Then, tests are done. The tests that are done depend on your own and your family's history.

Rarely, the cells don't grow. Then, the procedure may need to be done again. This does not mean that the fetus has a problem.

Results

It may take about 2 weeks for enough cells to grow and tests to be performed. The chromosomes within the cells are studied under a microscope. The number and shape of the chromosomes are checked. Also, special tests for specific genetic diseases can be done on the cells.

Tests of the amniotic fluid itself are another way to find some defects. One such test is the alpha-fetoprotein (AFP) test. AFP is a protein made by a growing fetus. Small amounts of AFP are passed into the amniotic fluid. Too much AFP in the amniotic fluid can be a sign of fetal defects, such as open neural tube defects or openings in the fetal abdomen.

One type of AFP test is a blood test. It checks the levels of AFP in the woman's blood. This test may help a woman decide whether to have amniocentesis.

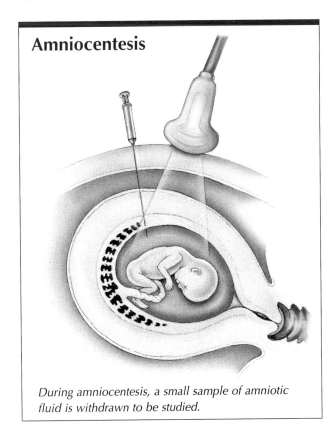

Amniocentesis

During amniocentesis, a small sample of amniotic fluid is withdrawn to be studied.

Risks

Although amniocentesis is fairly safe, there is some risk involved. Side effects that may occur include:

- Cramping
- Bleeding
- Infection
- Leaking of amniotic fluid after the procedure
- Miscarriage

Injury to the fetus from amniocentesis is rare.

All pregnancies have some chance of ending in a miscarriage—whether a test is done or not. Very early in pregnancy, the risk of natural miscarriage is higher. Later in pregnancy, it is lower. The normal risk of miscarriage at the time when amniocentesis would be done is 2–3%. The risk of miscarriage is increased very slightly with amniocentesis—less than 1 in 200 women who have the test will have a miscarriage that they would not have had otherwise.

▶ ANEMIA

Anemia is a disorder in which the blood has a low number of red blood cells. When you are anemic, you often feel very tired. You may also have headaches or feel dizzy. There are three main causes for anemia:

1. Lack of iron in diet

2. Blood loss, through menstruation or bleeding

3. Failure of the body to make enough normal red blood cells

To treat anemia, a change in diet or taking iron pills may be needed. Red meat, dried beans and peas, enriched cereals, and prune juice are some foods rich in iron.

Vitamin C helps your body absorb the iron in food. Calcium, however, can block absorption. Thus, don't take iron and calcium at the same time. It's a good idea to take iron in the morning with orange juice and calcium before you go to bed.

Women who are anemic in pregnancy are less able to cope with bleeding, infections, and other problems that may occur at the time of birth. The fetus may suffer because less oxygen is passed to the placenta. Getting plenty of iron when you're pregnant is a must. Women need more iron in their diet during pregnancy to support the growth of the fetus and to produce extra blood.

Talk with your doctor about whether you need extra iron. An iron supplement or a prenatal vitamin with iron will help boost your intake. Be aware, though, that iron pills can cause constipation, bloating, and black stools. If you are taking an iron supplement, keep it away from children (as with all medication).

▶ ANESTHESIA

Pain-relieving drugs fall into two categories—analgesia and anesthesia. Analgesia is the relief of pain without total loss of feeling. A person getting an analgesic stays conscious (awake). Although analgesics do not always stop pain completely, they do lessen it.

Anesthesia refers to the total loss of feeling. Some forms of anesthesia cause you to lose consciousness, whereas others remove all feeling of pain from parts of the body while you stay conscious.

Not all hospitals are able to offer all types of pain relief medications. An anesthesiologist may work with your health care team to pick the best method for you. Certain types, such as the epidural block, are used more often than others for childbirth.

Systemic Analgesia

Systemic analgesics are often given as injections into a muscle or vein. They lessen pain but will not cause you to lose consciousness. They act on the whole nervous system, rather than on one exact area. Sometimes other drugs are given with systemic analgesics to relieve tension or nausea.

Like other types of drugs, this type of pain medicine can have side effects. Most are minor, such as feeling drowsy or having trouble concentrating.

Local Anesthesia

Local anesthesia is given by injection into the area where the doctor will operate. It does not numb as large an area as does a regional anesthetic. Like regional anesthesia, local anesthesia eliminates pain, but not feelings of pressure. You may be familiar with this type of anesthesia from visits to the dentist.

Pudendal Block

A pudendal block is injected shortly before delivery of a baby to block pain in the perineum. It is especially helpful for numbing the perineum before birth. It relieves pain you may have around the vagina and rectum as the baby moves through the birth canal. Pudendal block is one of the safest forms of anesthesia. Serious side effects are rare.

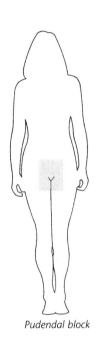

Pudendal block

Epidural Block

Epidural block, a regional anesthetic, affects a larger area than the other kinds of pain medicine. It causes some loss of feeling in the lower half of the body. The extent of the numbness depends on the drug and dose used.

An epidural block is injected into the lower back. The drug is placed into a small space (the epidural space) outside the spinal cord. This is where the nerves that get signals from the lower body pass to reach the spinal cord. The epidural helps ease the pain of contractions and the pain in the vagina as the baby comes out. In larger doses, epidural blocks are used to ease the pain during cesarean birth.

The procedure itself should cause little discomfort. Your back will be washed with an antiseptic, and a tiny area of the skin will be numbed with a local anesthetic. After the epidural needle is in place, a small tube (catheter) is usually inserted through it, and the needle is withdrawn. That way, small doses of the drug can be given through the tube later, or the drug can be given continuously without your needing another injection. Low doses are used because they are less likely to cause side effects for you and the baby.

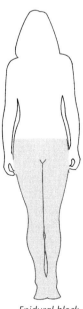

Epidural block

Epidural block can have some side effects. It may cause the mother's blood pressure to decrease temporarily, which in turn may slow the baby's heartbeat. To prevent these problems, the mother is usually given fluids through an intravenous (IV) line in her arm before the drug is injected. She may also be asked to lie on her side to help her blood circulate.

Serious problems with epidurals are rare. If the covering of the spinal cord is pierced, you can get a severe headache that can last for days or weeks if it's not treated. If the drug enters the spinal fluid, the muscles in your chest can be temporarily affected, making it hard to breathe. If the drug enters a vein, you could get dizzy or, rarely, have a seizure. In the rare case that a seizure does occur, there is usually no permanent damage.

Spinal Block

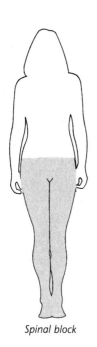

Spinal block

A spinal block—like an epidural block—is an injection in the lower back. While you sit or lie on your side in bed, a small amount of drug is injected into the spinal fluid to numb the lower half of the body. After the drug is given, you have to stay in bed. It brings good relief from pain and starts working fast, but it lasts only an hour or two.

A spinal block is usually given only once during labor, so it is best suited for pain relief during delivery. A spinal block can be used for cesarean birth. It is also useful in a vaginal birth if the baby needs to be helped out of the birth canal with forceps or by vacuum extraction. Spinal blocks can sometimes cause the same side effects as epidural blocks, which are treated in a similar way.

A saddle block is a form of a spinal block, but the medicine is allowed to drop to the lower part of the spine. The part of your body that loses feeling is the part that sits in a saddle— your buttocks, perineum, and vagina.

General Anesthesia

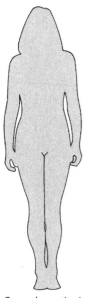

General anesthesia

General anesthesia makes you completely unconscious. First you may be given oxygen through a mask placed over your nose and mouth. The anesthetic is then given through your IV line. After you are asleep you will continue to receive the anesthesia through the IV line, the mask, or a tube that is placed into your mouth and down your windpipe. This tube will be removed shortly after the operation is over.

A rare but serious problem with general anesthesia occurs when food or acid from the stomach enters the windpipe and lungs and causes injury. Because of this, you may be told not to eat. You may be given an antacid to help prevent stomach acids from getting into your lungs.

Regional Anesthesia

Regional anesthesia, unlike general anesthesia, does not make you unconscious. Rather, it works by blocking out feeling in a region of the body. You may still feel a sense of pressure in this part of your body during the operation. Regional anesthesia for surgery in the pelvic area is given as an injection into the lower back, where nerves that carry feeling from the lower body meet the spinal cord. To receive regional anesthesia, you will be positioned either sitting up or on your side. You'll need to be completely still while the needle is placed.

Any anesthesia carries some risks, but the drugs and techniques used today are generally safe. If you are concerned, talk to your doctor or anesthesiologist. The choice of anesthesia will depend on the types available, the type of operation, the state of your health, your wishes, and other factors.

◗ ASSISTED REPRODUCTIVE TECHNOLOGIES

◗ See also *Infertility*

Assisted reproductive technology (ART) includes treatments that involve a lab using human eggs and sperm or embryos to help an infertile couple conceive a child. Doctors may suggest ART procedures when basic infertility treatments, such as medication or surgery, do not work.

Infertile couples have many options. Following are some of the ART treatments available to couples trying to conceive.

Insemination

Insemination is a procedure in which sperm is placed in a woman's vagina by means other than sex. In most cases, the sperm are treated in a lab to increase the chances for fertilization. Around the time of ovulation, the sperm are placed in the vagina, cervix, or uterus.

The woman's partner or a donor may provide the sperm for insemination. It depends on the nature of the problem. Semen from a donor is frozen while the donor is checked to be sure he is free of genetic disorders and some sexually transmitted diseases (STDs), including acquired immunodeficiency syndrome (AIDS).

Biochemical Pregnancy

In ART programs, the pregnancy rate is not always the same as the live birth rate. In some programs, a positive pregnancy test is counted as a pregnancy. In other programs, an amniotic sac must be seen with ultrasound before a pregnancy is confirmed. A so-called "biochemical pregnancy" is fairly common after IVF. It is when a pregnancy is confirmed by blood and urine tests, but no fetus is seen on ultrasound. Including biochemical pregnancies in the count will increase the pregnancy rate.

In Vitro Fertilization

In vitro fertilization (IVF) is a procedure in which eggs from the woman and sperm from a man are fertilized outside the body in a lab. The fertilized egg then is placed in the woman's uterus to grow.

For IVF, the eggs are removed from the ovary just before ovulation occurs. Medication most often is used to cause more than one egg to mature. Eggs may be removed by laparoscopy or by inserting a needle into the ovary. Ultrasound is used to guide the needle, which is inserted through the vagina. The eggs are withdrawn through the needle. Pain relief or a sedative may be given.

The eggs are then combined with sperm and watched to see if fertilization occurs. Either your partner's or a donor's sperm is used. The sperm is obtained through masturbation.

A few days later, one or more fertilized eggs (embryos) are placed in the woman's uterus through her vagina. This is called embryo transfer. The unused fertilized eggs can be frozen and stored for later use. You should talk with your doctor about the number of eggs transferred so you understand the pros and cons.

The success rate of IVF depends on the woman's age and the reason for the infertility. IVF is costly. Its possible side effects are the same as those from ovulation medications or procedures.

Gamete Intrafallopian Transfer

Gamete intrafallopian transfer (GIFT) is an option similar to IVF. During laparoscopy, a mix of eggs and sperm is injected into the fallopian tube, where fertilization may result. It has about the same success rates as IVF. It is more costly, though.

Intracytoplasmic Sperm Injection

Intracytoplasmic sperm injection is a procedure in which one sperm is placed directly into an egg to fertilize it. First, sperm are removed from the semen, which is obtained by masturbation. One sperm is injected into each egg's center. They are checked to see if the eggs are fertilized. Once fertilized, the eggs are placed in the woman's uterus to grow, or they are frozen for later use.

Zygote Intrafallopian Transfer

Zygote intrafallopian transfer (ZIFT) is a variation of IVF and GIFT. As in IVF, the egg is fertilized in a dish before placement in the tube.

Sex Selection

Sex selection is the use of medical techniques to choose the sex of an embryo. Some parents-to-be want to choose the sex of their child because they are carriers of a genetic disorder that occurs only in one sex (such as hemophilia or muscular dystrophy, which are both most common in boys). There also are many social, economic, cultural, and personal reasons for selecting the sex of children. In cultures in which males are valued over females, sex selection has been practiced to ensure that children will be male. This use of sex selection is not supported by ACOG or the medical community.

Fertilization with Assisted Reproductive Technology

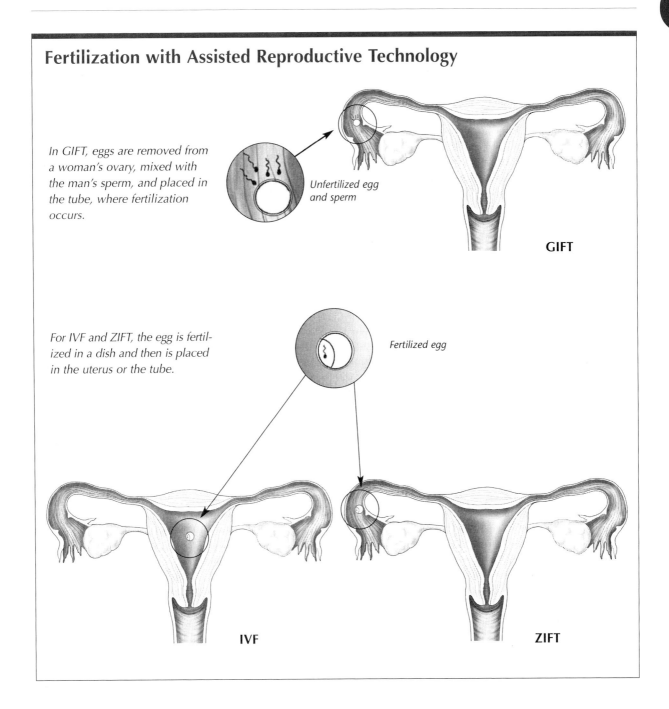

In GIFT, eggs are removed from a woman's ovary, mixed with the man's sperm, and placed in the tube, where fertilization occurs.

Unfertilized egg and sperm

GIFT

For IVF and ZIFT, the egg is fertilized in a dish and then is placed in the uterus or the tube.

Fertilized egg

IVF

ZIFT

▶ ASTHMA

Asthma is a chronic disease of the lung airways. During normal breathing, the airways to the lungs are fully open. This allows air to move in and out easily. With asthma, the airways are inflamed, or swollen, and make more mucus than normal. This clogs the airway, making it harder for air to move in and out freely. Certain things that do not bother most people, such as exercise or pollen, cause problems in people with asthma. These are called triggers.

Asthma triggers vary from person to person. Some of the most common triggers include:

- Allergens, such as dust mites, pollens, molds, pet hair, and cockroaches

- Smells or irritants in the air, such as cigarette smoke, wood fires, charcoal grills, or strong fumes or odors like household cleaners, perfume, and scented soap

- Respiratory infections, such as a cold, flu, sore throat, and sinus infection

- Exercise or any activity that makes you breathe harder

- Weather, such as dry wind, cold air, or quick changes in temperature

Common symptoms of asthma include:

- Wheezing

- Coughing

- Shortness of breath

- Chest tightness

Although the symptoms in a person with asthma may come and go, the condition does not go away. It must be kept under control to keep well. When symptoms get worse, it is called an asthma attack.

If you have asthma, you can help get and keep it under control if you:

- Know what triggers your symptoms

- Watch for early symptoms and respond quickly

- Avoid things that make your asthma worse

- Take your asthma medications as described by your doctor

- Work closely with your health care team

- See your doctor on a regular basis

If you have any symptoms but do not know if you have asthma, visit your doctor for a complete checkup. A number of tests may be needed to find the cause of the problem. They include spirometry (to measure if your airways are open), a chest X-ray, an electrocardiogram (to check for heart disease), or a blood test.

Between 12 and 15 million people, including close to 5 million children, in the United States have asthma. Allergic diseases are the sixth leading cause of chronic disease in the United States.

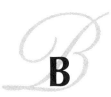

▶ BACK PAIN

Back pain affects almost everyone at some time. For most people this pain occurs in the lower region of their back. Lower back pain is a common problem for women older than the age of 35.

Most back pain lasts for a short amount of time, usually a few days to several weeks. Half of the women with back pain are better within 1 week. Almost all are better within 90 days. Back pain may require some time off work until the pain improves.

Often, within a few days, the pain goes away without treatment. This is called acute back pain. If you do have problems with your lower back, it is important to keep in mind it will probably feel better soon.

If your back pain does not go away you should see your doctor. This is called chronic back pain and may be a symptom of another problem.

Causes and Symptoms

The main causes of acute back pain are sudden tears or strains of the muscles and tendons of the back. The cause of these tears and strains are often unknown, although bad posture and the repeated lifting of heavy objects may play a role.

Weakness of the abdominal muscles can also cause back pain. The abdominal muscles normally support the spine and play an important role in the health of the back.

An unhealthy lifestyle also may cause back pain. For example, women who are not in good shape or do work that includes long periods of sitting or standing are at greater risk for lower back problems.

Back pain may spread to the buttocks or thighs. Some women may also feel stiff all over, not just in their lower back. Symptoms of acute back pain often do not occur right after strain or injury. You may not feel the pain until hours or even days afterward. Lower back symptoms can keep you from doing your normal activities or things that you enjoy.

Diagnosis

To diagnose acute back pain, your doctor may ask you about your medical history. In many cases, this is more helpful than an exam. Muscle strains or tears cannot be found simply by looking at your back.

Some doctors use a pain questionnaire to assess back pain. The questions measure the level of back pain and its effect on your body. Some of these questions may include:

 ▶ When did your back pain start?

 ▶ Which of your daily activities are you not able to do because of your back pain?

 ▶ Have you noticed any problems with your legs?

Tell your doctor what seems to cause the pain to worsen. This will help your doctor decide the best treatment for you.

Treatment

Acute back pain was once treated with rest alone. Doctors now know that exercise and movement help the pain go away. Symptoms improve quickly with treatment in most patients.

For most women, NSAIDs (nonsteroidal anti-inflammatory drugs), such as aspirin or ibuprofen, work well to control pain and discomfort. You can buy most NSAIDs, over the counter. If these do not relieve your pain, talk to your doctor. He or she may prescribe some stronger medications.

NSAIDs work best when they are taken at the first sign of pain. You usually need to take them only for 1 or 2 days. Do not take more pills than the package suggests. You should avoid taking NSAIDs while drinking alcohol. Women with bleeding disorders, liver damage, stomach disorders, or ulcers should not take NSAIDs.

During the first 48 hours of treatment, your doctor may advise you to get more rest. Many times the pain can be relieved by simply lying flat in bed. Placing a pillow between the legs helps.

Heating pads, ice packs, or whirlpools (if possible) may provide short-term relief of pain. Massage also may help improve symptoms. Your doctor may also suggest simple exercises to stretch and strengthen your back muscles.

While waiting for your back to improve, you may be able to ease back pain if you:

 ▶ Wear comfortable, low-heeled shoes.

 ▶ Make sure your work surface is a good height for you.

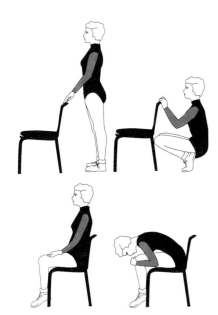

Simple stretches can relieve back strain.

- Use a chair with good lower back support that may recline slightly.

- Try using a pillow or rolled-up towel behind your lower back while driving, especially if you must drive long distances. Also, be sure to stop often and walk around for a few minutes.

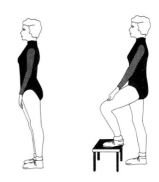

While standing, raising one leg may help relieve your pain.

Prevention

Acute back pain is less likely to occur again if you are in good shape. There are exercises that help relieve back pain. Stretching exercises, aerobic workouts, and swimming are good choices. Having a doctor advise you on your fitness programs usually can help to reduce the risk of injuries.
Ways to prevent back pain include:

- Strengthening back muscles

- Losing weight

- Avoiding lifting while twisting, bending forward, and reaching

- Standing with one foot on stool or bench

- Sitting with one or both knees raised above the hips

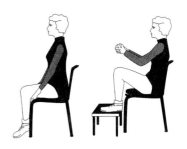

Sitting with your knees raised above your hips may help relieve pain.

Using a small pillow to relieve back strain while sitting also helps. Avoid wearing high-heeled shoes—they can increase your pain. Learn how to walk, stand, sit, and lie in positions that will decrease your back strain. The figures show ways that you can stand and sit to prevent problems.

▶ BACK PAIN DURING PREGNANCY

Back pain is one of the most common discomforts during pregnancy. As your baby grows during pregnancy, your uterus expands to as much as 1,000 times its original size. This amount of growth—centered in one area—affects the balance of your body and may cause discomfort.

What Causes Back Pain

Back pain in pregnancy has many possible causes. It usually is caused by strain on the back muscles. In midpregnancy, when your uterus becomes heavier, it changes your center of gravity.

You then slowly begin to change your posture and the ways that you move. Most women begin to lean backward in the later months of pregnancy—making their back muscles work harder.

Weakness of the abdominal muscles can also cause back pain. The abdominal muscles normally support the spine and play an important role in the health of the back. The hormones of pregnancy cause the muscles to relax and become loose. This may cause some back pain. It can also make you more prone to injury when you exercise.

What You Can Do

To help prevent or ease back pain, try to be aware of how you stand, sit, and move. Here are some tips that may help:

▶ Wear low-heeled (but not flat) shoes with good arch support.

▶ Ask for help when lifting heavy objects.

▶ When standing for long periods, place one foot on a stool or box.

▶ If your bed is too soft, have someone help you place a board between the mattress and box spring.

▶ Don't bend over from the waist to pick things up—squat down, bend your knees, and keep your back straight.

▶ Sit in chairs with good back support, or use a small pillow behind the lower part of your back.

▶ Try to sleep on your side with one or two pillows between your legs for support.

▶ Apply heat or cold to the painful area or massage it.

Doing special exercises for the back can also help lessen backache. They can help strengthen and stretch muscles that support the back and legs and promote good posture—keeping the muscles of the back, the abdomen, the hips, and the upper body strong. These exercises not only will help ease back pain but also will help prepare you for labor and delivery.

If back pain continues to be a problem, your doctor may suggest that you wear a maternity girdle, special elastic sling, or back brace. These devices help support the weight of your abdomen and ease the tension on your back. On rare occasions, mild pain medications, bed rest, or physical therapy may be suggested by your doctor.

Don't try to treat yourself. Back pain can also be caused by other problems. Back pain is one of the main symptoms of preterm labor. If it continues or gets worse, call your doctor. You should also call your doctor if you are having fever, burning during urination, or vaginal bleeding.

To help prevent back pain, keep things within reach. Put objects that you use often in close reach. This way, you won't have to bend or stretch to grab them.

Exercises for a Healthy Back

Diagonal Curl

This exercise strengthens the muscles of your back, hips, and abdomen. If you have not already been exercising regularly, skip this exercise. Sit on the floor with your knees bent, feet on the floor, and hands clasped in front of you. Twist your upper torso to the left until your hands touch the floor. Do the same movement to the right. Repeat on both sides 5 times.

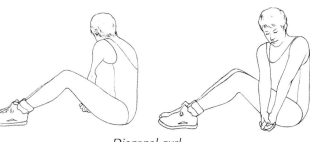

Diagonal curl

Forward Bend

This exercise stretches and strengthens the muscles of your back. Sit in a chair in a comfortable position. Keep your arms relaxed. Bend forward slowly, with your arms in front and hanging down. If you feel any discomfort or pressure on your abdomen, do not push any further. Hold this position for a count of 5, then get up slowly without arching your back. Repeat 5 times.

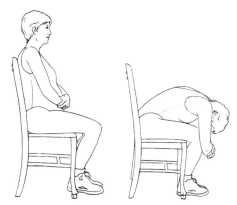

Forward bend

Upper Body Bend

This exercise strengthens the muscles of your back and torso. Stand with your legs apart, knees bent slightly, with your hands on your hips. Bend forward slowly, keeping your upper back straight. You should feel a slight pull along your upper thigh. Repeat 10 times.

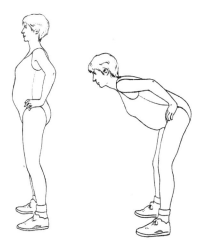

Upper body bend

Trunk Twist

This exercise stretches the muscles of your back, spine, and upper torso. Sit on the floor with your legs crossed, with your left hand holding your left foot and your right hand on the floor at your side for support. Slowly twist your upper torso to the right. Do the same movement to the left, after switching your hands (right hand holding right foot and left hand supporting you). Repeat on both sides 5–10 times.

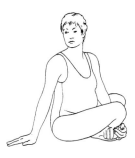 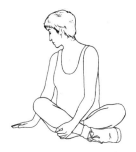 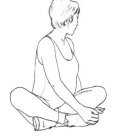 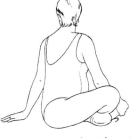

Trunk twist

(continued)

Exercises for a Healthy Back *(continued)*

Backward Stretch

This exercise stretches and strengthens the muscles of your back, pelvis, and thighs. Kneel on hands and knees, with your knees 8–10 inches apart and your arms straight (hands under your shoulders). Curl backward slowly, tucking your head toward your knees and keeping your arms extended. Hold this position for a count of 5, then come back up to all fours slowly. Repeat 5 times.

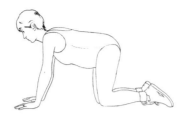
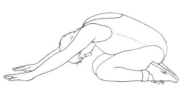

Backward stretch

Back Press

This exercise strengthens the muscles of your back, torso, and upper body and promotes good posture. Stand with your feet 10–12 inches away from a wall and your back against it. Press the lower part of your back against the wall. Hold this position for a count of 10, then release. Repeat 10 times.

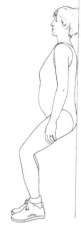

Back press

Leg Lift Crawl

This exercise strengthens the muscles of your back and abdomen. Kneel on hands and knees, with your weight distributed evenly and your arms straight (hands under your shoulders). Lift your left knee and bring it toward your elbow. Straighten your leg without locking your knee. Extend your leg up and back. Do this exercise to a count of 5. Move slowly; don't fling your leg back or arch your back. Repeat on both sides 5–10 times.

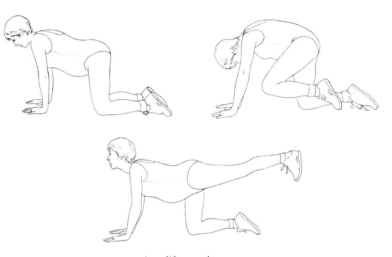

Leg lift crawl

Rocking Back Arch

This exercise stretches and strengthens the muscles of your back, hips, and abdomen. Kneel on hands and knees, with your weight distributed evenly and your back straight. Rock back and forth, to a count of 5. Return to the original position and curl your back upward as much as your can. Repeat 5–10 times.

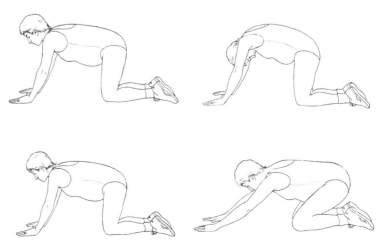

Rocking back arch

▶ BARRIER METHODS OF CONTRACEPTION

▶ See also *Birth Control, Cervical Cap, Condom, Diaphragm, Emergency Contraception, Reproductive Process* in *"Women's Bodies," Spermicide*

Barrier methods are some of the oldest and safest forms of contraception (birth control). These methods work by acting as barriers to keep the man's sperm from reaching the woman's egg. Some methods also may protect against certain sexually transmitted diseases (STDs).

About Barrier Methods

The use of barrier methods goes back 3,500 years. Today, barrier methods are safe and effective ways to prevent pregnancy. The types of barrier methods used in the United States include:

▶ Spermicides (vaginal creams, jellies, foams, films, and suppositories)

▶ Diaphragm

▶ Cervical cap

▶ Condom (male or female)

Barrier methods work by keeping the sperm from reaching the woman's fallopian tubes. The diaphragm, cervical cap, and condom (male and female) act as physical barriers. Only use water-based lubricants when you use any of these methods. Do not use any oil-based lubricants such as petroleum jelly. The oil can damage the rubber.

Spermicides act as chemical barriers. Physical and chemical barrier methods often are combined to provide more protection.

Effectiveness

Barrier methods are effective when used the correct way and every time you have sex. However, even one act of sex without birth control can result in pregnancy.

Barrier methods are not as effective as some other birth control methods, such as birth control pills or the intrauterine device (IUD). When two barrier methods are used together (such as a diaphragm and a condom), though, they become a highly effective form of birth control.

Backup Methods

If a woman has sex without any type of birth control or if she thinks her barrier method has failed (for instance, a condom broke), she may use emergency contraception. In the most common method, high doses of certain birth control pills are taken within 72 hours (3 days) of sex without birth control. The high dose of hormones in emergency contraception disrupt normal hormone patterns in the menstrual cycle that trigger ovulation. This helps prevent pregnancy.

The IUD is another type of emergency contraception. The IUD must be inserted within 5–7 days of having unprotected sex. A benefit of the IUD is that is can be left in for long-term use.

You can obtain emergency contraception from your doctor, a family planning clinic, or a hospital emergency room. Talk to your doctor right away if you think you might need this protection.

If you use emergency contraception within 72 hours of unprotected sex, your chance of getting pregnant is greatly reduced. There is still a chance you could become pregnant, though. Emergency contraception does not work as well as using birth control on a routine basis.

▶ See also *Breast Problems, Cervical Disorders, Pap Test* in *"Women's Wellness"*

▶ BIOPSY

A biopsy is a minor procedure to remove a small piece of tissue that is then studied under a microscope. Your doctor may be able to find the exact nature of a problem by studying cells from it or taking a sample of it. He or she will look at the structure of the tissue removed as well as the structure of the cells within it to help find the cause of a problem. To check a solid mass or a suspicious area in the breast, cervix, or vulva, your doctor may advise a biopsy.

Techniques

There are a number of types of biopsies. Your doctor may use one of the following methods:

▶ *Cone biopsy:* A cone-shaped wedge of tissue is removed from the cervix. This type of biopsy is used if a larger sample is needed.

▶ *Core biopsy:* A hollow needle removes a core of tissue.

▶ *Endocervical curettage:* A sample is removed from the inside part of the cervix with a small device shaped like a spoon.

▶ *Excisional biopsy:* The entire mass is removed.

▶ *Needle biopsy:* A small sample of cells from the mass is withdrawn through a needle.

- *Loop electrosurgical excision procedure (LEEP):* A thin wire loop carrying an electric current is used to remove abnormal areas of the cervix.

- *Punch biopsy:* A small sample of the cervix is removed with a special device.

The method used depends on the area of the body where the tissue is being removed. Because abnormal areas are removed, sometimes a biopsy also will serve as a method of treatment.

Biopsy Areas

Breast

A biopsy of the breast may be done if there is any unexplained lump in the breast of a female at risk of breast cancer. This may be done even if a mammogram (X-ray of the breast) is normal. It also may be done for any abnormal mammogram results.

After the breast lump is removed, cells taken from it are looked at under a microscope. Results will be negative (no cancer) or positive (cancer). Your doctor will discuss the results with you and determine what type of treatment is best.

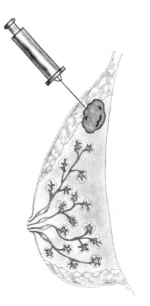

Needle biopsy

Cervix

When abnormalities of the cervix are seen by colposcopy, a biopsy may be done to diagnose the problem. In this procedure, small pieces of cervical tissue are removed for study. A biopsy is done in the doctor's office or clinic in most cases. You may have some mild cramping or a pinching sensation. The results of a biopsy may not be available for several days.

Vulva

Biopsy also is used to diagnose some diseases of the vulva. A portion biopsy and an excisional biopsy are the most common types of biopsy used.

▶ BIRTH CONTROL

Most women can become pregnant from the time they are in their early teens until they are in their late 40s. About half of all pregnancies are unplanned. Birth control (or contraception) helps a woman plan her pregnancies. Some methods of birth control also help protect against sexually transmitted diseases (STDs), including acquired immunodeficiency syndrome (AIDS). Today, there are many choices of birth control for women and men.

▶ See also *Barrier Methods, Birth Control Pills, Emergency Contraception, Hormone Implants, Hormone Injections, Intrauterine Device, Natural Family Planning, Sterilization*

How Birth Control Works

To understand how birth control works, you should know what happens during reproduction. A woman has two ovaries, one on each side of the uterus. Each month, one of the ovaries releases an egg into a fallopian tube. This release of an egg is called ovulation. In a woman with a regular menstrual cycle, ovulation occurs 12–14 days before the start of her next period.

A woman can get pregnant if she has sex around the time of ovulation. During sex, the man ejaculates sperm into the vagina. The sperm travel up through the cervix, through the uterus, and out into the tubes.

If a sperm meets an egg in the fallopian tube, fertilization (the joining of egg and sperm) can occur. The fertilized egg then moves down the fallopian tube to the uterus. It then attaches to the uterus and grows into a fetus.

Birth control methods work in a number of ways. They may:

▶ Block the sperm from reaching the egg

▶ Kill sperm

▶ Keep eggs from being released each month

▶ Change the lining of the uterus

▶ Thicken the mucus in the cervix so sperm cannot easily pass through it

Methods

According to a 1995 report by the National Academy of Sciences, 6 out of 10 pregnancies in the United States are unplanned.

There are many methods of birth control. Each method has good points as well as side effects. The greatest benefit of effective birth control is that it allows a woman to plan her family—both the size and the spacing.

Certain types of birth control have added benefits to your health. Discuss the pros and cons with your doctor.

The birth control pill, implants, injections, intrauterine device (IUD), diaphragm, and cervical cap require a prescription. Condoms, spermicides, and sponges do not.

More than one method may be used at the same time. For instance, a barrier method may be used with any other method. Using a barrier method with another method increases the effectiveness. It also may help protect against STDs.

Hormones

With hormonal birth control, a woman takes hormones like those her body makes naturally. These hormones prevent ovulation. When there is no egg to be fertilized, pregnancy cannot occur. They also cause other changes in the cervical mucus and uterus that help prevent pregnancy. Hormonal pills, injections, and implants are all very effective. They do not protect against STDs, though.

Birth control pill. The most commonly used method of hormonal birth control is the birth control pill (oral contraceptive). Most birth control pills contain the hormones estrogen and progestin. A few contain just progestin. The pill is safe and highly effective when taken each day. For most women, the risk of serious complications is small. The pill may pose a risk for women older than 35 who are heavy smokers. Birth control pills help protect against certain types of cancer, such as cancer of the ovary and endometrium (lining of the uterus). The menstrual period most often is lighter and easier to predict. Cramps occur less often, too.

Implants. With implants, match-size, soft plastic tubes are placed just under the skin of the upper arm. This is done through a small cut (incision). The woman is given local anesthesia. After the tubes are inserted, nothing else needs to be done to prevent pregnancy. Implants provide birth control for up to 5 years. They can be removed when a woman wishes to stop using them. Or, they can be replaced with new implants after 5 years. The hormones in implants may make your periods irregular. You may spot at any time in your cycle.

Injection. One injection of hormonal birth control provides birth control for 3 months. This means a woman needs only four injections each year. During the time that the injection is

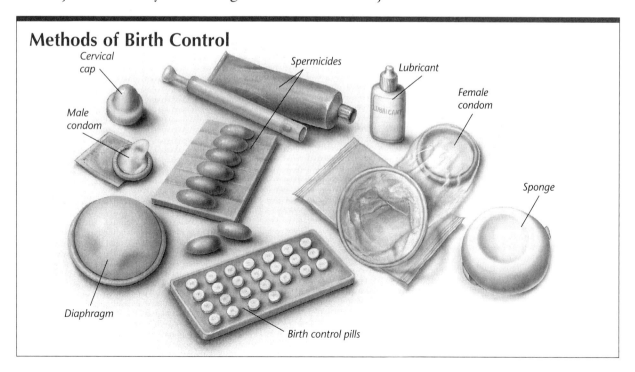

Methods of Birth Control

Cervical cap

Spermicides

Lubricant

Female condom

Male condom

Sponge

Diaphragm

Birth control pills

Emergency contraception greatly reduces the chance that a woman will become pregnant. It is not as effective as using birth control on a regular basis, though. Talk to your doctor right away if you think you might need this protection.

effective, you don't have to do anything else to prevent pregnancy. You may have irregular periods.

Emergency contraception. If a woman has sex without any type of birth control, she may be able to use a type of backup birth control called emergency contraception. This method also can be used if a birth control method fails, such as a condom slips or breaks. In this method, high doses of certain birth control pills are taken within 72 hours (3 days) of sex without birth control. The high dose of hormones in emergency contraception causes changes in the lining of the uterus that help prevent pregnancy.

Intrauterine Device

The IUD is a small, plastic device that contains copper or hormones. It is inserted and left in the uterus. The presence of the IUD prevents the egg from being fertilized in the tubes or from attaching to the wall of the uterus.

Barrier Methods

Barrier methods include the diaphragm, cervical cap, condom (male and female), sponge, and spermicides:

▶ The diaphragm is a round rubber dome that fits inside the woman's vagina and covers her cervix.

▶ The cervical cap is a small rubber cup that fits over the cervix and stays in place by suction.

▶ The male condom is a thin sheath made of latex (rubber) or animal membrane worn by the man over his penis.

▶ The female condom is a thin plastic pouch that lines the vagina. It is held in place by a closed inner ring by the cervix and an open outer ring at the opening of the vagina.

▶ The sponge is a doughnut-shaped device that is coated with spermicide. It is pushed up in the vagina to cover the cervix.

▶ Spermicides are chemicals that kill sperm. They are placed in the vagina close to the cervix. They include creams, jellies, foams, suppositories, and films.

The diaphragm, cervical cap, sponge, and male and female condom act as physical barriers. They keep the sperm from getting to the egg. To be effective, barrier methods must be used each time you have sex.

These methods are used with spermicides to further lower the risk of pregnancy. Spermicides and latex condoms also help protect against some STDs. Condoms made of animal membranes do not provide the same protection against STDs. Other types of condoms are being tested. Ask your doctor about your options.

Some couples use two barrier methods at the same time to increase effectiveness. Couples also may use different methods at different times.

Withdrawal

The withdrawal method prevents pregnancy by not allowing sperm to be released in the woman's vagina. This requires the man to take his penis out of the woman before he ejaculates. For this method to work, he must withdraw every time the couple has sex. Drawbacks are that sperm can be present in the fluid produced by the penis before ejaculation and some men fail to withdraw completely or in time.

Each year, 85% of the women who do not use any method of birth control during sex become pregnant. The only way to completely prevent pregnancy is to not have sex.

Natural Family Planning

Natural family planning also is called periodic abstinence or the rhythm method. This method can work only if you do not have sex during those times in your menstrual cycle when your chances of becoming pregnant are greatest. By knowing when you ovulate, you and your partner know when you should not have sex. There are a number of ways to predict ovulation:

▶ Check for changes in cervical mucus (ovulation method)

▶ Check for changes in body temperature (when combined with checking cervical mucus, this is the symptothermal method)

▶ Count days during the menstrual cycle (calendar method)

▶ Use an ovulation predictor kit

These methods often are combined to prevent pregnancy. For this method to work, the couple must know how to use the method, pay close attention to the woman's cycle, and not have sex near ovulation. Your doctor can refer you to groups that teach this method.

Sterilization

Sterilization for women and men works by permanently blocking the pathways of egg and sperm. This is done by surgery.

For women, both fallopian tubes are closed by tying, banding, clipping, or cutting them or by sealing them with electric current. This is called tubal ligation. The surgery is performed under general anesthesia in most cases. Some women have this done right after the birth of a baby.

For men, vasectomy involves clamping, cutting, and sealing the tubes that carry sperm to the penis. This prevents the release of sperm. In most cases, the man is given local anesthesia. Surgery is done in the doctor's office or a clinic.

Sterilization is meant to be a permanent form of birth control. If there is a chance you may want to have a baby later, you should choose another method to prevent pregnancy.

Choosing a Method

At any given time, a couple may find one method of birth control suits their needs better than others. Most women and couples use different methods over their lifetime. Here are some things to think about when choosing a method:

▶ How well the method works

▶ How likely you are to use it

▶ How safe it is

▶ How much it costs, month by month and over time

▶ Whether it helps protect against STDs

All methods have a chance of failure. When a method is used correctly and each time, the failure rates are lower (Table 10).

Most birth control failures result from not using birth control correctly each time. Any method of birth control described here can work well if it is used correctly. Choose a method you will be able to use on a regular basis.

You also should think about preventing STDs when choosing a method. You are at higher risk for STDs if you have had more than one sexual partner or if your partner has had more than one sexual partner. Use of condoms can help prevent some STDs. Condoms can be used along with other methods, such as the pill, injections, or implants.

Table 10. Contraceptive Failure Rates*

Method	Typical Use (%)	Perfect Use (%)[†]
No method (chance)	85	85
Spermicides	26	6
Periodic abstinence	25	
Calendar		9
Ovulation Method		3
Sympto-thermal		2
Post-ovulation		1
Cervical cap		
Women who have had children	40	26
Women who have not had children	20	9
Sponge		
Women who have had children	40	20
Women who have not had children	20	9
Diaphragm	20	6
Withdrawal	19	4
Condom		
Female	21	5
Male	14	3
Pill		5
Estrogen plus progestin		0.1
Progestin only		0.5
IUD		
With hormones	2.0	1.5
With copper	0.8	0.6
Contraceptive injections	0.3	0.3
Contraceptive implants	0.05	0.05
Female sterilization	0.5	0.5
Male sterilization	0.15	0.10

* The failure rate is the estimated percentage of all women using the method who will have an unplanned pregnancy in the first year of use.

† Using the method the correct way and every time you have sex makes birth control more effective.

Modified from Hatcher RA, Trussell J, Stewart GK, Kowal D, Guest F, Cates W Jr, et al. Contraceptive technology. 17th rev ed. New York: Irvington Publishers, 1998:800–801

▶ BIRTH CONTROL PILLS

▶ See also *Birth Control, Emergency Contraception*

Birth control pills (also called oral contraceptives or "the pill") are used by millions of women in the United States to prevent pregnancy. The pill contains synthetic (man-made) hormones that are like the ones made by your body. The hormones in the pill prevent an egg from being released from the ovaries. Without an egg, pregnancy cannot occur.

The pill is one of the most popular and effective birth control methods:

▶ It is easy to use.

▶ It is convenient. You do not need to do anything else before sex to prevent pregnancy.

▶ It is reversible. When you stop taking the pill, you are not protected against pregnancy.

▶ It has other health benefits, such as protection against some cancers.

How the Pill Works

The ovaries produce two hormones that affect a woman's menstrual cycle: estrogen and progesterone. Most pills contain synthetic estrogen and progesterone. They prevent eggs from being released from the ovaries. Without an egg, pregnancy cannot occur. At the end of a cycle, the menstrual period starts. Women taking the pill still have their periods, but they often are shorter, lighter, and more regular.

Birth control pills work very well. When women use them perfectly, less than 1 in 100 will get pregnant over 1 year. However, about 3 in 100 typical users will become pregnant. This is because women may forget to take the pill.

Most women who take the pill take a combination pill, which contains a mix of estrogen and progestin (the synthetic form of progesterone). There are many different brands. Most contain doses of hormones that are much lower than earlier pills. If the side effects of one type bother you, tell your doctor. He or she may be able to help.

Some women take a pill that has only progestin. It is called the minipill. It is a better choice for women who have certain health problems (for example, blood clots) and cannot take pills with estrogen. Minipills also are a good choice if you are breastfeeding because there is no estrogen which would cut down on your milk supply.

Although the pill is one of the most effective methods of birth control, to be effective, the pill must be taken as prescribed. This is true for all methods of birth control.

It is slightly less effective than the pill with both hormones. It may not offer the health benefits that pills with estrogen do.

The minipill comes in packs of 28 pills. Take one pill at the same time each day. All the pills in the pack contain hormones. It is very important not to miss a pill.

Women who use the minipill often bleed between periods. This is not serious, but it may be annoying.

Benefits of the Pill

Because the pill now contains much lower doses of hormones than it first did, it is much safer to use than it used to be. Usually, the health benefits of the pill far outweigh the risks.

The pill helps to keep your periods regular, lighter, and shorter. Because your periods are lighter and shorter, you are less likely to have anemia (iron-poor blood). Women who use the pill get cramps less often. In addition, the pill helps protect against benign breast disease and cancers of the ovary and endometrium. The pill also reduces your risk of ectopic pregnancy.

Many women have heard or believe things about the pill that are not true. Table 11 lists some common myths and facts about the pill.

Table 11. Myths About the Birth Control Pill

Myth	Fact
Taking the pill is risky.	The risks of having a baby, smoking, or driving a car are much higher than taking the pill. The pill may be risky for women older than 35 who smoke. For almost all women, the benefits of the pill far outweigh any possible risks.
Taking the pill causes weight gain.	As many women lose as gain weight while taking the pill.
Taking a break from the pill now and then is a good idea.	There is no health benefit to taking a break from the pill. Taking a break may increase a woman's chances of an unwanted pregnancy.
The pill causes cancer.	Most studies show that the pill does not increase the risk of cervical or breast cancer. It decreases the risk of ovarian and endometrial cancer.

Getting the Pill

Your doctor or nurse will examine you and ask you questions to see if the pill is a good birth control method for you. You will be asked about your lifestyle and health. This is to make sure that the pill is right for you. You may be asked:

▶ Your age

▶ Whether you smoke

▶ Whether you have had certain conditions or diseases

▶ Whether you take any medicines

This also is a good time to ask any questions you may have about taking the pill. Many women have heard or believe things about the pill that are not true.

This is a good opportunity for you to see your doctor for other health reasons, too. In addition to a general physical exam, including a pelvic and a breast exam, you may have other tests based on your age or your health.

Most healthy women who do not smoke can use the pill. This includes teenagers and women older than age 40. Some reasons why a woman may not be able to use the pill include:

◗ A history of blood clots in veins deep inside the legs

◗ A history of stroke or other disease of the blood vessels

◗ Active liver disease

◗ Unexplained bleeding from the vagina

◗ Breast cancer

◗ Smoking in women older than age 35

How To Take the Pill

When you start taking the pill will depend on the type of pill you are taking. Many pill instructions suggest starting to take the pill on the Sunday after your period starts. You can start even if you are still bleeding. If your period begins on Sunday, start taking the pill that day. Unless your period begins on Sunday, use another birth control method for the next 7 days of the first cycle as a backup method. Condoms that also protect against STDs and foam (spermicides) are a good choice. This is the only time you will need to use a backup method unless you forget to take your pills. Women who start to take pills on a Sunday will usually have their periods in the middle of the week.

You can also start taking the pill on the first day of your period. You will not need a backup method of birth control. Birth control pills alone, however, do not protect against STDs. Using condoms with your pills will help protect against STDs.

You will start each new pack of pills on the same day of the week as you started the first pack. It is a good idea to have an extra pack of pills and a backup method on hand in case you miss some pills or lose your pack.

Taking the Pill

Pills come in packs of 21 or 28 pills. They are both very effective when taken correctly.

21 Pills. If your pack has 21 pills, take one pill at the same time each day for 21 days. Then, wait 7 days before starting a new pack. During the week you are not taking the pill, you will have your period. Remember, you will start your new pack of pills on the same day of the week as you started the first pack.

28 Pills. If your pack has 28 pills, take one pill at the same time each day for 28 days. When you finish all the pills in the pack, start a new pack the next day. The last seven pills in the 28-day pack do not contain any hormones. They are in the pack so that you can take a pill every day. This may make taking the pill easier for you. During the week you are taking the last seven pills, you will have your period.

Do not skip pills for any reason. Pills only work if you take them as prescribed. Do not skip pills even if you bleed between periods or feel sick to your stomach (nausea). Call your doctor or nurse if you are concerned. Even if you do not have sex very often, it is important to keep taking the pill.

Your pills may not work well if your body does not absorb them. This may happen if you vomit or have diarrhea. In these cases, you should use a backup method for the rest of your cycle.

Each new pack of pills comes with facts about the pill. Read this carefully. Be sure to ask about anything that is not clear to you.

If You Miss a Pill

Most women forget to take a pill once in a while. If you forget to take one pill, take it as soon as you remember. Take the next pill at the normal time. It is okay if you have to take two pills in the same day. It is normal to feel a bit queasy if you do this.

If you forget to take two or more pills, use a backup method and call your doctor or nurse. Ask what you should do.

If you miss some pills, you may have some spotting or light bleeding even if you make up the missed pills. These side effects are not harmful.

If you have a 28-day pill pack and forget to take one of the last seven "reminder" pills (pills without hormones), do not worry. Throw away the reminder pills you missed. Keep taking one pill a day until the pack is empty. Remember, you should start your new pack of pills on the same day of the week as you started your first pack.

Side Effects of the Pill

There are some common side effects of the pill that can be annoying. These side effects are not usually harmful. Most go away within 3 months. If they do not go away or are severe, see your doctor. Switching to another type of pill may help.

Common side effects include:

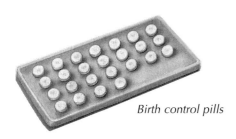

Birth control pills

▶ Nausea (many women find that taking the pill with a meal or before bed helps)

▶ "Spotting" or bleeding between periods

▶ Headaches (taking over-the-counter products for pain relief usually helps)

Missing a period is another common side effect. If you miss one period and have taken the pill correctly, you should keep taking the pill. If you have forgotten some pills and miss one period, call your doctor, but keep taking the pill.

Risks

The pill can cause severe illness in some women, although this is rare. The most serious problem is cardiovascular disease, such as blood clots in the legs, heart attack, or stroke. The risk is high for women who are older than age 35 and who smoke. They should not take the pill. The risk of this stops when pill use is stopped. There is no increased risk of heart attack or stroke for women who are healthy and do not smoke.

Other rare problems may occur. They include high blood pressure, gallbladder disease (in women already at risk for it), a very rare form of liver cancer, and liver tumors that are not cancer.

If any of the signs of a severe problem occur, see your doctor right away. These signs include:

▶ Severe abdominal pain

▶ Sudden, unexplained chest pain or shortness of breath

▶ Severe headaches

▶ Blurred or double vision

▶ Swelling or severe pain in one leg

▶ Slurred speech

▶ Tingling or weakness on one side of your body

Special Concerns

Sexually Transmitted Diseases

The pill does not protect a woman from STDs. These include human immunodeficiency virus (HIV), the virus that causes acquired immunodeficiency syndrome (AIDS); gonorrhea; chlamydia; human papillomavirus, which can cause genital warts; syphilis; and genital herpes. Using latex (rubber) condoms can help protect both a woman and her partner against

> **Backup Methods of Contraception**
>
> You should use a backup method of contraception, such as a sponge, condom, or spermicide, when:
>
> ▶ Your period begins on a day other than Sunday just before you begin taking a Sunday-start pill. Use a backup method for the first 7 days that you take the pill.
>
> ▶ You have vomiting or diarrhea. Your body may not absorb the pill. Use a backup method for the rest of your cycle.
>
> ▶ You forget to take two or more pills. Call your doctor or nurse and ask what you should do.

Most studies have not found increased risks of breast and cervical cancer for women who take the pill. For almost all women, the benefits of the pill outweigh the possible risks.

STDs. Using both the pill and condoms will help protect a woman from pregnancy and STDs.

Future Pregnancies

The pill is a good choice for women who may want to get pregnant later. If you could get pregnant before you took the pill, you should be able to after stopping it. It may take you a little longer to get pregnant than if you had not been on the pill, though. If your periods were irregular before you went on the pill, they may be so again.

See also *Genetic Disorders, Maternal Serum Screening*

▶ BIRTH DEFECTS

Birth defects can affect a baby's health, ability to function, or the way he or she looks. Some birth defects can be prevented. Out of 100 newborns, 2 or 3 have major birth defects. If a defect occurs, often it can be treated with medication or surgery.

What Is a Birth Defect?

A birth defect is a mental or physical problem that results in an error in the way bone, brain, skin, or tissue developed. Many birth defects can be seen right away. Others appear later in life although they were present at birth. A disorder may or may not be inherited—that is, passed from parent to child through genes and chromosomes.

Causes of Birth Defects

Some birth defects are inherited. Just as a baby gets certain traits from his or her parents, he or she can get certain diseases or conditions. These types of birth defects are called genetic disorders. Your doctor may ask you questions to see if you are at risk for certain genetic disorders.

Birth defects also can result from being exposed to harmful things during pregnancy. Sometimes, a mix of inherited traits and exposure during pregnancy is the cause of a birth defect. In as many as 50% of cases, the reason for a birth defect isn't known.

Prevention

Some birth defects can't be prevented. But you can decrease your risk of some birth defects by taking care of yourself and not being exposed to certain substances.

If you are thinking about getting pregnant, visit your doctor first for counseling. Your doctor or a counselor can help you determine your risk of having a baby with birth defects. There may be things you can do before you are pregnant that can help:

▶ Take a folic acid supplement

▶ Get vaccines to protect against infection

▶ Don't drink alcohol or use illegal drugs

▶ Avoid being exposed to harmful substances

▶ Ask your doctor about any medications you are taking

If you miss your period or suspect you are pregnant, visit your doctor. Tell your doctor as much as you can about your diet. Be sure to list any prescription or other medications you are taking. Tell your doctor about any concerns you have about your workplace or hobbies.

Harmful Agents

A baby can be born with a birth defect because the mother was exposed to infections or harmful substances during pregnancy. Agents that can cause birth defects when a woman is exposed to them during pregnancy are called teratogens.

Teratogens can affect normal development. They can cause physical and mental defects. Their effect depends on the type of agent, amount of the mother's exposure, and when she was exposed during pregnancy. It also depends on the genetic makeup of the mother and fetus.

Harmful Agents During Pregnancy

▶ Alcohol

▶ Androgens and testosterone derivatives (eg, danazol)

▶ Angiotensin-converting enzyme (ACE) inhibitors (eg, enalapril, captopril)

▶ Coumarin derivatives (eg, warfarin)

▶ Carbamazepine

▶ Cocaine

▶ Diethylstilbestrol (DES)

▶ Folic acid antagonists (methotrexate and aminopterin)

▶ Infections

▶ Lead

▶ Lithium

▶ Organic mercury

▶ Phenytoin

▶ Radiation

▶ Streptomycin and kanamycin

▶ Tetracycline

▶ Thalidomide

▶ Trimethadione and paramethadione

▶ Valproic acid

▶ Vitamin A and its derivatives (eg, isotretinoin, etretinate, and retinoids)

Vaccines

Vaccines help prevent diseases caused by infection. Although some vaccines are safe to receive during pregnancy, it's best to have all needed immunizations before you become pregnant. Women should have the following immunizations:

3 months before pregnancy

▶ Measles–mumps–rubella vaccine (once if not immune)

1 month before pregnancy

▶ Varicella vaccine*

Safe during pregnancy

▶ Tetanus–diphtheria booster (every 10 years)

▶ Hepatitis A vaccine*

▶ Hepatitis B vaccine*

▶ Influenza vaccine (if will be in the second or third trimester of pregnancy during flu season)

▶ Pneumococcal vaccine*

*These immunizations are given as needed based on risk factors. If you don't know whether you need one, check with your health care provider.

Infections

Infections are caused by germs that invade the body and then spread. When you have an infection, you develop antibodies in your blood to fight it. Testing for antibodies can help you find out if you have been exposed to a disease. In most cases, once antibodies to the disease are made, you will not get the disease in the future. Some infections can harm the fetus if the mother is exposed to them during pregnancy.

Medications

Some medications can be harmful to the fetus. It may be safer for the mother to take these medications than to risk not taking them. If you are taking any medication, talk with your doctor about its use during pregnancy. The box on the previous page includes medications that are known to be harmful during pregnancy.

Hazards

Some people are exposed to substances that can harm a fetus. Heavy metals, such as mercury and lead, are harmful. Radiation, such as that used in high doses to treat cancer, also can harm a fetus. The smaller doses used for most tests and procedures usually are not harmful.

People are exposed to many substances at work or while doing a hobby. For many of these substances, the risks of exposure are not known. If you think you may be exposed to a harmful agent at work, talk to your employer about it. You may be able to move to another job for a while or take steps to protect your fetus. If you have questions about whether a substance could be harmful, ask your doctor.

Alcohol and Other Drugs

Alcohol use during pregnancy is a leading cause of mental retardation in children. It is not clear how much, if any, alcohol is safe to drink during pregnancy.

Some babies exposed to large amounts of alcohol during pregnancy develop fetal alcohol syndrome. This is a pattern of physical, mental, and behavioral problems. Babies with fetal alcohol syndrome are shorter, weigh less than normal, and do not catch up, even after special care. They also may have problems with joints and limbs, abnormal facial features, or heart defects.

Many illegal drugs are harmful to the fetus. Most have not been studied enough to know which birth defects might result. It is known that cocaine—a highly addictive drug that can be snorted, injected, or smoked—is harmful during pregnancy.

Multifactorial Disorders

Many disorders are thought to come from a mix of factors (multifactorial). The exact cause is unknown. Some of these disorders can be found during pregnancy. They often can be corrected with surgery. The most common disorders include:

- *Congenital heart disease*—a condition that occurs when a baby is born with a heart defect.

- *Neural tube defects*—a fetal birth defect that results from improper development of the brain, spinal cord, or their coverings (such as spina bifida and anencephaly).

- *Cleft lip*—a congenital defect in which a gap or space occurs in the lip.

- *Cleft palate*—a congenital defect in which a gap or space occurs in the roof of the mouth.

- *Clubfoot*—a misshaped foot twisted out of position from birth.

- *Pyloric stenosis*—a disorder in which the opening between the stomach and intestine is blocked.

- *Abdominal wall defect*—a disorder in which the muscle and skin that cover the wall of the abdomen is missing or the bowel sticks out through a hole in the abdominal wall.

Birth defects of the heart and circulatory system (arteries and veins) affect more infants than any other type of birth defect. About 1 in 115 infants born every year has a heart or circulatory defect.

Testing

Many babies with birth defects are born to couples with no risk factors. The risk of birth defects is higher when certain risk factors are present. Testing can be done during pregnancy to detect some defects. During prenatal care, some tests are offered to all women (screening tests) and some are offered only to those with known risk factors (diagnostic tests). These tests, along with genetic counseling, will tell patients about their risk of a problem.

Choosing whether to have a test done is up to you. Some couples choose not to be tested for birth defects. Other couples find that testing and counseling can help them decide whether to become pregnant or continue a pregnancy.

No test is perfect. Your fetus may have a birth defect even if a test result is negative (doesn't show a problem). If a test result is positive (suggests a problem), further tests may be needed after birth to fully assess the problem.

Screening Tests

Screening tests are done even when a woman has no symptoms or known risk factors. A positive screening test suggests that you may want to think about having diagnostic tests to check your baby's health. Screening tests include:

▶ Blood tests

▶ Ultrasound exam

The results of a screening test may require further testing.

Diagnostic Tests

Diagnostic tests most often are offered after a screening test raises concerns. If a woman is already at an increased risk of having a baby with a disorder, she may be offered a diagnostic test first. Diagnostic tests include:

▶ Amniocentesis

▶ Chorionic villus sampling

▶ Fetal blood sampling

▶ Detailed ultrasound exam

For more information on birth defects contact:

March of Dimes
1275 Mamaroneck Ave
White Plains, NY 10605
Phone: 888-MODIMES

▶ See also *Ectopic Pregnancy, Miscarriage, Molar Pregnancy, Placental Disorders*

The Next Steps

For some tests, it may take a while to receive the results. This time is stressful. You may need to make choices and think about your options. Your doctor can help you do this.

▶ BLEEDING DURING PREGNANCY

Vaginal bleeding in pregnancy has many causes. Some are serious and some are not. Some causes result in bleeding early in pregnancy. Others result in bleeding later. Slight bleeding often stops on its own. Sometimes, though, bleeding may pose a risk to you or your fetus. You should call your doctor or seek medical advice if bleeding occurs.

Early Pregnancy

Many women have vaginal spotting or bleeding in the first 12 weeks of pregnancy. If you are bleeding in early pregnancy, your doctor may do a pelvic exam. A blood test may be done to measure human chorionic gonadotropin (hCG). It is a substance produced during pregnancy. You may have more than one test because hCG levels increase as the pregnancy progresses.

Ultrasound may be used to find the cause of the bleeding. Sometimes the cause is not found.

If you have bleeding during pregnancy, you may need special care. You have a higher chance of going into labor too early (preterm labor) or having an infant who is born too small.

Miscarriage

Bleeding doesn't mean that miscarriage is certain, but it can occur. About half of the women who bleed do not have miscarriages. If there is a problem with the pregnancy, fetal death usually results in the passage of tissue, and the pregnancy ends.

Miscarriage can occur at any time during the first half of pregnancy. Most occur during the first 12 weeks. Miscarriage occurs in about 15–20% of pregnancies.

Signs of miscarriage include:

▶ Vaginal bleeding

▶ Cramping pain felt low in the stomach (often stronger than menstrual cramps)

▶ Tissue passing through the vagina

Many women who have vaginal bleeding have little or no cramping. Sometimes the bleeding stops and pregnancy goes on. At other times the bleeding and cramping may become stronger. Then miscarriage occurs.

If you think you have passed fetal tissue, take it to the doctor's office so it can be examined. If some tissue stays in the uterus, bleeding often continues. The tissue that remains may be removed by a procedure called dilation and curettage (D&C). The tissue also may be removed by a suctioning device. This is called suction curettage.

Most miscarriages cannot be prevented. They are often the body's way of dealing with a pregnancy that was not normal. There is no proof that exercise or sex causes miscarriage. Having a miscarriage doesn't always mean that you can't have more children or that something is wrong with your health. If you have two or three miscarriages in a row, your doctor may suggest that some tests be done to look for a cause.

The cause of some miscarriages is not known. Miscarriage is the body's way of dealing with a pregnancy that may not be growing as it should.

Ectopic Pregnancy

Another problem that may cause pain and bleeding in early pregnancy is ectopic pregnancy. If pregnancy occurs in a fallopian tube, it may burst. There may be internal bleeding also. Blood loss may cause weakness, fainting, or even shock. A ruptured ectopic pregnancy needs prompt treatment.

Women who have had an ectopic pregnancy have a 7–15% chance of it happening again. They should be sure to see their doctor regularly if they are trying to conceive so they can be more closely monitored for problems.

Ectopic pregnancies are much less common than miscarriages. They occur in about 1 in 60 pregnancies. Women are at a higher risk if they have had:

▶ An infection in the tubes (such as pelvic inflammatory disease)

▶ A previous ectopic pregnancy

▶ Previous tubal surgery

Molar Pregnancy

A rare cause of early bleeding is molar pregnancy. It is also called gestational trophoblastic disease (GTD) or simply a "mole." It is the growth of abnormal tissue instead of an embryo. A molar pregnancy may require treatment with suction curettage or with drugs.

Late Pregnancy

The causes of bleeding in the second half of pregnancy differ from those in early pregnancy. Common conditions that cause minor bleeding include an inflamed cervix or growths on the cervix.

Late bleeding may pose a threat to the health of the woman or the fetus. It may require treatment in a hospital. Heavy vaginal bleeding usually involves a problem with the placenta. The two most common causes of bleeding in late pregnancy are placental abruption and placenta previa. Preterm labor can also cause vaginal bleeding.

Placental Abruption

The placenta may detach from the uterine wall before or during labor. This may cause vaginal bleeding. Only 1% of pregnant women have this problem. It usually occurs during the last 12 weeks of pregnancy. Stomach pain often occurs, even if there is no obvious bleeding.

When the placenta becomes detached, the fetus may get less oxygen. This can pose a danger to the fetus.

Those at high risk include women who:

▶ Have already had children

▶ Are age 35 or older

▶ Have had abruption before

▶ Have sickle cell anemia

Placental abruption has been linked to:

▶ High blood pressure

▶ Blows or other injuries to the stomach

▶ Cocaine use

▶ Smoking

Placenta Previa

When the placenta lies low in the uterus, it may partly or completely cover the cervix. This is called placenta previa. It may cause vaginal bleeding. Placenta previa is serious and requires prompt care.

Placenta previa occurs in 1 woman in 200. It is more common in women who have had more than one child, who have had a cesarean birth or other surgery on the uterus, or who are carrying twins or triplets. Bleeding often occurs without pain. Women with placenta previa may need to have a cesarean delivery.

Preterm Labor

Late in pregnancy, vaginal bleeding may be a sign of labor. A plug that covers the opening of the uterus during pregnancy is passed just before or at the start of labor. A small amount of mucus and blood is passed from the cervix. This is called "bloody show." It is common. It is not a problem if it happens within a few weeks of your due date. If it happens earlier, you may be going into preterm labor. You should talk to your doctor right away.

Preterm labor can lead to preterm birth. About 1 of every 10 babies born in the United States is born preterm. The earlier the baby is born, the greater the risk of a problem.

Other signs of preterm labor include:

▶ Vaginal discharge
—Change in type (watery, mucus, or bloody)
—Increase in amount

▶ Pelvic or lower abdominal pressure

▶ Low, dull backache

▶ Stomach cramps, with or without diarrhea

▶ Regular contractions or uterine tightening

Taking Action

Call your doctor if you have bleeding in late pregnancy. You may need to be admitted to the hospital to find its cause. Ultrasound may be advised. You may have to stay in the hospital for a few weeks. A blood transfusion may be required.

Conditions that cause bleeding in late pregnancy pose a risk to both mother and fetus. They may be serious enough to require early delivery of the baby, sometimes by cesarean birth.

▶ See also *Rh Factor*

▶ BLOOD TYPES

Everyone's blood is one of four major types: O, A, B, or AB. These blood types are determined by special proteins, called antigens, which blood cells carry. Antigens are substances that produce an immune response and cause the production of an antibody. Type A has only A antigens. Type B has only B antigens. Type AB has both antigens. Type O has neither.

Blood types are passed on from parents to their children. Most of the time it makes no difference what type of blood a person has. But when someone needs a blood transfusion (the transfer of new blood into the body), the blood donor must have a blood type that matches (Table 12). If not, a bad reaction could occur. Knowing your blood type can be helpful, but if you donate blood or need to get blood, your blood type will be checked. Learn more about donating blood by taking the quiz in the box.

Table 12. Blood Type Compatibility

Your blood type	The blood type(s) your body will accept
A	A and O
B	B and O
AB	A, B, AB, and O
O	O

Check Your Blood I.Q.

The following "true-or-false" statements test what you know about blood. The correct answers are on the following page.

T F 1. Just one pint of your blood can help save the lives of several people.

T F 2. Giving blood is a simple process.

T F 3. Artificial or animal blood can now be used in place of human blood.

T F 4. Filling out the blood donor forms honestly and completely is a very important part of the process of giving blood.

T F 5. You cannot get AIDS or any other disease by donating blood.

T F 6. Most donors are paid money for their blood.

T F 7. It is best to wait until a friend needs blood before donating.

T F 8. Some people can donate blood for their own use.

T F 9. The nation's blood supply is safer now than ever before.

T F 10. Giving blood more than once a year will make you weak.

T F 11. The chance of getting AIDS from blood transfusions is very low.

(Continued)

Check Your Blood I.Q. *(continued)*

Answers to the Blood I.Q. Quiz

1. *True.* The pint of blood you donate often is split into several parts to meet the needs of different patients. For instance, your platelets may give a child with leukemia a chance to live, while your red cells may help an accident victim get well. Your single donation can help many patients.

2. *True.* Giving blood is simple and easy. You can expect to follow four steps: registration, medical history, donation, and snacks. The actual blood donation takes less than 10 minutes and is painless except for a little hurt at the very start. The entire process, from when you sign in to the time you leave, takes about 45 minutes.

3. *False.* There is no substitute for human blood. Human blood cannot be manufactured; animal blood cannot replace it. People are the only source of blood. Much of today's medical care depends on a steady supply of blood provided by healthy donors. The gift of blood is the gift of life.

4. *True.* It is very important to complete the blood donor forms honestly. People who should not donate need to be identified before the blood is taken. All information given by the donor is treated confidentially.

5. *True.* There is no risk of getting AIDS or any other disease from giving blood. A brand new needle is used for each blood donation. Once it is used, the needle is destroyed.

6. *False.* Volunteers now provide almost all of the nation's blood supply. This is a huge increase in volunteer donations over the past 10 years. People donate blood out of a sense of duty and community spirit, not to make money.

7. *False.* Many tests must be done before blood can be used. For emergencies, there is no time to collect, test, and process the blood from friends. Having enough blood on hand when we need it is possible only if healthy volunteers donate blood regularly.

8. *True.* For planned surgery, it is often possible to donate your own blood ahead of time so that it will be ready to use during your operation if needed. It also may be possible for a surgeon to collect blood from a wound during an operation and return it to the patient. Both are forms of autologous transfusion. It is the safest kind of transfusion, but most patients needing blood cannot provide their own. Therefore, there remains a great need for healthy people to donate blood for others. For information on whether you can donate blood for your own use, ask your doctor.

9. *True.* The risk of getting unsafe blood from a transfusion has been greatly reduced. Blood collection centers help to protect the blood supply by constantly improving safety measures. For instance, they:

   - Inform donors about high-risk behaviors and conditions that are not safe for blood donation;

   - Allow anyone to indicate confidentially that their blood should not be used for the general blood supply;

   - Take a medical history to check that donors are healthy;

   - Collect blood using sterile methods under medical supervision; and

   - Test blood for certain diseases.

10. *False.* Giving blood will not decrease your strength. Your body won't miss the one pint of blood you donate. Healthy donors can give blood as often as every eight weeks. If all blood donors gave at least twice a year, it would greatly strengthen the nation's blood supply.

11. *True.* The risk of getting AIDS from blood transfusion is extremely low. Necessary blood transfusions can save lives; therefore, the benefits are much greater than the risks. Ask your doctor for more information about blood transfusions.

National Blood Resources Education Program. Coordinated by the Office of Prevention, Education, and Control. "Check Your Blood I.Q.," Factsheet. Bethesda, Maryland: U.S. Department of Health and Human Services, Public Health Services, National Institutes of Health, National Heart, Lung, and Blood Institute, 1988; NIH Publication No. 88-2991

▶ See also *Hormone Replacement Therapy, Menopause, Osteoporosis*

Hormone replacement therapy can help slow bone loss in women. If a post-menopausal woman is at risk for osteoporosis and is not taking hormone replacement therapy, her doctor may suggest bone mineral density testing. A normal X-ray cannot detect early osteoporosis.

▶ BONE MINERAL DENSITY TEST

Bone mineral density tests are used to assess the strength and mass of your bones. These tests are helpful for people at risk for osteoporosis. Osteoporosis is a condition in which bones become so fragile that they break more easily. It is most common in older women who have gone through menopause. Men also may be affected. Osteoporosis can lead to serious hip and spine fractures that cause pain, disability, or death. When osteoporosis is detected, treatments that may help include exercise, changes in diet, hormone replacement therapy, and drugs that slow or prevent bone loss.

Bone mineral density tests measure bone mass in the heel, spine, hip, hand, or wrist. Measuring an area, such as your heel, can give your doctor a good sense of your bone density in other parts of your skeleton. The devices used for the tests vary, but all involve X-rays or beams from other energy sources. You may be asked to lie on your side or back for the X-ray, or you may sit and place your hand or foot into a cylinder. The tests can take as little as 1 minute or as much as 40 minutes.

Your doctor might give you a bone mineral density test if you have some of these risk factors:

▶ A small, thin frame

▶ Advanced age (65 years and older)

▶ A family history of osteoporosis

▶ Early or premature menopause (can occur when a woman's ovaries suddenly stop working or are removed before age 40)

▶ An eating disorder

▶ A diet low in calcium

▶ Use of certain medicines that can affect bone mass

▶ An inactive lifestyle

▶ Smoking

▶ Heavy drinking (more than two drinks a day)

A bone density test can help detect problems before a fracture occurs. It can also confirm a diagnosis of osteoporosis, help determine the rate of bone loss, and monitor whether treatment is working.

▶ BOWEL CONTROL PROBLEMS

▶ See also *Colorectal Cancer, Constipation, Diarrhea, Hemorrhoids, Irritable Bowel Syndrome*

Bowel control problems are very common. They affect at least 1 million people in the United States. Loss of normal control of the bowels is called fecal incontinence. This leads to leakage of solid or liquid stool (feces) or gas when you do not mean to or did not expect it. Bowel control problems occur up to eight times more often in women than in men. The problem also is more common in older people or in women who have just given birth. However, it can occur at any time in a person's life.

Many women are not comfortable talking about bowel control problems. If you talk with your doctor about it, he or she can help. Treatments are very effective.

Normal Bowel Control

Stool is the solid waste that is formed inside the large intestine. Stool is stored in the rectum—the last few inches of the large intestine. When the rectum is full, nerve messages send a signal to the brain that it is time to have a bowel movement. Stool leaves the body through the anus—the opening at the end of the rectum.

Normally, the rectum can store stool until a person can get to the bathroom. A pair of muscles—the anal sphincters—tighten (contract) around the anus and squeeze it closed. The anal sphincters prevent stool from leaving the rectum until you are ready to have a bowel movement.

Normal bowel function requires healthy muscles and nerves in the rectum. Problems in this area can lead to loss of bowel control. Common problems include:

▶ Injury to the anal muscles—this can cause stool or gas to leak from the rectum.

▶ Loss of feeling in the rectum—this can make it hard to tell when it is time to have a bowel movement.

▶ Inability of the rectum to stretch and store stool—this may make it hard to hold a bowel movement until you can get to the bathroom.

Questions Your Doctor May Ask You

If you know or think you have a bowel control problem, your doctor will ask you a series of questions. Your answers can help your doctor find the cause of your problem. Some questions you may be asked include:

▶ How often do you leak and when?

▶ Do you leak gas or liquid or solid stool?

▶ Do you use a pad?

▶ Do you have any other symptoms, such as diarrhea, abdominal pain, or an urgent need to move your bowels?

▶ Does the condition have an impact on your lifestyle?

▶ Do you take any prescription medications or over-the-counter products such as enemas, laxatives, or herbal remedies?

▶ Do you find certain foods make the condition better or worse?

▶ Have you had anal intercourse?

Causes of Bowel Control Problems

The most common cause of bowel control problems is childbirth. As the baby passes through the vagina, the muscles or the nerves near the rectum may be stretched or torn.

Some women have short-term loss of bowel control right after childbirth. It likely will improve within a few days. In other cases, bowel control problems do not show up until many years later. As a person ages, the anal muscles may weaken. A minor problem in a younger woman can become worse in later life.

Bowel control problems can be linked to:

▶ Stools that are too loose (diarrhea)

▶ Stools that are too hard (constipation)

▶ Certain medications

▶ Certain illnesses such as diabetes, multiple sclerosis, or a stroke

▶ Problems with the gastrointestinal system, such as inflammatory bowel disease, colitis, or cancer of the rectum

▶ Surgery or radiation therapy to the pelvic area

▶ Certain sexual practices, such as anal intercourse

Symptoms

A woman with a bowel control problem may have gas or leak liquid or solid stool. Other symptoms may include:

▶ A strong or urgent need to have a bowel movement

▶ Stool spotting on underwear or pads

▶ Diarrhea

▶ Constipation

The frequency of bowel movements among healthy people varies from three a day to three a week. But, you may fall outside both ends of this range and still be normal and healthy.

Problems may occur often or only once in a while. Your doctor may ask you to keep a symptom diary to describe your bowel movements and record when they occur. Be sure to write in your diary when you leak gas or stool.

In some women, fecal incontinence occurs with urinary incontinence (not being able to control urine). Some treatments for bowel problems also will help urine problems.

Diagnosis

To try to find the cause of your problem, your doctor will ask you questions about your medical history. Describe your symptoms clearly. Be open and honest. Tell your doctor about any prescription or over-the-counter products or herbal remedies you may be taking. This will help your doctor find the best treatment for you.

The doctor will examine your vagina, anus, and rectum. He or she will look for signs of problems, such as loss of normal nerve reflexes or muscle tone.

Tests may be needed to help find the cause:

▶ A scope may be used to see inside the rectum.

▶ Anorectal manometry may be used to test the strength of the anal muscles. A small sensing device is placed into the anus. The device records changes in pressure as you relax and tighten the anal muscles.

▶ A special test may be done to check if the nerves to the rectum and anus are working as they should.

▶ Ultrasound pictures from inside the rectum may be done to check the anal muscles.

Treatment

Once the cause of the problem is known, you and your doctor can discuss the best treatment for you. The type of treatment depends on the cause. Your doctor may suggest certain lifestyle changes to help you control your bowels. For instance, the problem may be treated by changes in your diet and simple home exercises to strengthen the anal muscles.

If a disease is causing the problem, proper treatment may improve symptoms. In some cases, surgery is needed to correct the problem.

Regular Bowel Habits

Having regular bowel movements helps to prevent diarrhea or constipation. If you have diarrhea, your doctor will help you find out if certain foods, such as dairy products, trigger loose stools. Not eating these foods may help prevent loss of control.

If you have constipation, your doctor may suggest more exercise. He or she also may suggest some changes in your diet, such as eating more fruits and vegetables and drinking plenty of water. You may need to slowly increase your fiber intake to 25–30 grams a day.

If a certain medication is causing diarrhea or constipation, your doctor may change your dosage or switch to another medication. In some cases, the doctor may prescribe a medication to prevent diarrhea or constipation and help you have regular bowel movements.

Muscle Exercises

Your doctor may suggest you do Kegel exercises. Kegel exercises strengthen the muscles that surround the openings of the rectum, urethra, and vagina. Your doctor can help ensure you are doing the exercises the correct way.

The average woman eats only half the amount of fiber she needs each day. To get your daily dose of fiber (25–30 grams), be sure to eat plenty of vegetables, fruits, and whole-grain cereals and breads. High-fiber foods are those that have at least 2 grams of fiber per serving.

Kegel Exercises

Kegel exercises tone your pelvic muscles. Just like doing sit-ups to flatten your abdomen, these exercises work only if the right muscles are used, the "squeeze" is held long enough, and enough repetitions are done. This is how they are done:

▶ Squeeze the muscles that you use to stop the flow of urine.

▶ Hold for up to 10 seconds, then release.

▶ Do this 10–20 times in a row at least 3 times a day.

After doing these exercises on a regular basis for at least 6 weeks, you should be able to better control the muscles that surround your rectum, urethra, and vagina.

Biofeedback Training

With biofeedback, you learn to contract the anal muscles with the help of a recording device. The device measures the strength of your contractions. A monitor shows you how well you are doing. Biofeedback can help you learn to tighten your anal muscles when you sense stool or gas in the rectum.

Surgery

In some cases, surgery may help correct loss of bowel control. Your doctor will help you decide if surgery may be an option for you and who may be the best person to perform it.

Skin Care

Leakage of stool can irritate the skin around the anus. Use a cleanser that is soap-free and doesn't irritate your skin. Make sure to keep the area dry. There are special creams, liquids, and powders for people with incontinence that can help protect skin.

If you develop a skin rash or irritation, tell your doctor. Also tell your doctor right away if you have any of the following signs:

▶ Warmth

▶ Swelling

▶ Redness

▶ Pain

▶ Severe itching of the skin

▶ See also *Breast Problems, Breast Self-Exam* in *"Women's Wellness,"* *Cancer, Mammography* in *"Women's Wellness"*

▶ BREAST CANCER

Breast cancer is the leading cause of death from cancer in women between ages 34 and 50. If breast cancer is found and treated early, most women can be cured. This is why routine breast self-exams, mammography, and checkups by your doctor are vital.

There are many factors that may affect the risk of breast cancer. Factors that may increase risk include the following:

▶ Breast cancer in the family, especially mother, daughter, or sister

▶ Older age

▶ No pregnancies or pregnancy later in life (after age 30)

▶ Early menarche—the time in a young woman's life when menstrual periods begin

▶ Late menopause

▶ Obesity, especially in older women

Factors that may decrease the risk of breast cancer include the following:

▶ Pregnancy early in life (before age 20)

▶ Ovaries removed before age 40

▶ Early menopause (before age 50)

Risk factors are not found in all women who have breast cancer. Many women have no risk factors.

Some women worry about a link between breast cancer and the hormones that are used in oral contraceptives (birth control pills) and hormone replacement therapy. It does not appear that oral contraceptives increase the risk of breast cancer in most women. It appears that the benefits of hormone replacement therapy, when taken in moderate doses to replace hormones no longer produced after menopause, greatly outweigh the risks.

Selective estrogen receptor modulators (SERMs) can reduce the risk of breast cancer in some women. Tamoxifen is a SERM that blocks the effects of the hormone estrogen in the body. It is used to treat breast cancer in women or men and may help prevent breast cancer in women who have a high risk.

▶ Breast Problems

Your breasts are always changing. They change during the menstrual cycle, pregnancy, breastfeeding, and menopause (when menstrual periods end). Along with these normal changes, problems can arise. Most of the problems are minor, but a few can be severe. One major problem, breast cancer, remains one of the leading causes of death in women.

Screening for Breast Problems

Screening tests are used to find a health problem early. If they are done on a routine basis, they may detect a problem even before symptoms appear. There are three screening exams for breast problems that can be done by you or your doctor:

1. Mammography

2. Breast self-exam

3. Doctor's exam of the breasts

For the best results, all three should be done. If any one of these tests shows a problem, even if the other results are normal, it should be checked out.

▶ See also *Biopsy, Breast Self-Exam* in *"Women's Wellness,"* *Fibrocystic Breast Changes, Mammography* in *"Women's Wellness"*

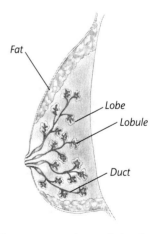

Breasts are made up of glands, fat, and fibrous tissue. Each breast has 15–20 sections, called lobes. Each lobe has many smaller lobules that end in tiny bulbs that can produce milk. These all are linked by thin tubes called ducts.

Mammography

Mammography is a way to detect changes in the breast tissue by X-ray. It is useful for finding tiny lumps before they can be felt. The test is more useful in women older than age 40. Older women's breasts are less dense, so it is easier to detect lumps. Also, breast cancer is more likely to occur as a woman gets older.

The Breast Self-Exam

Most breast lumps (about 90%) are found through breast self-exams. That is why it is key to examine your breasts every month. Self-exams help you learn the normal feel and shape of your breasts and make it easier to notice any changes. It is best done a few days after your menstrual period starts, when your breasts are not tender or swollen. It may help to do the exam at the same time each month.

The breast self-exam is one of the best things you can do for your health. Keep doing the self-exam even after you've reached menopause. Routine exams become even more important after menopause because the risk of breast cancer increases with age. About 85% of women with breast cancer are older than age 40.

If you have breast implants of any type, you still need to do a breast exam, especially around the chest wall. Ask your doctor how to examine your breasts.

Breast self-exams are vital for women with breast implants. A monthly exam can help to reveal not only any lumps, but also any problems that might be due to the implants

The Doctor's Exam of the Breasts

Your doctor will examine your breasts during your routine checkups. Most women should be examined at least once a year. A breast exam by a doctor takes only a short time. The breasts are first checked for any changes in size or shape. The doctor also looks for puckering, dimpling, or redness of the skin. You should tell your doctor if you have noted any discharge from your nipples. He or she then will check each breast for signs of a problem.

If you have noticed a change in your breasts at any time, you should have your doctor examine them. He or she will review when you started having symptoms and how long they have lasted. Then your doctor will look at your medical past to check for other factors that could point to an increased risk of breast cancer.

Breast Problems in Women

Benign Breast Problems

Most breast problems, especially in younger women, are benign growths (not cancer). This includes lumps (which may be felt in one exact place or throughout the breast), discharge from the nipple, and tender places.

The most common breast problem is a benign condition called fibrocystic changes. These changes include lumpy breasts and thickened (fibrous) and tender areas. They may include cysts. A cyst is a small sac filled with fluid. It can be almost any size, from a fraction of an inch to about the size of a golf ball. Cysts occur most often in women between the ages of 25 and 50.

Often cysts will vary in size, changing with the menstrual cycle. In many cases, they decrease in size after a menstrual period or at the time of menopause. Most women who have fibrocystic changes do not have a greater chance of getting breast cancer.

Symptoms of fibrocystic change include pain and tenderness, often in both breasts. It occurs most often in the upper, outer part of the breast and is most severe 7–14 days before a menstrual period. You should inform your doctor of any symptom of breast problems right away.

Some women are bothered by caffeine. Some find that cutting out or cutting down on drinks that contain caffeine (for instance, coffee, tea, and colas) may help.

Fibroadenomas are another common type of breast lump. They are solid, benign lumps that occur most often in young women.

Breast Cancer

Breast cancer is the leading cause of death from cancer in women between ages 34 and 50. If breast cancer is found and treated early, most women can be cured. This is why routine breast self-exams, mammography, and checkups by your doctor are vital.

Breast cancer is one of the most common types of cancer among women in the United States. Each year, more than 180,000 women in the United States learn they have breast cancer.

Tests

If you have found a lump in your breast or the results of your mammography are not normal, other tests may be used to help diagnose breast problems. Sometimes, these tests are done by your doctor. Other times, you will be referred elsewhere.

Ultrasound

In ultrasound, sound waves are used to create pictures of the inside of some body organs or tissues, like the breast. This painless method can tell your doctor about certain types of breast lumps. These pictures can show whether the lumps are solid or filled with fluid, such as with a cyst.

Aspiration

Sometimes, when the doctor suspects you have a cyst, fluid or tissue is withdrawn through a needle to be examined. This is called needle aspiration. If the fluid is clear and the cyst goes away, it is likely that no more tests will be needed. Aspiration also can be used to drain a cyst. Ultrasound may be used to help guide the needle. The sample may be sent to a lab to be checked.

Biopsy

The only way your doctor can find out the exact nature of a lump is to study cells from it or take a sample of it. To check a solid mass or a suspicious area, your doctor may advise a biopsy. A biopsy may be done if a lump feels abnormal, even if a mammogram is normal. In a needle biopsy, a small sample of cells from the mass is withdrawn through a needle.

Two other types of biopsy involve a surgical incision (cut). With a portion biopsy, part of the mass is removed. In an excisional biopsy, all of it is removed.

When a needle biopsy is needed, it often can be done in a doctor's office. A surgical incision biopsy most often is done in a surgical clinic or a hospital. After the breast lump is removed, cells taken from it are looked at under a microscope. Results will be negative (no cancer) or positive (cancer). Your doctor will discuss the results with you and determine what type of treatment is best.

Treatment

Benign breast disease often goes away on its own over time. If not, it often can be treated with medication or minor surgery.

The treatment of breast cancer depends a great deal on:

▶ The type of cells

▶ The size and location of the tumor

▶ How much the cancer may have spread

Most first treatments include either removal of the lump (lumpectomy) plus radiation treatment (with X-rays) or complete removal of the breast and the lymph nodes in the armpit (modified radical mastectomy). Treatment with either lumpectomy and radiation or modified radical mastectomy is now standard for breast cancer in early stages. Radical mastectomy, in which the chest muscles are also removed, is rarely done.

In some cases, cancer also may be treated with medication (chemotherapy) once the lump has been removed. For instance, some patients may receive chemotherapy after surgery and radiation are complete. This is especially true in younger women whose cancer has spread to the lymph nodes in the armpits.

More than one treatment may be needed. Chemotherapy may help prevent the cancer from coming back. Sometimes, hormones, such as tamoxifen, may be used.

Although more than 80% of all breast lumps biopsied are not cancerous, it is vital to check your breasts regularly.

Ductal carcinoma in situ is a precancerous condition in which breast cells show some changes, but they have not yet invaded nearby tissues. Most women with ductal carcinoma can be cured. Having a yearly mammogram greatly increases the chances of finding the cancer at this stage.

A woman who has all or part of a breast removed will begin a program of exercise to help her return to daily tasks. Some women consider having plastic surgery.

▸ BREASTFEEDING

Breastfeeding—or nursing—can be one of the most rewarding experiences in a mother's life. Many women find it a loving, convenient, and inexpensive way to feed their babies. You decide whether breastfeeding is right for you. Factors such as lifestyle, attitude, and personal choice are involved in making this decision. Feel free to discuss any questions with your doctor or nurse, your partner, or friends who have breastfed. You may also find it helpful to talk with a lactation specialist, who you can find through your doctor or hospital.

During pregnancy, your body prepares to breastfeed whether or not you plan to nurse your baby. By 6–8 weeks of pregnancy, your breasts may be much larger. This is because the fat layer of your breasts is getting thicker and the number of milk glands is increasing.

Your breasts will slowly increase in size and weight. They will feel firm and tender. You will also notice that the nipples and areolas (darker skin around your nipples) will become darker. Your nipples may stick out more now. Your areolas also grow larger.

Facts About Nursing

Breasts are glands. Inside are tiny sacs that contain cells that make milk. These sacs are clustered together into lobes. Each lobe has a single milk duct that carries milk to the nipple.

Around the fourth or fifth month of pregnancy, the nipple may sometimes drip a tiny amount of colostrum, a thick yellowish liquid. Colostrum is also the first milk secreted after the baby is born.

It contains proteins and other substances to nourish the newborn as well as antibodies to protect against infection. Within a few days after delivery, the colostrum will change to mature milk.

Commonly Asked Questions About Breastfeeding

Are my breasts too small for breastfeeding?
Breast size makes no difference. The amount of milk a woman's breasts make does not depend on their size or shape.

Do I have to prepare my nipples?
Nipple size and shape do not affect the ability to nurse. A woman who has flat or inverted (turned in) nipples is still able to breastfeed if her nipples can become erect. You can try wearing plastic breast shells during the last several weeks of pregnancy to make the nipples stick out. Once a woman starts to breastfeed, she can also wear the shells between feedings.

Will my breasts sag or be uncomfortable?
Breastfeeding itself will not make your breasts sag. Each pregnancy, however, does cause some change as the breasts enlarge and prepare to make milk. The increase in breast weight during pregnancy or nursing can stretch the ligaments that support the breasts. Wearing a good support bra will help you feel more comfortable.

What if I couldn't breastfeed last time?
If you have given birth before and had trouble breastfeeding, that does not mean you cannot breastfeed this baby.

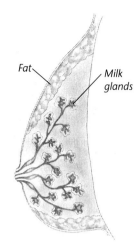

Normal breast

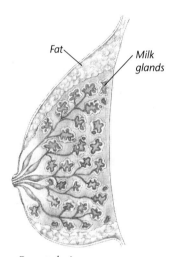

Breast during pregnancy

During pregnancy (bottom), the fat layer of your breasts thickens and the number of milk glands increases. This makes them larger than before pregnancy (top).

When your baby starts to nurse at the breast, the nerves in your nipples send a message to the brain. This causes hormones to be released that tell ducts in the breasts to "let down" milk from the nipple. This is known as the "let-down" reflex. It usually occurs about 2–3 minutes after the baby starts sucking. The let-down reflex may be slowed by embarrassment, pain, anxiety, or stress. It can be triggered by hearing the baby cry, looking at the baby, or even thinking about the baby.

Benefits of Breastfeeding

Mother's milk is the best food for any infant. It has the right amount of all the nutrients the baby needs, such as sugar, protein, vitamins, and fat. Breast milk contains antibodies that help protect the baby from disease. Infants who are breastfed tend to be less constipated and have fewer infections and allergies.

Breastfeeding is basically free and costs much less than bottle feeding. Breast milk does not have to be prepared and is ready at anytime, wherever you may be.

Breastfeeding is good for the mother, too. The baby's sucking releases hormones that contract the uterus, helping it return to its normal size more quickly. At first, this cramping may cause discomfort. If this occurs, you can take mild pain medication to relieve it.

How to Breastfeed

The very first feeding should occur as soon after birth as possible, when the baby is alert, awake, and ready to suck. During your pregnancy, tell your doctor or nurse that you would like to breastfeed your baby. When you're at the hospital, remind the delivery room staff that you want to start right away.

Before you start to breastfeed, take time to find a comfortable position. If you are in a good position, you should be able to hold the baby for some time without feeling cramped or stiff. Incorrect positioning of the baby while breastfeeding can cause nipple discomfort.

Most healthy, full-term babies will take to the breast. A baby is born with all the reflexes needed to nurse, such as the rooting reflex—a baby's natural instinct to look for the nipple and nurse. When you're ready to begin, stroke the baby's lower lip with your nipple. Your baby will respond by opening his or her mouth wide (like a yawn) and begin to suck. The most important skill for you to learn is getting the baby on the breast correctly. At first, this may require some practice for you and your baby.

It was once believed that newborns should be limited to just a few minutes of nursing at each breast per feeding. It is now known that this can result in poor emptying of the breast. This also means the baby may not get enough milk. As you breastfeed, the more milk the baby takes, the more milk the breast produces.

All babies set their own nursing patterns. Many newborns nurse for about 10–20 minutes on each breast. Your baby will let you know when he or she is finished by letting go of the breast. Most milk is taken in during the first 5–15 minutes of nursing.

You can tell your baby is hungry when he or she begins to nuzzle against your breast, make sucking motions, or cry. It's best to follow these signals, rather than the clock, to decide when to

Finding a Good Position

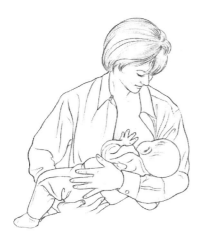

Cradle hold: Sit as straight as possible and cradle the baby in your arm—his or her stomach against yours. Let the baby's head rest in the bend of your elbow so that he or she is facing your breast.

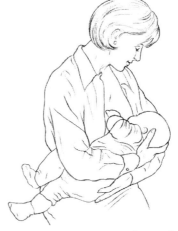

Cross-cradle hold: As in the cradle hold, place the baby's stomach against yours, but hold him or her with the opposite arm, so that your hand supports the back of the neck.

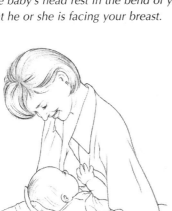

Football hold: In this hold you tuck the baby under your arm like a football. Sit the baby up at your side at about the level of your waist, so he or she is facing you. Support the baby's back with your upper arm, your hand holding his head at the level of your breast. This hold is good for nursing twins and for mothers who had cesarean births, since the baby doesn't lie across the stomach.

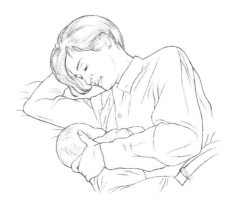

Side-lying position: Lie on your side with the baby lying facing you. Place your fingers beneath the breast and lift upward to make it easier for the baby to reach the nipple. This position is good for night feedings or if you're uncomfortable sitting up.

nurse. A baby who wants to nurse for a very long time (say, 30 minutes on each side) may be having trouble getting enough milk. If this happens every time you breastfeed, tell your doctor.

You may breastfeed as long as you like. Any breastfeeding is good for the baby. When your baby is about 6 months old, solid food can be used. Talk with your baby's doctor about a healthy diet for the baby.

When you decide to stop breastfeeding, it is easier and more comfortable to do it slowly. Every few days you can replace one feeding with a bottle. Take several weeks to change the breast-feedings to bottle feedings. Your milk supply will decrease at the same time.

Is My Baby Getting Enough?

After the first week, your baby should gain weight steadily. This is a sign that the baby is getting enough to eat. Your baby's diapers will also provide clues. During the first month your baby should wet at least six diapers and have at least two to three bowel movements each day. Most breastfed infants pass a stool after each feeding. It is normal for breastfed babies to have stools that are loose and yellowish in color.

Back to Work

If a woman returns to work soon after a baby is born, it does not have to be the end of breastfeeding. Many mothers continue to nurse their babies after returning to work. Some women express milk from their breasts by hand or by breast pump to be given to the baby later. This allows them to leave the milk with the baby's caregiver while they are away. Other women just breastfeed a few times a day and use a formula for the baby's other feedings.

Breast Pumps

Breast pumps can be rented or bought. An electric pump may be faster than a manual pump, although it is more costly. Electric pumps offer a range of benefits:

- Easy to use
- More closely mimic a nursing baby
- Work better at emptying the breast

If you buy a manual pump, avoid the kind with a rubber bulb at one end that looks like a bicycle horn. The milk can flow back into the bulb, which is hard to clean and can invite germs.

Breastfeeding rates decreased in the past half century as formula feeding gained popularity. In 1971, about 25% of mothers left the hospital breastfeeding. Recently these rates have been increasing. In 1998, almost 64% of women left the hospital breastfeeding.

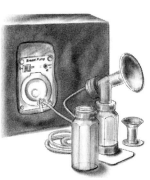

Breast pump

Storing Breast Milk

Breast milk can be stored in the refrigerator—in sterile glass or plastic containers—for up to 48 hours. Or it can be kept in a regular freezer for 2–4 weeks, or in a deep freeze for several months. Frozen milk can be thawed quickly under running water or gradually in the refrigerator. It should not be left out at room temperature for a long time, exposed to very hot water, or put in the microwave. Once milk has been thawed, it can be kept in the refrigerator for up to 24 hours.

Clean containers are a must when storing breast milk. Screw cap bottles, hard plastic cups with tight caps or special heavy nursery bags that can be used to feed your baby are all good choices. Do not use regular plastic storage bags or formula bottle bags for storing milk.

Your Diet

A nursing mother needs extra food to produce milk for her baby. Calcium is particularly important for nursing mothers. Calcium is found in milk and other dairy products such as yogurt and cheese. If you cannot digest milk products, you can buy calcium supplements. Your doctor may suggest you continue taking your prenatal vitamins while you breastfeed.

You will need about 500 more calories per day than you needed before you were pregnant. It's important to have a well-balanced diet, with a variety of foods. That means daily servings of fruits and vegetables; whole-grain or enriched breads and cereals; milk and milk products; and high-protein foods such as fish, beans, meat, and poultry. You should drink a lot of extra fluids, and you may notice that you're often thirsty. This is normal.

Nursing mothers must also avoid or limit their intake of certain substances. Some medications (prescription or over-the-counter) can pass through breast milk and harm your baby. Be sure to tell your doctor you are breastfeeding when seeking treatment for a health problem. Illegal drugs such as cocaine and marijuana are harmful and should not be used. You also shouldn't smoke cigarettes around your baby. Ask your doctor if it is all right to have an occasional drink.

Breastfeeding and Birth Control

Although you may not have menstrual periods while you are breastfeeding, you can become pregnant. Up until your baby is 6 months old, your chances of getting pregnant are lower than those of women who do not breastfeed. But, you shouldn't rely on breastfeeding as a form of birth control. If you don't want to become pregnant during this time, you will need to use birth control. Talk with your doctor about what form of birth control is right for you. What you were using before pregnancy might not be good now.

Breast Problems

There are a few minor problems that may occur while breast-feeding. Usually, these can be treated easily.

Engorgement and Blockage

When your milk comes in—usually about 2–5 days after delivery—the breasts may become full and tender ("engorged"). You may even have a low fever. If your fever persists longer than 6 hours, call your doctor.

Nursing often is the best treatment for engorgement. You can also help relieve any discomfort by massaging your breasts and taking a hot shower or applying hot packs to your breasts.

Warmth may not help severe engorgement. Applying cold packs to your breasts between feedings may help relieve your discomfort and reduce swelling.

Sore Nipples

Most new mothers have some nipple tenderness in the first few weeks of nursing. To avoid or reduce the soreness:

- Learn proper breastfeeding technique and change positions while nursing.
- Make sure that both the areola and the nipple are placed in the baby's mouth.
- Avoid excessive washing of nipples.
- Keep nipples dry and exposed to air between feedings.
- Don't use plastic bra liners or irritating soaps or perfumed creams.
- Nurse from the less tender breast first.

Blocked Ducts

If a milk duct becomes clogged, you may develop a tender lump in the breast. Call your doctor if breast soreness doesn't go away in a few days or if you develop a fever. In the meantime, try following these methods to open the duct:

- Nurse longer and more often.
- Nurse from the breast with the blocked duct first.
- Pump out or express by hand any milk that remains after each feeding.
- Take warm showers and hot soaks before feeding.
- Massage the affected area.

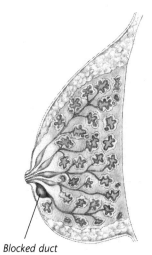

Blocked duct

If a duct gets clogged with unused milk, a hard, tender knot will form in your breast.

Mastitis

If your breast is swollen, painful, and feels hot, you may have a breast infection called mastitis. Other symptoms include fever and a general sense of feeling ill. If you have these symptoms, contact your doctor immediately.

Mothers with Special Problems

Chronic Illnesses

Most mothers who have a chronic illness can still breastfeed. However, you may need to make certain changes. For instance, nursing mothers who have diabetes will need to eat a little more than usual. Those who take insulin may need to change the amount. If you have a chronic illness, consult your doctor for advice about breastfeeding.

An exception to this is mothers who have the human immunodeficiency virus infection (HIV). Because breast milk can carry HIV and pass the infection to the baby, these women should not breastfeed.

Breast Surgery

Women who have had breast surgery can often nurse without a problem. The removal of cysts and other benign lumps rarely affects a woman's future ability to breastfeed.

Silicone implants to enlarge the breasts can rupture and cause scarring that interferes with milk production and release. If you are concerned that silicone from a ruptured implant may appear in your breast milk, the milk can be examined in a laboratory. Breastfeeding is safe as long as the silicone implant is intact.

Whether to breastfeed is one of many decisions you will make about the care of your new baby. If you are well-informed, you will be better able to make the choice that is right for you. Talk with your doctor, nurse, or partner. Talk to other women with children. You may also find it helpful to contact local groups that provide information about breastfeeding, such as La Leche League.

For more information on breastfeeding, contact:

La Leche League
1400 N Meacham Rd
Schaumburg, IL 60173-4018
Phone: 847-519-7730
Web Address: www. laleche
league.org

▶ BREECH PRESENTATION

Most babies move into the normal, head-down position in the mother's uterus a few weeks before birth. But if this doesn't happen, the baby's buttocks, or buttocks and feet, will be in place to come out first during birth. This is called breech presentation, and it occurs in about 3 out of every 100 full-term births.

Although most breech babies are born healthy, they do have a higher risk for certain problems than babies in the normal position do. Your doctor may advise cesarean birth (when the baby is born through a surgical cut in the mother's abdomen and uterus) instead of vaginal delivery, or try to turn the baby into the proper position. Problems can arise during and after delivery, though, and are often not related to how the baby is born.

If your baby is in the breech presentation near the end of your pregnancy, you should be aware of what this entails. You can then understand and take a more active part in your doctor's plan for the best way to manage your labor and delivery.

Breech Positions

By 3–4 weeks before a mother's due date, most babies move into the head-down, or vertex, presentation. Most of the babies who don't turn by then will be in a breech presentation when it's time for delivery. The baby will appear to be sitting in the uterus, with its head up and its buttocks, feet, or both down at the entrance of the birth canal, ready to emerge first. There are three main positions of a baby that is in a breech presentation:

1. *Frank breech*—The baby's buttocks are at the top of the birth canal, and the legs extend straight up in front of the body, with the feet up near the head

2. *Complete breech*—The buttocks are down, with the legs folded at the knees and the feet near the buttocks

3. *Footling breech*—One or both of the baby's feet are pointing down

Diagnosis

One way for the doctor to tell what position the baby is in is to carefully feel the baby through the mother's abdomen and uterus. Placing his or her hands at certain points on your lower abdomen, the doctor can try to make out the general position of the baby's head, back, and buttocks.

If the doctor thinks that the baby may be in a breech presentation, ultrasound may be used to confirm the diagnosis. In this procedure, a microphone-like device is moved across the mother's abdomen, producing sound waves that create an image of the baby that can be seen on a TV-type screen.

Your doctor may also order special X-rays. This is one of the few times X-rays are used during pregnancy. These X-rays can not only confirm the baby's position, they can also be used to measure the pelvis to help the doctor decide whether vaginal delivery of a breech baby may be attempted.

Because your baby may keep moving around up until the end of pregnancy, your doctor may not be able to tell for sure whether your baby has settled into a breech presentation until labor has begun.

Breech Positions

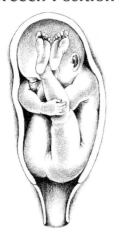

Frank breech

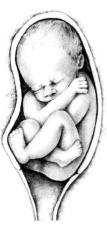

Complete breech

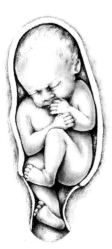

Footling breech

Related Factors

The causes of breech presentation are not completely clear. It is known, though, that breech presentation is more common when other factors are present:

- The mother has had more than one pregnancy

- There is more than one fetus (twins or more) in the uterus

- The uterus holds too much or too little amniotic fluid (the liquid that surrounds the baby inside the uterus)

- The uterus is not normal in shape or has abnormal growths, such as fibroids

- The placenta (the tissue inside the uterus that is connected to the baby) partly or fully covers the opening of the uterus—a condition known as placenta previa

Premature babies (those born 3 or more weeks early and weighing less than 5½ pounds) are also more likely to be breech. Early in pregnancy, the shape of the uterus and the shape of the baby's head and body are such that breech presentation is more common. Birth defects are also more common in breech babies and may account for why these babies have not turned into the proper position before delivery.

Can a Breech Presentation Be Changed?

In some cases, the baby's position can be changed by a method called external version. This technique consists of manually moving or turning the baby into the head-down position. It does not involve surgery. The doctor places his or her hands at certain key points on your lower abdomen and then gently tries to push the baby into the head-down position, much as if the baby were doing a slow-motion somersault inside the uterus. Often a drug is given to the mother first to relax her uterus.

Version may be tried if there are no problems that make this technique risky and if certain conditions are present. Also, several safeguards are used in case problems arise. An ultrasound exam done in advance allows the doctor to better examine the condition and position of the baby, the location of the placenta, and the amount of amniotic fluid in the uterus. Before, during, and after version, your baby's heartbeat will be checked closely. If any problems arise, efforts to turn the baby will be stopped right away. Most attempts at version succeed, but some babies will shift back into a breech presentation. If that happens, your doctor may try again, but version tends to be harder to perform as the time for delivery grows closer.

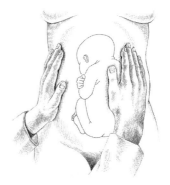

In a procedure called external version, the doctor manually shifts a baby from the breech position into the vertex position.

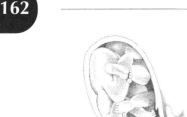

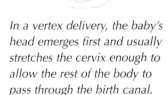

In a vertex delivery, the baby's head emerges first and usually stretches the cervix enough to allow the rest of the body to pass through the birth canal.

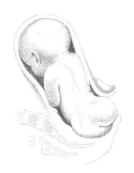

In a breech birth, where the lower body is delivered first, there may be less room for the head to be guided out.

Vaginal Delivery: Risks and Complications

At the time of birth, the baby's head is the largest part of its body, as well as the firmest. When the baby is in the normal, head-down position, the largest part of the body is born first, and the rest can usually be guided out through the birth canal. In a breech birth, though, the baby's head is the last part to emerge, and it may be harder to ease it through the birth canal. Sometimes special instruments called forceps are used to help guide the baby's head out.

Breech presentation can pose especially serious risks for premature babies. Because they are so small and fragile, and because the head is relatively larger, their bodies don't stretch the cervix as wide as full-term babies do during birth. This means that there may be less room for the head to emerge. For this and other reasons, breech babies who are premature are often delivered by cesarean birth.

Another problem is called cord prolapse. This means that the umbilical cord—the cordlike structure that connects the baby to the placenta and supplies nourishment—slides to the bottom of the uterus, towards the birth canal, during delivery. As the baby's buttocks and legs move down into the birth canal, the cord can get squeezed, slowing the baby's supply of oxygen and blood. A baby in any breech presentation is harder to deliver than a baby in the normal, head-down position. But vaginal delivery is usually easier for babies in the frank breech presentation (when the legs extend straight up) than for babies in other breech presentations.

Vaginal Versus Cesarean Delivery

It would be nice to know well in advance if your breech baby will be born vaginally or by cesarean birth. Your doctor may not be able to decide this, though, until you are in labor. Some of the factors that need to be present for vaginal birth to be tried are as follows:

▶ The baby is full-term (not premature) and in the frank breech presentation.

▶ Your doctor estimates that the baby is not too big or your pelvis too narrow for the baby to pass safely through the birth canal.

▶ You are in a setting where anesthesia is available and a cesarean delivery can be performed on short notice.

▶ The baby does not show signs of distress as its heart rate is closely checked.

▶ The progress of your labor is smooth and steady—the cervix is widening and the baby is moving down.

> You are willing and able to help during labor, especially during delivery, when you'll need to keep pushing down.

Even if these conditions apply, though, it's important to realize that vaginal delivery of a breech baby still carries more risk than vaginal delivery of a baby in the normal position.

If a vaginal delivery is tried, electronic fetal monitoring will be used to monitor your baby's heartbeat throughout labor. Electronic sensors will be placed either on your abdomen, on the fetus, or on both. If there are any signs that the baby may be in trouble, your doctor may consider cesarean delivery.

In many cases, cesarean deliver may be safer than vaginal delivery of a breech baby. Still, this is a major operation that carries its own risks for both mother and baby. These risks include infection, excessive bleeding, and complications from the anesthesia. Breech babies are harder to deliver, even by cesarean birth. You should also keep in mind that cesarean delivery won't solve all of the problems, such as prematurity and birth defects, that are linked to breech presentation.

▶ CANCER

Each year, several thousand women die from cancer. Many of these lives could be saved if the cancer is detected and treated early. In some cases, cancer can be prevented by avoiding possible causes. A healthy lifestyle can go a long way toward preventing cancer. Prevention and early detection—which gives a better chance for cure—are the key.

> See also *Breast Cancer, Cervical Cancer, Colorectal Cancer, Lung Cancer, Ovarian Cancer, Skin Cancer, Uterine Cancer, Vaginal Cancer, Vulvar Cancer*

What Is Cancer?

Normally, healthy cells that make up the body's tissues grow, divide, and replace themselves on a regular basis. This keeps the body in good repair. Sometimes, however, certain cells develop abnormally and begin to grow out of control. Too much tissue is made, and growths or tumors begin to form. Tumors can be benign (not cancer) or malignant (cancer).

Malignant tumors can invade and destroy nearby healthy tissues and organs. Cancer cells can also spread (or metastasize) to other parts of the body and form new tumors.

It is important for your doctor to find out as early as possible if a tumor is benign or malignant. As soon as a malignant tumor is found, your doctor can begin treatment to control the disease. Cancer is much easier to treat and cure if it has not spread to other parts of the body.

Screening

A screening test looks for possible signs of disease in people who do not have symptoms. For some types of cancer, use of screening tests has proven to be an effective way to find cancer. Regular physical exams and talking with your doctor can serve as effective screening methods, too. Screening tests include:

▶ *Colon and rectal exam*—A rectal exam may be performed at the time of a pelvic exam. Beginning at age 50, stools should be tested for blood every year and a sigmoidoscopy should be performed every 3–5 years.

▶ *Mammography*—Women aged 40–49 should have a mammogram every 1–2 years. Women aged 50 or older should have one done every year.

▶ *Pap test*—All women who have been sexually active or who have reached age 18 should have a Pap test and a pelvic exam every year. After three or more normal tests in a row, the doctor may decide to perform the Pap test less frequently.

Warning Signs of Cancer

It is important to notice signs of cancer as early as possible. The American Cancer Society gives seven warning signs for cancer:

1. Change in bowel or bladder habits

2. Sore that does not heal

3. Unusual bleeding or discharge

4. Thickening or lump in the breast or elsewhere

5. Indigestion or difficulty in swallowing

6. Obvious change in a wart or mole

7. Nagging cough or hoarseness

None of these warning signs is a sure sign of cancer, but they are clues that something could be wrong. If you have one of

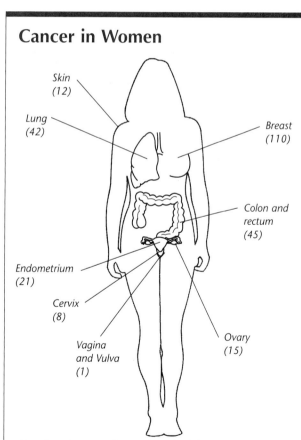

Cancer in Women

Skin (12)

Lung (42)

Breast (110)

Colon and rectum (45)

Endometrium (21)

Cervix (8)

Vagina and Vulva (1)

Ovary (15)

Numbers in parentheses show incidence rates—number of people per 100,000 who develop cancer of this site (from the American Cancer Society and the National Cancer Institute).

these warning signs, see your doctor. Pain is seldom an early sign of cancer. Don't wait for pain if other symptoms don't go away.

Prevention

Many cancers are linked to your lifestyle. By being aware of things that can cause cancer, you can make changes that will help prevent it:

▶ Limit your intake of fat

▶ Eat high-fiber foods

▶ Don't smoke

▶ Get regular exercise

▶ Use sun block when you go outside

▶ Pay attention to your body

If you or any of your family members have had cancer, this may increase your risk. Be sure to ask other family members details about cancer. This is an important part of your history for you and your children.

▶ CERVICAL CANCER

▶ See also *Cancer, Cervical Disorders, Pap Test* in *"Women's Wellness"*

Over time, diseases of the cervix can develop into cancer. Cancer that has spread beneath the top layer of the cervix or to other parts of the body is called invasive. In the United States, it accounts for nearly 2.4% of all cancers in women. There are about 12,800 new cases of invasive cervical cancer and 4,800 deaths from this disease each year.

Cancer results when cells grow out of control and can no longer perform their normal functions. Only malignant (cancerous) cells spread. They travel through the body in blood and lymphatic fluid (a yellow liquid derived from tissue fluids found throughout the body). They also spread directly through the tissue next to the cervix. If cancerous cells are found before they have spread, treatment is more likely to succeed.

Because cervical cancer usually develops after abnormal cells have been present for several years, it tends to affect older women. Although invasive cervical cancer can occur at any age, it is most common in women between the ages of 35 and 50. Risk factors for cervical cancer are similar to those for dysplasia. You may be at risk if you:

▶ Have or have had genital warts

▶ Have more than one sexual partner (or male partners who have more than one partner)

▶ First had sex at a young age

▶ Smoke

Chemoradiation

Recent studies have shown that women with invasive cervical cancer have better rates of survival when they receive low-dose chemotherapy that includes the drug cisplatin and 5-fluorouracil (5-FU) along with radiation therapy. Chemotherapy helps radiation work more effectively. This type of therapy has fewer and less severe side effects than traditional chemotherapy. Until now, surgery or radiation alone has been considered standard treatment for this form of cancer.

These women should be alert for symptoms of cancer and get regular checkups.

Often there may be no symptoms of cervical cancer. When symptoms do occur, the first sign may be abnormal bleeding, spotting, or discharge from the vagina. With advanced cancer, there may be pain, problems urinating, and swelling in the legs. These symptoms do not necessarily mean that you have cancer. If you have any of them, however, you should see your doctor without delay.

If tests show that a woman has cancer, her doctor will determine the size of the tumor and the extent (if any) to which it has spread. This is referred to as its stage. Stages range from I to IV. Stage I is the earliest stage and is treated most easily. Stage IV is the most advanced stage and means that cancer has spread to other parts of the body.

Earlier stages of cancer have a greater chance of successful treatment. The cure rate for Stage I cancer is 85–90%. The chance of a cure decreases to as low as 5–10% for Stage IV cancer.

Your doctor may consult with, or refer you to, a gynecologic oncologist—a specialist in treating cancer in women—or a radiation oncologist—a specialist in using radiation to treat cancer. They will work together in a team approach to choose treatment that meets your needs. Your doctors will keep in mind not only the extent of the disease, but also your age, your general health, and other personal factors. There is no one approach that is right for all women. Your doctors will discuss with you what they feel is best. Together you can decide on a course of treatment.

Any woman who has had cervical cancer is at risk for having the cancer return. A new cancer may also begin growing somewhere else in the body. For this reason, regular checkups are important, even after successful treatment. Your doctor will work with you to set up the needed follow-up visits.

▶ See also *Barrier Methods of Contraception, Diaphragm*

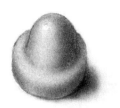

Cervical cap

▶ CERVICAL CAP

A cervical cap is a thimble-shaped rubber or plastic dome. It is smaller than a diaphragm and fits tightly over the cervix. Like the diaphragm, it is obtained with a doctor's prescription and is always used with a spermicide. The combination of cervical cap and spermicide acts as both a physical and a chemical barrier. As with the diaphragm, oil-based lubricants such as petroleum jelly should not be used.

One advantage to the cervical cap is that it can remain in place longer than the diaphragm—up to 36 hours. Other advantages are that less spermicide is used with the cervical cap, and you do not need to add more spermicide before each act of intercourse. For some women, however, it may be harder to learn how to place the cap correctly. Also, it must not be worn during the menstrual period.

Cervical caps come in different sizes. You will need to be examined and fitted to find the right size for you. Then, you will be taught how to insert and remove it. Inserting a cervical cap is a lot like inserting a diaphragm. Spermicide is placed inside the cap, which is then squeezed between your fingers and inserted into the vagina. The cap is then pressed onto the cervix until the cervix is completely covered. Before each act of intercourse, the cervix should be checked to make sure it is covered by pressing on the dome of the cap with your finger. After sex, the cap should be left in place for at least 6 hours, but not longer than 36 hours. Cervical caps sometimes cause irritation or odor in the vagina, especially if left in too long.

▶ CERVICAL DISORDERS

▶ See also *Biopsy, Cervical Cancer, Colposcopy, Cryotherapy, Pap Test* in *"Women's Wellness"*

Disorders of the cervix are common. They range from fairly mild problems, such as infection and inflammation, to more serious ones, such as cancer. Many types of cervical disorders can develop into cancer or can make it more likely for a woman to develop cancer. The Pap test is the best way to find changes early—before they become serious.

The Cervix

The cervix is the lower, narrow end of the uterus. It opens into the vagina. The cervix is covered by a thin layer of tissue (like the skin inside your mouth). As with all cells, the cells that make up this tissue grow all the time. During this growth, the cells at the bottom layer slowly move to the surface of the cervix. When these cells reach the surface, they are shed. During this process, some cells can become abnormal.

Types of Cervical Disorders

Cervicitis

Cervicitis is an inflammation of the cervix that may or may not cause symptoms. It is common in women during their childbearing years. Causes of cervicitis include:

▶ Infections, especially with an organism that can be passed through sex
   —Bacteria such as those that cause gonorrheal or chlamydial infections

—Viruses such as the ones that cause herpes or genital warts

—Trichomonas, an organism that can cause vaginal infection

▶ Irritation from a foreign body

—Intrauterine device (IUD)

—Forgotten tampon

—Pessary (a device placed in the vagina to hold sagging pelvic organs in place)

In some cases, the cause of cervicitis cannot be found.

When symptoms of cervicitis do occur, they include a vaginal discharge that may have a bad odor. A tender feeling or pain in the pelvic region may occur. Slight bleeding between periods or after sex also may occur.

Polyps

Polyps are benign (not cancer) growths or tumors that often appear on the cervix. Polyps vary in size and may cause vaginal bleeding. They often can be found during a pelvic exam or with colposcopy. In most cases, polyps can be removed in the office. Anesthesia is not needed in most cases.

Genital Warts

Human papillomavirus (HPV) cannot be cured, but it can be treated. Although warts may go away on their own, the virus can remain.

Genital warts, also called condyloma, are spreading growths that are caused by some types of human papillomavirus (HPV). The virus is most often passed during sex. Some types of HPV are linked to cancer. Women who have had genital warts should have regular checkups that include Pap tests.

Dysplasia

Dysplasia is a type of cervical disorder that occurs when there is a change in the cells on the surface of the cervix. Normal, benign cells are replaced by abnormal cells. It is not cancer. The abnormal cells can turn into cancer cells if they are not treated, though.

Dysplasia often can be diagnosed and treated with success. Dysplasia is found in women of all ages, but it is more common in young women and teens. The box lists risk factors for dysplasia.

The range of dysplasia includes mild, moderate, and severe dysplasia and carcinoma in situ (CIS). CIS is not a true form of cancer. It is the most likely to develop into cancer if not treated, though.

Other terms may be used to report cervical changes on a Pap test. These include squamous intraepithelial lesion (SIL) and cervical intraepithelial neoplasia (CIN). SIL is a term that is used to refer to Pap test results only. The terms dysplasia and CIN can be used when your doctor refers to the result of a Pap test or a biopsy.

There are three grades of CIN:

1. CIN 1 includes mild dysplasia

2. CIN 2 includes moderate dysplasia

3. CIN 3 includes severe dysplasia and CIS

SIL may be low-grade or high-grade. Low-grade SIL includes mild dysplasia (CIN 1) and changes linked to HPV. High-grade SIL includes moderate and severe dysplasia (CIN 2 and 3) and CIS.

> **Risk Factors for Dysplasia and Cervical Cancer**
>
> You may be at risk for dysplasia or cervical cancer if you:
>
> ▶ Have or have had genital warts
>
> ▶ Have more than one sexual partner (or male partners who have more than one partner)
>
> ▶ First had sex at a young age
>
> ▶ Smoke

Invasive Cervical Cancer

The cancer is invasive when it moves into deeper tissue layers or spreads to other organs. Risk factors for cervical cancer are much like those for dysplasia. Women at special risk should be alert for symptoms of cancer and get regular checkups.

Diagnosis of Cervical Disorders

The key to successful treatment of disorders of the cervix is finding them early. Some disorders, such as dysplasia, may precede cancer by some years. The earlier the stage when they are found, the more likely it is that treatment will succeed. Finding problems early depends on getting regular exams. This includes a pelvic exam and Pap test. Some of the methods used to diagnose cervical disorders also may be used to treat them at the same time.

The Pap Test

For most women, a Pap test done each year, starting at age 18 or sooner if they are sexually active, is the best screening method for finding changes in the cervix. The Pap test is a screening test. It is used to detect problems when there is no sign of disease. The Pap test can detect changes in the cells of the cervix at an early stage. Some types of genital warts, dysplasia, cervicitis, and cancer of the cervix can be detected by the Pap test.

If the Pap test shows abnormal cells, your doctor will explain the results to you. You may be advised to have further tests to diagnose the problem.

Colposcopy

Colposcopy is the next test performed if a Pap test is abnormal. It is a way of looking at the cervix through a special magnifying instrument called a colposcope. It lets your doctor detect problems of the cervix that cannot be seen with the eye alone.

Colposcopy often is used to diagnose cervical cancer, dysplasia, genital warts on the cervix, cervicitis, and benign growths such as polyps.

Biopsy

When abnormalities of the cervix are seen by colposcopy, a biopsy may be done to diagnose the problem. In this procedure, small pieces of cervical tissue are removed for study. A biopsy most often can be done in the doctor's office or clinic. You may have some mild cramping or feel a pinch. The results of a biopsy may not be ready for several days.

Methods of Treatment

Treatment of cervical disorders depends on the type of problem. For instance, mild cervicitis may be treated with medicines such as antibiotics.

Minor surgery may be used to treat genital warts, dysplasia, and early stages of cancer. With surgery, the affected tissue is removed. A new layer of normal cells then grows over the affected area.

Types of surgery that may be performed include:

▶ *Cryotherapy:* A probe coated with freezing agents is applied to the cervix.

▶ *Electrosurgery:* Heat destroys the affected cervical tissue.

▶ *Loop electrosurgical excision procedure (LEEP):* Abnormal growths are removed using a thin wire loop and electrical energy.

▶ *Laser treatment:* A high-intensity beam of light is used to remove abnormal tissue or growths.

▶ *Conization:* A cone-shaped wedge of tissue is removed from the cervix.

Most cases of dysplasia, including CIS, may be treated with one of these methods. Sometimes a hysterectomy (removal of the uterus) may be done to treat CIS if the patient no longer wants to have children or if there are other gynecologic problems. Women who wish to remain able to have children should discuss their options with their doctor.

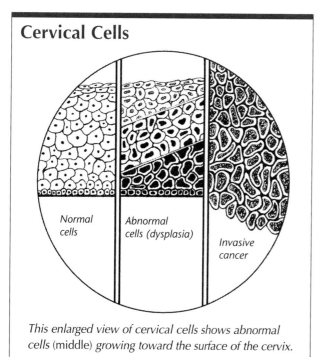

Cervical Cells

Normal cells

Abnormal cells (dysplasia)

Invasive cancer

This enlarged view of cervical cells shows abnormal cells (middle) growing toward the surface of the cervix.

▶ CESAREAN BIRTH

▶ See also *Labor, Vaginal Birth After Cesarean Delivery*

The natural way for babies to be born is through the mother's vagina. Sometimes, however, it isn't possible. In such cases, cesarean birth may be performed. Cesarean birth is the birth of a baby through surgical incisions (cuts) made in the abdomen and uterus.

Reasons for a Cesarean Birth

There are many reasons why a cesarean birth may be the best way to deliver your baby. It may be the safest way for both you and your baby. A cesarean delivery may be planned in advance when certain conditions are known. Sometimes, the decision is made during labor if problems arise.

If you have a cesarean delivery, it may take a while for you to feel like yourself again. You are recovering not only from labor and delivery but also from major surgery.

A Large Baby

Sometimes a baby does not fit through the mother's vagina and the surrounding bones (pelvis). This is known as cephalopelvic disproportion. Women with certain medical conditions, such as diabetes, tend to have larger babies. Larger babies are also born today because of better nutrition.

Multiple Pregnancy

Women having two or more babies may need cesarean birth. Although many women having twins are able to have vaginal birth, the risk increases with the number of babies.

Failure of Labor to Progress

About one third of cesarean births are done because labor stops. Contractions may not open the cervix enough for the baby to move through the vagina. Sometimes, the doctor can speed up labor with medication if labor is moving slowly. Labor may progress slowly before it is clear that it has stopped. Because of this, doctors may watch for several hours before deciding a cesarean birth is needed.

Concern for the Baby

The baby could be having trouble during labor and may need to be delivered by cesarean birth. One reason may be that the umbilical cord is pinched or compressed or not enough blood is flowing to the baby from the placenta. Fetal monitoring may detect an abnormal heart rate. If this problem cannot be corrected, a cesarean delivery may become necessary.

Problems with the Placenta

Placenta previa is a condition in which the placenta is below the baby and covers part or all of the cervix. This will block the baby's exit from the uterus. Another problem that may arise is abruptio placenta. This is when the placenta separates before the baby is born and cuts off the flow of oxygen to the baby. Both of these conditions can cause heavy bleeding.

Medical Conditions

Women with certain medical conditions are more likely to have a cesarean birth. For example, if a woman has diabetes or high blood pressure, there may be times when a vaginal birth cannot happen safely. If the mother has an active herpes infection on her genitals, a cesarean delivery may be needed.

Previous Cesarean Birth

Sometimes, having had a cesarean birth before can play a part in whether you will need to have one again. Many women, however, who have had a cesarean birth before can try to deliver vaginally. There is some risk of rupture of the uterus with vaginal birth after cesarean delivery, and it is not a good option for some women.

In deciding if you can have a vaginal birth after having a cesarean, one factor is the type of incision in the uterus—not in the skin—used in your previous cesarean. Sometimes, a vertical incision is used and you may have a higher risk of the scar tearing or rupturing.

The Procedure

In most hospitals, your birth partner may stay with you in the operating room for the cesarean birth. This depends on whether you are awake for the surgery and how urgent the surgery is. In some cases, cesarean birth may be done as an emergency and there isn't time to prepare in advance. The hospital and staff are equipped to respond quickly to your needs.

Preparation

Before you have a cesarean delivery, the nurse prepares you for the operation. You may be given a medication that will help dry secretions in your mouth and upper airway and reduce acid in your stomach. Your abdomen will be washed and may be shaved.

A catheter (tube) is then placed in your bladder. Keeping the bladder empty lowers the chance of injuring it during surgery. An intravenous (IV) line will be put in a vein in your arm or hand. This allows you to get fluids and medications during the surgery.

The scar from your cesarean delivery may not be the same on your uterus as it is on your abdomen.

Anesthesia

Anesthesia will be given so that you do not feel any pain during surgery. You will be given either general anesthesia, an epidural block, or a spinal block. If general anesthesia is used, you will not be awake during the delivery.

An epidural block numbs the lower half of the body. An injection is made into a space in your spine in your lower back. A small tube may be inserted into this space so that more of the drug can be given through the tube later, if needed. That way, you don't need another injection, and the baby is exposed to as little of the drug as possible.

A spinal block is similar to the epidural block. It also numbs the lower half of your body. You receive it the same way, but the drug is injected directly into the spinal fluid.

The type of anesthesia used depends on many factors, including your well-being and that of your baby. The doctor will talk with you about the types of anesthesia and will take your wishes into account.

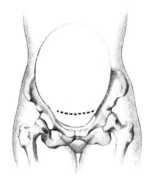

Transverse

Delivery

The doctor will make an incision through your skin and the wall of the abdomen. Another will be made in the wall of the uterus. The one in the abdomen may be transverse (horizontal) or vertical, just above the pubic hairline. The incision in the wall of the uterus may be transverse or vertical.

When possible, the transverse incision is preferred because it is done in the lower, thinner part of the uterus and it results in less bleeding. It also heals with a stronger scar. Sometimes, however, a vertical incision is needed—for example, if you have placenta previa or if the baby is in an unusual position.

The baby will be delivered through the incisions, the umbilical cord will be cut, and then the placenta will be removed. The uterus will be closed with stitches that will dissolve in the body. Stitches or staples are used to close your skin.

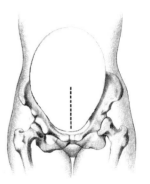

Low vertical

Complications

Like any major surgery, cesarean birth involves risks. These problems occur in a small number of women and usually are easily treated:

- The uterus, nearby pelvic organs, or skin incision can get infected.

- You can lose blood, sometimes enough to require a blood transfusion.

- You can get blood clots in the legs, pelvic organs, or lungs.

- Your bowel or bladder can be injured.

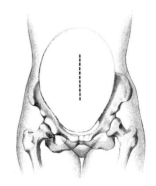

High vertical

The incision made in the uterine wall for cesarean birth may be transverse (top), low vertical (middle), or high vertical (bottom).

After Delivery

If you are awake for the surgery, you can probably hold your baby right away. You will be taken to a recovery room or directly to your room. Your blood pressure, pulse rate, breathing rate, and abdomen will be checked regularly.

You may need to stay in bed for a while. The first few times you get out of bed, a nurse or other adult should help you.

Soon after surgery, the catheter is removed from the bladder. You will receive IV fluids for 1–2 days, until you are able to eat and drink. The abdominal incision will be sore for the first few days. Your doctor can prescribe pain medication for you to take after the anesthesia wears off.

A hospital stay after cesarean birth is usually 4 days. The length of your stay depends on the reason for the cesarean birth and on how long it takes for your body to recover. When you go home, you may need to take special care of yourself and limit your activities.

After cesarean delivery, be sure to ask your doctor which type of cut was made on your uterus—transverse or vertical. This affects how you will deliver your next child. You can't tell what type of scar you have on your uterus by looking at your skin.

After You Go Home

It will take a few weeks for your abdomen to heal. While you recover, you may have:

▶ Mild cramping, especially if you are breastfeeding

▶ Bleeding or discharge for about 4–6 weeks

▶ Bleeding with clots and cramps

▶ Pain in the incision

Help yourself heal. For a few weeks after the cesarean birth, you should not place anything in your vagina or do any strenuous activity. Call your doctor if you have a fever or the pain gets worse.

▶ See also *Condoms, Gonorrhea, Pelvic Inflammatory Disease, Sexually Transmitted Diseases*

▶ CHLAMYDIA

One of the most common sexually transmitted diseases (STDs) in both women and men is chlamydia. This infection is passed from person to person through sex. It is similar in many ways to gonorrhea, and they often occur together. The factors that place a person at risk for both are the same. They also infect the same sites in a woman's reproductive tract. For these reasons, the two are often diagnosed and treated together.

Chlamydia can cause serious health problems if it is not treated. One of these problems is pelvic infection. If a pelvic infection is not treated, it can damage the fallopian tubes and make ectopic pregnancy more likely. A woman who has had a severe infection may not be able to become pregnant. She may also have problems during pregnancy or after birth that pose risks to herself and her baby.

What Is Chlamydia?

Chlamydia infects about 3 million to 5 million women and men each year. It is one of the most common STDs in women in the United States. Chlamydia usually infects a woman's cervix.

Chlamydia that is not treated can spread into the uterus and fallopian tubes. It can also spread to the urethra, causing urethritis. The rectum, throat, and even the lining of the eye can also become infected. In both women and men, chlamydia may occur without causing symptoms. The box lists symptoms that may occur.

Health Risks

If not treated, chlamydia can pose serious, long-term risks to your health. The sooner this disease is found and treated, the lower the chance that serious problems will develop.

Pelvic Inflammatory Disease

Chlamydia can cause pelvic inflammatory disease (PID) if it is not treated. PID is an infection of the uterus, fallopian tubes, and other structures inside a woman's pelvis. It is the most common serious infection in women between ages 16 and 25.

PID almost always results from an untreated infection that spreads upward into the pelvic area. It is the most common preventable cause of infertility in the United States. It can lead to long-term pelvic pain.

A woman who has had PID may have problems getting pregnant. This is because the infection may have scarred the fallopian tubes, blocking them partly or completely. When this happens, an egg released by an ovary may not be able to move through the tube to the uterus.

Problems During Pregnancy

Chlamydia can cause problems for a pregnant woman and her baby, both during

Symptoms of Chlamydia

Many women and men with chlamydia have few or no symptoms when they are first infected. When they do occur, symptoms may appear anywhere from 2 days to 3 weeks after contact with an infected partner.

The most common symptoms in women include:

▶ A yellowish vaginal discharge

▶ Painful or frequent urination

▶ Burning or itching in the vaginal area

▶ Redness, swelling, or soreness of the vulva

▶ Pain in the pelvis or abdomen during sex

▶ Abnormal vaginal bleeding

The most common symptoms in men include:

▶ Discharge from the penis

▶ Pain and burning during urination

None of these symptoms in either sex is a sure sign of chlamydia. Any of them, though, should prompt you to see your doctor.

pregnancy and after birth. Chlamydia increases the risks of preterm birth (birth before 37 weeks) and premature rupture of membranes (in which the sac that surrounds the fetus breaks before labor begins).

Chlamydia can be passed from a pregnant woman to her fetus before birth. The baby of an infected mother has a 40% chance of developing an infection of the lining of the eye (conjunctivitis). This is the most common problem in babies born to infected mothers. It can be easily treated with drops of medicine in the eye, which is routine in most hospitals. Other problems in the newborn can be more serious. About 10–20% of babies of infected mothers develop pneumonia, which can require special care in the hospital.

Because of the risks posed to both mother and baby by this infection, tests for chlamydia are offered to pregnant women who are at risk for these diseases. Some states require that all pregnant women be tested for certain STDs. There is less risk to the baby when the mother is treated for chlamydia during pregnancy.

Many women have no symptoms of chlamydia. They may learn they have chlamydia only when their sexual partners are found to have the disease or if they are tested during pregnancy.

Risk Factors

Like other STDs, chlamydia is passed on by sexual contact. The risk of getting this infection is high if you have sex—vaginal, anal, or oral—with someone who is infected.

Anyone who has sex can get this disease. But the risk is higher in young women and those who:

▶ Have more than one sexual partner

▶ Have sex with someone who has or has had more than one partner

▶ Began sexual activity at an early age

▶ Have other types of STDs, either now or in the past

▶ Have had gonorrhea before

▶ Use illegal drugs

Diagnosis

If you have any of the risk factors described here, or if you think you may have been exposed to someone with this infection, contact your doctor to get tested. Lab tests can be done to find out if you have chlamydia.

It is possible to have more than one STD at the same time. Your chances of having another STD are higher if you have chlamydia. The same factors that place you at risk for this infection also increase your risk of having others. For this reason, your doctor may also test you for other STDs, such as gonorrhea, genital herpes, syphilis, or human immunodeficiency virus (HIV) infection.

Because the most common site of chlamydia in women is the cervix, diagnosis is usually done by a pelvic exam and culture of the cervix. During the exam, your doctor will look at your cervix and any discharge. A sample of cells will then be taken from the cervix. These cells will be tested. Other sites that may be cultured are the rectum, urethra, and throat.

Treatment

To treat chlamydia, your doctor may prescribe antibiotics that can be taken by mouth. Treatment may last for up to 7 days.

For treatment to work, it's important to follow these guidelines:

▶ Finish all of your medicine. Even if your symptoms go away before you finish all the medicine your doctor prescribes, you can still be infected. If you stop taking the medicine, the infection may progress silently. Remember, many women have this infection with no symptoms at all.

▶ Your sexual partner should also be tested and treated. If your partner is infected and does not get treatment, the disease can be passed back to you.

▶ Don't have sex until you are fully cured. Chlamydia can be passed to your sexual partner while you are being treated. If this happens, you may end up passing the infection back and forth, and you could be reinfected. After you and your partner have completed treatment, you can resume having sex.

Prevention

Even if you have already had chlamydia, there are things you can do to keep from getting it again. These safeguards can also help protect against other STDs:

▶ *Limit your sexual partners.* Your risk of getting STDs increases with the number of your sexual partners. The only sure way to prevent most STDs is to not have sex. Having sex with only one partner who in turn has sex only with you will lower your risk.

▶ *Know your partner.* Ask about your partner's sexual history and whether he or she has had STDs. Your partner's sexual history can place you at risk. Even if your partner has no symptoms, he or she may still be infected and can pass on an infection to you during sex. It can be hard to be sure you are safe. It is up to you to protect yourself.

Because condoms are regulated as medical devices, they are tested at random by the U.S. Food and Drug Administration. Also, each latex condom made in the United States is tested electronically for holes before it is packaged. Condom breakage rates are low in the United States—no more than 2 per 100 condoms used.

> *Use a condom.* Both male and female condoms are sold over the counter in drug stores. Neither is 100% foolproof, but they do offer protection against STDs, such as gonorrhea, chlamydia, and HIV. For the best protection against STDs, use a condom every time you have sex.

> *Use a spermicide containing nonoxynol 9.* Most spermicides, as well as vaginal sponges and inserts, contain a chemical called nonoxynol 9. This is an agent that may provide some protection against certain STDs, such as chlamydia. Many brands of condoms are also treated with this substance.

> *If you think you may be at risk, get tested.* In this case, what you don't know can hurt you. If you have had sexual contact with someone who may be at risk for STDs, see your doctor. These diseases will do the least harm to your health if they are caught early. Getting prompt treatment and protecting yourself against reinfection are the best ways to take care of your health.

▶ CHOLESTEROL

Cholesterol is a natural substance that has an important function in your body. It serves as a building block for cells and hormones. But, too much cholesterol is bad for you. Excess cholesterol can stick to the walls of blood vessels, making it harder for blood to move through them. Sometimes cholesterol completely blocks an artery. If that happens, the body part served by the artery cannot receive needed nutrients or oxygen. A heart attack can occur if an artery is blocked in the heart. If the blockage is in the brain, a stroke can result.

A high level of cholesterol in your blood puts you at risk for heart attack, heart disease, and stroke. This risk is as serious for women as it is for men. In fact, half of all U.S. women will die of cardiovascular disease (diseases of the heart and blood vessels).

The female hormone estrogen tends to protect a woman from the effects of too much cholesterol. But after menopause, the level of estrogen decreases. Then, a woman's risk of cardiovascular disease begins to increase. Hormone replacement therapy after menopause can reduce this risk.

High blood cholesterol has no symptoms. That is why every adult should have his or her cholesterol level checked. A simple blood test can show whether your level is normal.

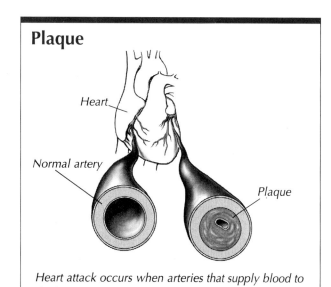

Plaque

Heart

Normal artery

Plaque

Heart attack occurs when arteries that supply blood to the heart are damaged by a buildup of plaque on their walls (right). *This cuts off the heart's supply of oxygen.*

Knowing how to keep a healthy cholesterol level through diet, exercise, and regular checkups will help you to lower your risk of cardiovascular disease.

How Cholesterol Works in the Body

Where It Comes From

Most of the cholesterol in your body is made by the liver. A small amount also comes from certain foods, such as meat, dairy products (such as butter, whole milk, and cheese), and eggs. The amount of cholesterol in your body depends partly on your diet and partly on factors passed on from your parents (heredity).

What It Does

The fat in the foods you eat is digested and sent to the liver. The liver then packages the fat into lipoproteins, which are made of cholesterol, other fats, and protein. Lipoproteins carry fat through your blood vessels for use or storage in other parts of the body. Without them, fat could not travel through the bloodstream. This is because blood is mainly made of water, and fat and water do not mix.

There are three kinds of lipoproteins:

1. VLDL (very-low-density lipoprotein)

2. LDL (low-density lipoprotein)

3. HDL (high-density lipoprotein)

Each lipoprotein has a job to do. First, the liver packages the fat into VLDL, which carries the fat through your blood vessels to your fat tissue. After the VLDL drops off some of the fat, but not its cholesterol, it becomes LDL. It is LDL, sometimes called "bad cholesterol," that can stick to the sides of blood vessels and even block arteries in vital organs such as the heart and brain.

HDL, sometimes called "good cholesterol," keeps cholesterol from building up in artery walls. It does this by picking it up and carrying it back to the liver. Then, the liver breaks it down so that it can be passed out of the body. A high level of HDL helps to lower the level of LDL. The goal of a healthy diet is to keep HDL high and LDL low.

What Happens When You Eat Too Much Fat?

A high-fat diet causes too much LDL, or bad cholesterol, in the bloodstream. This can make it hard for the HDL, or good cholesterol, to do its job.

Eggs Are OK in Moderation

It was once believed that eggs caused heart disease because they contain a high amount of cholesterol. Doctors advised patients to limit the number of eggs they ate to 3–4 per week. Studies now show that dietary fat may be more of a factor in raising cholesterol levels than dietary cholesterol. So, if you don't have high cholesterol levels, eating one egg a day should not increase your risk of heart disease or stroke.

Too much cholesterol can clog blood vessels. This causes deposits that form a substance called plaque. Over the years, the plaque narrows and hardens the arteries. This is called atherosclerosis.

Testing for Cholesterol Levels

The amount of total cholesterol in your blood can be found by a simple blood test. Total cholesterol is the sum of VLDL, LDL, and HDL. In general, the lower your cholesterol level, the better.

A lipoprotein analysis may be done if the blood test shows that your cholesterol level is more than 200 mg/dL. This test breaks down the total cholesterol into LDL and HDL. Your level of VLDL may be tested, too. Even if your cholesterol level is less than 200 mg/dL, you may need a lipoprotein analysis if you have one of the following risk factors:

▶ History of parent, brother, or sister with a cholesterol level of 240 mg/dL or higher

▶ History of brother, sister, parent, or grandparent with heart disease before age 55

▶ Diabetes

▶ Cigarette smoking

You may also have your triglycerides tested. They are a type of fat. Recommended levels of cholesterol and triglycerides are shown in Table 13.

The most important value is LDL cholesterol. When it's too high, your risk of heart attack, stroke, or other cardiovascular disease is increased. If you have high cholesterol, take steps to bring your level down. Eat a low-fat, low-cholesterol diet and exercise regularly. Your doctor may prescribe medicine if these things don't work and will check your cholesterol on a regular basis.

All women should have their cholesterol levels checked. Women with a normal cho-

Table 13. Cholesterol and Triglyceride Levels*

Level (mg/dL)	Result
Total cholesterol	
<200	**Desirable**
200–239	Borderline
≥240	High
HDL cholesterol	
<35	Low (undesirable)
35–59	**Normal**
≥60	High (desirable)
LDL cholesterol	
<130	**Desirable**
130–159	Borderline high risk
≥160	High risk
Triglycerides	
<200	**Normal**
200–400	Borderline high
400–1,000	High
>1,000	Very high

*Recommended levels are shown in bold type

Please note that the most common cholesterol screening tests give you your total cholesterol level, not a complete breakdown of types and levels as is listed here.

Data from Expert Panel on Detection, Evaluation, and Treatment of High Blood Cholesterol in Adults. Summary of the second report of the National Cholesterol Education Program (NCEP) Expert Panel on Detection, Evaluation, and Treatment of High Blood Cholesterol in Adults (Adult Treatment Panel II). JAMA 1993; 269: 3015–3023

lesterol level should have the test repeated about every 5 years. Women who should be tested every 1–2 years are those who:

‣ Have had high cholesterol or cardiovascular disease

‣ Have a family history of high cholesterol or cardiovascular disease

‣ Smoke

‣ Have diabetes

A woman with high cholesterol should be tested at least once a year.

Risk Factors for Atherosclerosis

The amounts of total and LDL cholesterol in the blood are the best ways to predict whether a person will develop atherosclerosis. Other risk factors, though, also have an effect:

‣ Age 55 or older in women

‣ Heart attack or sudden death before age 55 in father or brother or before age 65 in mother or sister

‣ Cigarette smoking

‣ High blood pressure

‣ Levels of HDL below 35 mg/dL

‣ Diabetes

‣ Inactive lifestyle

‣ Obesity

Some risk factors for artherosclerosis you cannot control—such as age and family history. However, the other risk factors listed can be controlled with changes in lifestyle, such as eating a healthy diet, stopping smoking, and exercising.

As the number of these risk factors increases, so does the risk of cardiovascular disease. Your doctor can make up a treatment plan to help you control some of these risk factors.

If you are extremely overweight or do not exercise enough, you add to your risk. Changes in your lifestyle can help you control some of these risk factors. The sooner you make changes, the better the chance you have to stay healthy.

Certain risk factors may be more key in women than in men. These include diabetes, high levels of triglycerides, and extremely low levels of HDL. If you have one of these risk factors as well as high cholesterol, your doctor may suggest you receive special care.

How High Cholesterol Affects Women

The leading causes of death in women are heart attack and stroke. In fact, cardiovascular disease causes twice as many deaths in women as cancer. The same number of women and men die from heart attacks, but women die at an older age.

Before menopause, estrogen protects most women from developing cardiovascular disease. Estrogen increases the amount of good (HDL) cholesterol and decreases the amount of bad (LDL) cholesterol. After menopause, though, a woman's body no longer produces as much estrogen. As a result, the risk of cardiovascular disease in women increases steadily after middle age. By age 65, women have nearly the same rate of heart disease as men. One way to reduce this risk is by taking hormone replacement therapy after menopause.

Hormones affect levels of cholesterol. Hormone replacement therapy after menopause lowers a woman's risk of heart disease. This is true partly because estrogen has a good effect on cholesterol levels. The levels of hormones used in birth control pills today have little effect on blood cholesterol.

Lowering Your Cholesterol

You can lower your cholesterol level by eating foods low in fat (Table 14)—especially low in saturated fat—and cholesterol and by losing weight. Exercise helps, too. It increases the level

Table 14. A Low-Fat Diet

For a balanced diet that is low in fat and cholesterol, choose from each of the following food groups each day. Use few fats, oils, and sweets. Check the following lists for examples of foods to select and avoid.

Food Group	Choose More Often:	Choose Less Often:
Fruits	Citrus fruits (oranges, grapefruit); apples, berries, pears	Coconut
Vegetables	Dark-green, leafy vegetables (spinach, collard, endive); yellow-orange vegetables (carrots, sweet potatoes, squash); cabbage, broccoli, cauliflower, Brussels sprouts	Vegetables prepared in butter, oil, cheese, or cream sauces
Bread, Cereal, Rice, and Pasta	Whole-wheat, rye, oatmeal, and pumpernickel breads; whole-grain and bran cereals; rice; pasta	Refined-flour breads and cakes; biscuits, croissants; crackers, chips; cookies, pastries; granola
Milk, Yogurt, and Cheese	Low-fat or skim milk; low-fat or nonfat yogurt and cheeses (ricotta, farmer, cottage, mozzarella); sherbet; frozen low-fat yogurt; ice milk	Whole milk; butter; yogurt made from whole milk; sweet cream, sour cream whipped cream, and other creamy toppings (including imitation); ice cream; coffee creamers (including nondairy); cream cheese, cheese spreads, Brie, Camembert, hard cheeses (Swiss, cheddar)
Meat, Poultry, Fish, Dry Beans, Eggs, and Nuts	Low-fat chicken or turkey without skin; fresh or frozen fish; water-packed canned tuna; lean meat trimmed of all fat; cooked dry beans and peas; egg whites	Beef, veal, lamb, and pork cuts with marbling, untrimmed of fat; duck, goose; organ meats, such as liver; luncheon meats, sausage, hot dogs; shellfish*; peanut butter, nuts, seeds; trail mix; tuna packed in oil; egg yolks, whole eggs

*Although shellfish are low in fat, they have at least as much cholesterol as meats and poultry.

of good (HDL) cholesterol in your blood, helps you lose weight, and lowers your blood pressure. The good news is that there is a two-for-one benefit: your risk of heart disease decreases 2% for each 1% that your cholesterol level decreases.

Change Your Diet

Making changes in your diet can help lower your cholesterol level. You should eat more soluble fiber (oats, beans, and fruit) and starches (grains and root vegetables such as carrots, turnips, and potatoes). Eat foods that are low in cholesterol. It's also important to eat foods low in saturated fat because this fat interferes with cholesterol breakdown in the body.

Saturated fat is solid at room temperature. It includes animal fats (butter and lard) and some vegetable fats (coconut, palm, and those listed on labels as "partially hydrogenated" oils).

Monounsaturated fats (olive, peanut, and canola oils) and polyunsaturated fats (safflower, sunflower, and corn oils) are better choices than saturated fats. Monounsaturated fats do not increase your cholesterol level as much as saturated fats.

If a food is labeled "cholesterol free," one serving has less than 2 milligrams of cholesterol and the saturated fat content must be 2 grams or less. If a food is labeled "low cholesterol," one serving contains 20 mg or less cholesterol and the saturated fat content must be 2 grams or less.

The best choice, though, is to limit all fats. Fat should make up less than 30% of the total calories in your diet. Based on a 2,000-calorie diet, this is about 65 grams of fat a day. Women who eat fewer calories should eat fewer grams of fat.

Low-fat cooking methods help, too. Broil, steam, braise, bake, or poach foods. Skim or cut all visible fat from food. A good way to reduce the amount of fat in your diet is to cut back on butter, heavy sauces, mayonnaise, rich desserts and baked goods, and fried foods. When you eat meat, choose lean cuts, or choose poultry without skin or fish. Choose low-fat dairy products.

Exercise Regularly

Aerobic exercise (such as walking, jogging, or swimming) increases your HDL (good cholesterol) level. It is best to exercise regularly, at least three times a week. Your doctor can help you choose a safe exercise plan.

Quit Smoking

Smoking lowers your HDL level and increases your risk of heart attack, heart disease, and stroke. It also increases your risk of lung cancer. If you smoke and are older than age 35, you should not use birth control pills. The combination greatly increases the risk of heart attacks, particularly in women older than 35 years.

Medical Treatment

If eating a healthy diet, exercising, and quitting smoking don't work after several months, your doctor may prescribe drugs to decrease your cholesterol level. While you are taking these drugs, you should still stick to a low-fat, low-cholesterol diet.

▶ See also *Amniocentesis, Birth Defects, Genetic Disorders*

▶ CHORIONIC VILLUS SAMPLING

Chorionic villus sampling (CVS) is a procedure used to test for birth defects during pregnancy. This test may help your doctor find chromosomal problems such as Down syndrome. It also may detect other genetic diseases such as cystic fibrosis, Tay–Sachs disease, and sickle cell disease.

Chorionic villus sampling can be done earlier in pregnancy than amniocentesis (another procedure to test for birth defects). In most cases, it is done about 10–12 weeks from the woman's last menstrual period. This allows for earlier detection of birth defects. Like amniocentesis, CVS is done in a hospital or the doctor's office.

Chorionic villus sampling is newer than amniocentesis. Fewer doctors are trained to perform CVS than are trained in amniocentesis. As a result, it isn't offered in all areas of the United States. You might need to travel to a center where it is performed.

The Procedure

With CVS, a small sample of cells is taken from the placenta where it is attached to the wall of the uterus. Chorionic villi are tiny parts of the placenta. Villi are formed from the fertilized egg. Therefore, they have the same genes as the fetus.

There are two ways to collect cells from the placenta: through the vagina or through the abdomen. To collect cells through the vagina, a speculum is inserted just as for a Pap test. Then, a very thin, plastic tube is inserted up the vagina and into the cervix. With ultrasound, the tube is guided up to the placenta. A small sample is removed. To collect cells through the abdomen, a slender needle is inserted through the woman's abdomen to the placenta, much like for amniocentesis.

The sample of chorionic villi then is sent to a lab. There the cells are grown and tested.

If you have an active sexually transmitted disease (STD), bleeding during pregnancy, or certain problems with the cervix,

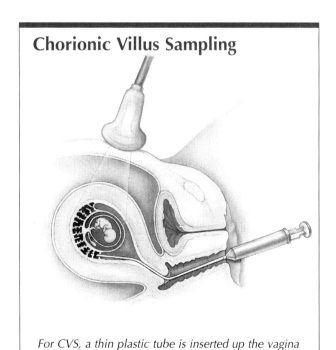

Chorionic Villus Sampling

For CVS, a thin plastic tube is inserted up the vagina and into the uterus. The cells removed can be tested for birth defects early in pregnancy.

you may be offered CVS through the abdomen. In other cases, neither type may be a good choice.

Results

Chorionic villus sampling can detect most of the same defects as amniocentesis. One defect that cannot be detected by CVS is open neural tube defects. If you have CVS, you may want to think about having a blood alpha-fetoprotein (AFP) test later in the pregnancy to screen for neural tube defects.

The results of CVS can be obtained earlier in pregnancy and more quickly than with amniocentesis. Most women get their results within 10 days.

AFP is a protein made by the fetus. Small amounts of AFP are passed into the amniotic fluid. Too much AFP in the amniotic fluid can be a sign of fetal defects, such as neural tube defects.

Risks

Chorionic villus sampling may carry a slightly higher risk of miscarriage than amniocentesis. The rate is higher than that for amniocentesis because CVS is done earlier. Infection also can occur with CVS. Limb defects in infants may occur, especially if CVS is done before 10 weeks. This is rare, though.

Options

Most of the time, tests show normal results. If your tests diagnose a major birth defect, you have tough choices to make. You may choose to continue the pregnancy and have the baby, or you may choose to have an abortion.

If you choose to have the baby, you may need to deliver at a special hospital. You also may need extra help after the baby is born.

If you choose to have an abortion, you should decide as soon as possible. The earlier an abortion is done, the safer it is for you.

Before you decide, get as much information about the defect as you can—from doctors, counselors, or parents of a child with the same type of defect. Ask friends or family for advice and support. Knowing as much as you can will help you to make the best choice.

▸ CIRCUMCISION, FEMALE

Female circumcision, or female genital mutilation, is any type of genital alteration performed on girls and young women for non-medical reasons. Female circumcision is estimated to have been done on more than 130 million females worldwide. Although it is mainly practiced in Africa, variations have been found in many other regions of the world, including Yemen, United Arab Emirates, Malaysia, Indonesia, Pakistan, and India. The practice is based on cultural beliefs and, in most cases, performed by a person with little or no medical training.

Female circumcision is performed on girls 8–12 years old in most cases. In most countries where female circumcision is practiced, it is a rite of passage from childhood to womanhood. In some cultures, it is performed several months after birth. In others, it is performed closer to marriage. In cultures that practice female circumcision, virginity is prized because it ensures marriageability. In these cultures, it is strongly believed that only a circumcised woman is desirable for marriage. Uncircumcised women are outcasts. Because marriage and bearing children are thought to be a woman's livelihood, it is believed that not circumcising one's daughter is denying her the opportunity to lead a fulfilled life.

This ancient rite is harmful to the woman's health. In the United States, federal law makes it a crime to perform female circumcision on a minor. Side effects of female genital mutilation may include infection, tetanus, shock, hemorrhage, and death.

▶ CIRCUMCISION, MALE

A layer of skin, the foreskin, covers the glans (head) of the penis. Circumcision is the surgical removal of this foreskin. If it is done, it's usually done soon after birth. Whether to have your son circumcised is your decision.

Making the Decision

Circumcision is an elective procedure. That means it is the parents' choice whether to have their son circumcised. In most cases, there is no medical reason for a circumcision. It is not required by law or by hospital policy.

Although many newborn boys in the United States are circumcised, it is much less common in Northern Europe and other parts of the world. Some parents have their sons circumcised for religious or cultural reasons. Moslems and Jews, for example, have circumcised their male newborns for centuries.

Some parents choose to have their sons circumcised for the sake of hygiene. Smegma—a cheesy discharge containing dead cells—can build up under the foreskin of males who are not circumcised. This can lead to odor or infection. A boy can be taught to wash his penis to get rid of smegma as a part of his daily bathing routine.

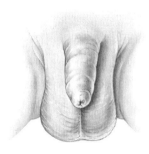

Uncircumcised penis

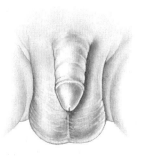

Circumcised penis

Some parents choose not to circumcise their sons because they are worried about the pain the baby feels or the risks involved with the surgery.

Some doctors feel that circumcision lowers the risk of sexually transmitted diseases (STDs). There is no proof of this, however. Others feel that circumcision helps prevent cancer of the penis, a rare condition in uncircumcised men. Circumcised infants appear to have less risk of infections of the urinary tract than uncircumcised infants. However, the risk in both groups is low.

The Procedure

Circumcision is done before the mother and baby leave the hospital. During the procedure, the baby is placed on a special table. The doctor may use local anesthesia to lessen the pain. Various surgical techniques are used, but they follow the same steps:

- The penis and foreskin are cleaned.
- A special clamp is attached to the penis and the foreskin is removed.
- Ointment and gauze often are placed over the cut to protect it from rubbing against the diaper.

The procedure is done quickly. The baby will cry during and for a short while afterward. The skin will heal in about 7–10 days.

Parents who want their sons circumcised must request it. If you choose to circumcise your son, you may want to ask about how your doctor feels about pain relief. Not all doctors routinely use pain relief, and some question its value.

Risks

Complications from a circumcision are rare. However, every surgery carries some risk. Complications that can occur are:

- Bleeding
- Infection
- Injury to the penis or urethra
- Scarring

Caring for Your Newborn

Circumcised Infants

If your baby boy is circumcised, a light dressing such as gauze with petroleum jelly may be placed over the head of the penis after surgery. Keep the area as clean as possible. Wash the baby's penis with soap and water every day. Change the diapers often so that urine and stool do not cause infection.

With one type of circumcision, a plastic ring is left on the penis. This ring will slip off when the edge of the circumcision is fully healed.

Uncircumcised Infants

Washing the baby's penis and foreskin properly is important. The outside of the penis should be washed with soap and water. Do not attempt to pull back the infant's foreskin. The foreskin may not be able to pull back completely until the child is about 3–5 years old. This is normal.

Teach your boy to wash his penis, including under the foreskin after it has begun to retract. Once he learns to do this, it will become part of his daily routine.

▶ See also *Cancer, Colonoscopy*

▶ COLORECTAL CANCER

Colon and rectal cancer—or colorectal cancer—is a disease that affects the large intestine and rectum. It is the third leading cause of cancer death of women in the United States. You may be at high risk for colorectal cancer if you:

▶ Have a family history of bowel problems

▶ Have had colon polyps (benign growths on the colon)

▶ Don't exercise regularly

▶ Eat a diet low in fiber

▶ Eat a diet high in fat

Colorectal cancer can have several warning signs:

▶ Bleeding from the rectum

▶ Blood in the stool

▶ Change in bowel habits

▶ Abdominal discomfort (bloating, cramps, or frequent gas pains)

▶ Stools that are more narrow than usual

Cancers of the colon and rectum are two of the most common cancers in the United States. These cancers occur in both women and men and most often are found in people older than age 50.

Having these symptoms does not confirm that you have cancer, however. They can also occur as a result of other less serious problems. Regular screening tests can help detect colon cancer early. Early detection is the key to effective treatment. Here are some guidelines to follow:

▶ Women aged 40 and older who have certain bowel problems or who have a family history of bowel problems should have an annual colonoscopy.

▶ Women aged 50 and older should have an annual rectal exam and fecal occult blood test.

▶ Women aged 50 and older should have a sigmoidoscopy every 3–5 years.

Colon and rectal cancer may also be linked to diet. Eating foods that are low in fat and high in fiber, such as fruits, vegetables, and whole-grain cereals, may help reduce the risks of getting the disease. You also can help prevent colorectal cancer by eating a balanced diet and exercising regularly.

▶ COLONOSCOPY

▶ See also *Colorectal Cancer*

A colonoscopy is an exam of the entire colon. A long, flexible, lighted tube called a colonoscope is used to find growths, ulcers, inflamed tissue, or signs of cancer. The scope is inserted into the rectum. Then it is slowly guided through the entire length of the colon (large bowel).

Your doctor may suggest a colonoscopy if you have pain, bleeding, or changes in bowel habits that cannot be explained.

The doctor can see the inside of your colon through the scope. Pictures of the colon's lining also can be seen on a video screen. The scope blows air into your colon to inflate it, which helps the doctor see it better. Tiny instruments can be passed through the scope to remove polyps (noncancerous growths) or bits of tissue for a biopsy.

For colonoscopy, you are given sedatives and pain relief to keep you comfortable during the exam. You may feel a bit of pressure, bloating, or cramping. Afterwards, you should be able to eat normally and resume normal activities.

You may be asked to follow a liquid diet for 1–3 days before the exam to be sure your colon is completely free of stool. To help clean out the colon, you will be prescribed special fluids to drink, laxatives, or enemas.

Although problems seldom occur with colonoscopy, there can be some complications. In rare cases, the scope may puncture or tear the colon wall, which may require surgery.

▶ COLPOSCOPY

▶ See also *Cervical Disorders, Pap Test* in *"Women's Wellness"*

Colposcopy is a way of looking at the cervix through a special magnifying device called a colposcope. It shines a light onto the vagina and cervix. It can enlarge the normal view by 2–60 times.

This allows the doctor to find problems that cannot be seen by the eye alone.

Reasons for Colposcopy

Colposcopy is done when a Pap test shows changes that could lead to cancer. It provides more information about the abnormal cells.

Colposcopy also may be used to further assess certain problems:

▶ Genital warts on the cervix

▶ Cervicitis (inflammation of the cervix)

▶ Benign (not cancer) growths, such as polyps

▶ Pain or bleeding

Sometimes colposcopy may need to be done again. It also can be used to check the result of a treatment.

The Procedure

Colposcopy is done like a Pap test in a doctor's office. You may be referred to another doctor or to a special clinic to have it done.

The procedure is best done when a woman is not having her period. For at least 24 hours before the test:

▶ Don't douche.

▶ Don't use tampons.

▶ Don't use vaginal medications.

▶ Don't have sex.

As with a pelvic exam, you will lie on your back with your feet raised and placed in stirrups for support. A speculum will be used to spread apart the vaginal walls so that the inside of the vagina and the cervix can be seen. The colposcope is placed just outside the entrance of your vagina.

A mild vinegar solution will be applied to your cervix and vagina with a cotton swab or cotton ball. This liquid makes abnormal areas on the cervix easier to see. You may feel a slight burning. With your permission, pictures of the vagina and cervix may be taken.

Biopsy

During colposcopy, the doctor may see abnormal areas. A biopsy of these areas may be done.

A Pap test is a good way to find changes that could become cancer. Colposcopy will give you even more information. In most cases, abnormal results are not cancer. Talk with your doctor about the results of your colposcopy and biopsy.

Colposcopy

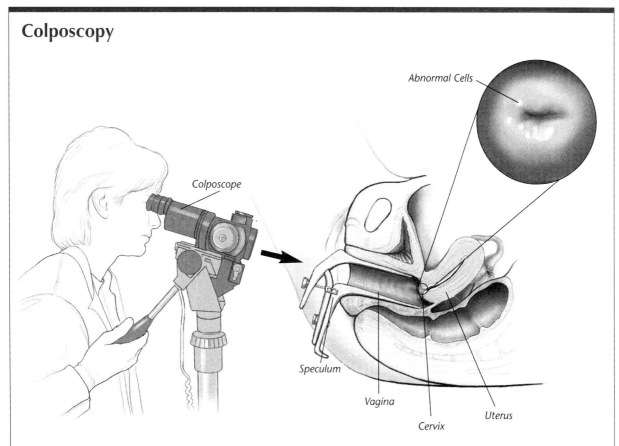

Abnormal Cells

Colposcope

Speculum

Vagina

Cervix

Uterus

Your doctor can look through the colposcope to check for any abnormal cells on your cervix (left). A special solution is applied to your vagina and cervix to help highlight any abnormal areas (right).

During a biopsy, a small piece of abnormal tissue is removed from the cervix. The sample is removed with a special device.

Cells also may be taken from the canal of the cervix. Because they are not easy to see by the colposcope, a special device is used to scrape the cells. This is called endocervical curettage (ECC).

Results

Normal results mean the cervix and vagina look normal. Abnormal results mean some problem was found. If a biopsy was taken, it must be studied in a lab. When biopsy results come back from the lab, your doctor will discuss them with you. Depending on the results, you may need to be checked more often or you may need further testing or treatments.

Recovery

If you have a colposcopy without biopsy, you should feel fine right away. You can do the things you normally do. You may have a little spotting for a couple of days.

If you had a colposcopy with a biopsy, your vagina may feel sore for a day or two. You also may have some vaginal bleeding and a dark discharge for a few days. You may need to wear a sanitary pad until the discharge stops.

While the cervix heals, do not put anything into your vagina for at least 1 week:

▶ Do not have sex.

▶ Do not use tampons.

▶ Do not use a douche.

Your doctor may suggest you limit your activity for a brief time. Call your doctor right away if you have any of these problems:

▶ Heavy vaginal bleeding (using more than one sanitary pad per hour)

▶ Severe lower abdominal pain

▶ Fever

▶ Chills

▶ Foul-smelling vaginal discharge

▶ COMPUTED TOMOGRAPHY SCANS

Like other X-rays, a computed tomography scan is painless. CT scans that require the patient to receive contrast dye may cause slight, short-term discomfort when the IV needle is placed.

Computed tomography, often called a CT scan or CAT scan, is a type of X-ray that shows "slices" of internal organs and structures in your body. The slices are then put together to show an image of the inside of the body, sometimes with movement.

CT scans clearly show the shape and location of organs, muscles, tissues, blood vessels, and bones. They help doctors evaluate abnormal growths, find injuries, and see how far cancer has spread.

During a CT scan you will lie very still on an examining table. The table passes through an X-ray machine shaped like a large doughnut. The machine rotates around you while it takes pictures of many thin segments of tissue. You may be given dye through an intravenous (IV) line or asked to drink a solution. This allows the area to show up more clearly in the picture. How long the exam takes depends on how large the area is that must be X-rayed.

A computer processes images from the X-rays to make a "computed tomogram." "Tomo" mean slice. Doctors view these images on a TV-like screen.

The amount of radiation you receive during a CT scan is slightly more than from a regular X-ray. In rare cases, people have a reaction to the dye injection. Overall, the risk from a CT scan is low.

▶ CONDOMS

Condoms are a form of barrier method to prevent pregnancy. Condoms act as physical barriers. They keep the sperm from getting to the egg. To be effective, condoms must be used each time you have sex. There are two types of condoms, a male condom and a female condom.

Male Condom

The male condom is a thin sheath placed over the man's erect penis. When semen is released, it stays inside the condom and does not pass into the woman's vagina. Besides sterilization, using condoms is the only effective method of contraception used by men. Condoms are also known as rubbers, prophylactics, and sheaths. They are simple to use and are effective when used correctly. Also, they are fairly inexpensive and widely available.

How to Use a Condom

If you have a new sexual partner or if you and your partner have not used condoms before, talk about it before you have sex. It is easier to talk about it at that time than it is in the heat of the moment.

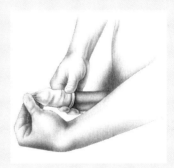

If your partner does not want to use a condom, explain the benefits to both of you. Proper condom use helps protect both of you from STDs. If your partner refuses to use a condom, you may want to not have sex rather than risk your health. A partner who refuses to use a condom may not have your best interest at heart. If you still want to have sex, use the female condom to protect yourself. Because it is new, not as much is known about its ability to prevent STDs. But, it may provide protection similar to that of the male condom.

To use the male condom, place the rolled-up condom over the tip of the erect penis. Hold the end of the condom to allow a little extra space at the tip. Then unroll the condom over the penis.

Right after ejaculation, grasp the condom around the base of the penis as it is withdrawn. The condom should then be thrown away—never reused.

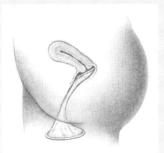

To use the female condom, squeeze the inner ring between your fingers and insert it into the vagina. Push the inner ring up until it is just behind the pubic bone. About an inch of the open end should be outside your body.

Right after ejaculation, squeeze and twist the outer ring and pull the pouch out gently. Like the male condom, it should then be thrown away—never reused.

Male latex condoms also help protect against some STDs. Condoms made of animal membranes do not provide the same protection against STDs. Women who are allergic to latex can use the female condom. Other types of condoms are being tested.

Most condoms are made of latex rubber. Latex condoms come in a variety of colors and may have shaped or contoured ends that provide a place to hold the semen. They are sold either dry or lubricated. Some contain spermicide.

Oil-based lubricants such as petroleum jelly should never be used with latex condoms because they can damage the rubber. Use only water-based lubricants. Condoms should be used for only one act of intercourse. They must never be reused.

Female Condom

The female condom is a thin plastic pouch that lines the vagina. It is held in place by a closed inner ring at the cervix and an open outer ring at the opening of the vagina. It comes with a lubricant. You can also use both oil- and water-based lubricants with it. Like the male condom, it should be used for only one act of intercourse.

◗ CONSTIPATION

Constipation is a common bowel problem. It is infrequent bowel movements with stools that are firm or hard to pass. Signs of constipation include:

◗ Swelling or bloating of the abdomen

◗ Straining during bowel movements

◗ Feeling full even after a bowel movement

Although constipation is uncomfortable, it usually is not a sign of a serious problem. You can help prevent constipation by:

◗ Drinking plenty of fluids—at least 8 glasses of water a day

◗ Eating a diet high in fiber (see Table 15)

◗ Increasing your physical activity

◗ Not holding your stool—use the bathroom when you feel the urge to have a bowel movement

If constipation continues, you may want to use an over-the-counter laxative. There are different types of laxatives, and they work in different ways:

Laxative Abuse

Laxatives are usually not necessary and can be habit-forming. The colon begins to rely on laxatives to bring on bowel movements. Over time, laxatives can damage nerve cells in the colon and make it hard for the colon to work properly. If you are taking laxatives on a regular basis, see your doctor for information on other ways to relieve constipation.

▶ Bulk-forming agents absorb water and expand, thus increasing the moisture in the stool and making it easier to pass (these are thought to be the safest and most natural laxatives).

▶ Stool softeners add liquid content to the stool to soften it.

▶ Stimulants provide a chemical irritant to the bowel that increases bowel activity, which moves the stool through the intestines.

Bulk-forming and stool-softening products can be used on a regular basis as part of your diet. Stimulants should be used with more caution. They are available as medication, enemas, and suppositories. You should stop using these products once your bowel movements become regular again. Overusing stimulants can cause your bowels to become dependent on them. People who have constipation may also develop hemorrhoids. Hemorrhoids are enlarged veins, which cause swelling and tenderness of the tissue inside or outside the rectum. If constipation persists after trying these remedies, you should see a doctor for further evaluation.

Table 15. Good Sources of Fiber

You should eat 25–30 grams of fiber each day. The average woman gets only half that amount. To get a daily dose of fiber, eat plenty of vegetables, fruits, and whole-grain cereals and breads. High-fiber foods are those that have at least 2 grams of fiber per serving.

Food	Serving Size	Total Fiber (grams)
Pinto beans	1/2 cup	7.4
Raisins	3/4 cup	4.7
Whole-wheat bread	2 slices	3.9
Brussels sprouts	1/2 cup	3.8
Apple (with skin)	1 medium	3.7
Sweet potato	1 medium	3.4
Orange	1 medium	3.1
Oat-bran cereal (cooked)	1/2 cup	2.9
Prunes	4	2.4

▶ CRYOTHERAPY

Cryotherapy, also know as "cold cautery," is a freezing technique used to destroy abnormal cells. It is often used to remove small growths and tumors on the skin. It also can be used to remove abnormal cells on the cervix (the opening of a woman's uterus). Cryotherapy is also a common way to treat genital warts.

Most of the time cryotherapy can be done right in the doctor's office or clinic. A probe is used to apply carbon dioxide to "freeze" the affected region. It takes only a few minutes. Afterward, there may be a little discomfort, but recovery time is short.

▶ See Also *Cervical Disorders, Chorionic Villus Sampling, Human Papillomavirus Infection*

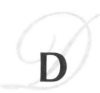

See also *Postpartum Depression*

Get Help!

Suicide kills more than 30,000 Americans a year— one person every 17 minutes. Women make up almost 20% of this total. Depression plays a major role in many of these cases. If you feel you could do harm to yourself or others, seek help right away.

D

▶ DEPRESSION

Depression is a common illness that can affect anyone. About 1 in 20 Americans—more than 11 million people—are affected by depression every year. The condition is found twice as often in women as in men. Depression is a medical problem that can be treated.

What Is Depression?

Depression is a medical disorder, like diabetes, high blood pressure, and heart disease. It is more than feeling sad for a short time or feeling grief after a loss. These feelings are hard to deal with, but they get better with time. Depression disrupts your daily life. It affects your thoughts, feelings, behavior, and physical health. It is not a weakness or a fault. Depression often does not get better without help.

Depression has many causes. The chemicals in the brain may not be balanced. A family history of depression may mean that you are more likely to have depression. Other illnesses may trigger it. About 10–15% of all depressions are triggered by other medical conditions (such as thyroid disease, cancer, or neurologic problems) or by medications. The use of drugs or alcohol can also cause depression.

In some people, depression can occur even though life is going well. In others, conditions such as extreme stress or grief may bring on depression. Stresses may include:

▶ Trying to raise children and work outside the home

▶ Trying to balance tasks at work and home

▶ Having a stressful job

▶ Being a single parent

▶ Having money problems

You may think you are depressed if you are under a lot of stress or if you have had a loss. Such feelings are often linked to a situation—that is, when the situation gets better, you feel better. For women, these feelings may occur around the time of certain reproductive events, such as menstruation, pregnancy, loss of a baby, birth of a baby (postpartum blues or postpartum depression), infertility, or menopause. These feelings are normal. Many women do not need treatment for these feelings. Depression linked to a situation can sometimes trigger true depression, though. If the feelings don't go away, they should be treated.

Symptoms of Depression

The time when you have the symptoms of depression is called an episode. An episode lasts at least 2 weeks. Often it lasts longer. People often have more than one episode. The symptoms that are used to diagnose depression are shown in the box.

You may have other physical or mental symptoms of depression as well. These may include:

▶ Headaches or other aches and pains

▶ Digestive problems

▶ Sexual problems

▶ Hopeless and negative feelings

▶ Prolonged worry or fear

Depression may be mild, moderate, or severe. If you have a mild depression, you will have only a few symptoms. It takes extra effort to do what you have to do, but you can often still do those things. Moderate depression means you have many symptoms. You may not be able to do things you need to do. If you have a severe depression, you have nearly all the symptoms of depression. This type of depression almost always keeps you from doing daily tasks.

Symptoms of Depression

People who are depressed have several of the following symptoms of the illness nearly every day, all day, for at least 2 weeks:

▶ Lack interest in things they used to enjoy

▶ Feel sad, blue, or "down in the dumps"

▶ Slow down or act restless and not able to sit still

▶ Feel worthless or guilty

▶ Have a change in appetite or lose or gain weight

▶ Have thoughts of death or suicide or try to commit suicide

▶ Have problems concentrating, thinking, remembering, or making decisions

▶ Sleep too much or are not able to fall asleep or to stay asleep

▶ Lack energy and feel tired all the time

If you have had at least five of these symptoms (including at least one of the first two), you may be depressed. If you are troubled by any of these symptoms, talk to your doctor.

Some kinds of depression are mild but chronic (long-lasting or recurring episodes). Even though they are mild, chronic symptoms need treatment, too.

Diagnosing Depression

Depression is diagnosed by a doctor. The doctor takes note of your physical and mental condition. He or she may diagnose and care for you or may refer you to a specialist.

In looking for the cause of your depression, the doctor will ask questions about your other medical problems, use of certain medications, and use of drugs or alcohol. If your doctor finds that one of these things may be causing your depression, treating that problem may get rid of the depression.

Treatment

You and your doctor need to work as a team to find the best treatment for you. Treatment may include antidepressant medication, psychotherapy, or both. It may include a hospital stay. Your doctor may refer you to a specialist for treatment. There are also things you can do to help cope with depression.

Some types of treatment work better for some disorders than for others. When talking about treatment options, make sure to get the answers to these questions:

▶ What are the chances of getting better?

▶ What are some risks and side effects?

▶ What are the costs?

SSRIs

Selective serotonin reuptake inhibitors or SSRIs are medications used to treat depression. They help relieve symptoms of depression by acting on serotonin, a neurotransmitter found in the brain. SSRIs seem to have fewer side effects than the older antidepressant medications. One side effect of SSRIs is that one third of the women who take these medications have problems reaching orgasm.

Antidepressants

Antidepressant medications are used to treat severe depression and bipolar disorder. These medications also may be useful for mild to moderate depression. Antidepressants relieve symptoms in more than half the people who take them. They work by changing the balance of chemicals in the brain. Most people who take them start to feel better after a few weeks.

There are many types of antidepressants. Your doctor will prescribe one based on your symptoms and your medical and family history. It may take some time to find the type that works best for you and has the fewest side effects. Like all medications, antidepressants work best if you:

▶ Take them as your doctor prescribes

▶ Report side effects that bother you

▶ Follow all parts of your treatment plan

All antidepressant medications can have some side effects. About half of the people who take them get some side effects early in their treatment (the first 4–6 weeks). Side effects almost always go away after this time. Common side effects include:

▶ A dry mouth

▶ Nausea

▶ Dizziness

▶ Constipation

▶ A skin rash

▶ Feeling sleepy or having trouble sleeping

▶ Gaining or losing weight

▶ Feeling restless

More serious side effects are rare. These may include trouble urinating, sexual problems, heart problems, seizures, or fainting. Tell your doctor if you have any side effects.

While you're taking antidepressants, do not drink alcohol or use any drugs your doctor has not prescribed. These can affect how well the medication works and may cause unsafe side effects.

Your doctor will want to see you often when you are starting treatment to check the dosage, watch for side effects, and see how the treatment is working. Once you begin to feel better, you may visit your doctor less often.

You may need to take the medication for a few months after you feel better. This helps to prevent the depression from coming back. If you have had three or more episodes of depression, you may need long-term treatment to stay well.

Psychotherapy

In psychotherapy, a therapist works with you to help you overcome your depression. Psychotherapy alone helps about half the people with mild to moderate depression. You can work with your doctor to find a therapist.

You may have one-on-one therapy (with just you and the therapist) or group therapy (with a therapist and other people with problems like yours). If you have family or marriage therapy, you and family members or your spouse may work with a therapist. Psychotherapy for depression often has a time limit, such as 8–20 visits.

Coping With Depression

If you are depressed, there are things you can do to make your daily life easier:

▶ Do not demand too much of yourself.

▶ Set a routine that is realistic. Don't expect to be able to do all the things you are used to doing.

▶ Avoid making any major life decisions. If you must make such a decision, ask someone you trust to help you.

▶ Avoid using alcohol and drugs that your doctor has not prescribed.

▶ Seek out people you trust and support groups for help. Emotional support is key to helping you get better.

▶ Follow your doctor's advice. Take medication correctly and keep all your appointments.

Bipolar Disorder

One type of depression is called bipolar disorder, or manic–depressive disorder. People with this disorder have extreme highs (mania) and severe lows (depression). These highs and lows can last days to months. In between the highs and lows, patients feel normal.

Bipolar disorder affects about one in 100 people. It can be inherited (passed from parents to children). It may also be caused by other medical problems, such as a head injury or neurologic (nervous system) conditions.

Symptoms of a manic episode include:

▶ Feeling happier or more irritable than is common for you

▶ Needing less sleep

▶ Talking a lot or feeling that you can't stop talking

▶ Being easily distracted

▶ Having many ideas in your head at the same time

▶ Doing things that may feel good but have bad effects, such as spending too much money, making poor choices about sex, or making unwise business investments

▶ Making lots of plans for activities (at work, school, or socially) or feeling that you have to keep moving

If you have had any four of these symptoms at one time for a week or longer, including the first symptom, you may have had a manic episode. See a doctor for care. Medicine is needed to treat bipolar disorder.

If psychotherapy does not work, another kind of treatment may be needed. Psychotherapy often is coupled with antidepressant medication to treat severe depression or bipolar disorder.

Antidepressants Plus Psychotherapy

Medication plus psychotherapy relieves the symptoms of depression in more than half of patients. It may take a couple of months for the treatment to work. This combined treatment may work best for long-term depression, for people with symptoms between episodes, or for people who do not respond fully to medicine or psychotherapy alone.

Light Therapy

Some people have mild or moderate seasonal depression (depression that comes during seasons with shorter days). Light therapy may help some of these people. With light therapy, people are exposed to broad-spectrum light to give the effect of having a few extra hours of daylight each day.

Hospital Treatment

Most people with depression are treated with visits to their doctor or therapist. People who don't get better or who are at risk of suicide may need to stay in the hospital. Being in the hospital removes the patient from daily stresses and offers more intense treatment.

◗ DIABETES

◗   See also *Hypertension, Preconceptional Counseling, Nutrition* in *"Women's Wellness"*

About 15 million Americans have diabetes mellitus—a chronic disease that causes high levels of glucose (sugar) in the blood. Health problems can arise if the glucose level becomes too high or is not well controlled. Only about half of the people with diabetes have been tested and diagnosed. Knowing the warning signs of diabetes and how to help prevent it is key to staying healthy.

What Is Diabetes?

Diabetes is a disease in which the body does not make enough insulin or does not use it as it should. Insulin is a hormone that helps balance the amount of glucose in your blood. Glucose is a sugar that is the body's main source of energy.

Normally, your body changes most of the food you eat into glucose. Then, glucose is carried to the body's cells with the help of insulin. If your body does not make enough insulin, or the insulin doesn't work as it should, the glucose cannot enter the body's cells. Instead, it stays in the blood. This makes your blood glucose level high.

There are two types of diabetes: type 1 and type 2. Diabetes can occur at any age. Some people develop diabetes as children or teens. Most cases—90%—of diabetes occur in adults aged 45 years or older.

Diabetes may first occur during pregnancy. This is called gestational diabetes. In most cases, gestational diabetes goes away after the baby is born. However, women who develop diabetes during pregnancy are at greater risk for type 2 diabetes later in life.

Type 1 Diabetes

Type 1 diabetes also is known as insulin-dependent diabetes. A person with type 1 diabetes needs to take insulin to survive because their body makes little or no insulin on its own. Type 1 accounts for 10% of all cases of diabetes.

Type 2 Diabetes

Type 2 diabetes also is known as non-insulin-dependent diabetes. In type 2 diabetes, some insulin is produced, but it either is not enough or it doesn't work as it should. Type 2 diabetes may occur as a result of other diseases or as a side effect of certain medications. People with type 2 diabetes may not need to take insulin. They may be able to control their blood glucose with proper diet,

New Treatment Available

Women with diabetes can receive insulin through an internal pump that acts like the pancreas and gives them a steady flow of insulin to control blood sugar. New pumps are in the works that can gauge the amount of insulin to blood sugar levels and adjust the dose as needed.

medication, or both. You may be able to prevent type 2 diabetes by taking certain steps now.

Symptoms

The symptoms of type 1 and type 2 diabetes often are alike. Type 2 diabetes is harder to detect than type 1. In some cases, there are no symptoms with type 2 diabetes, or symptoms can be so mild that they are not noticed. If symptoms occur, it often is because blood glucose levels are very high.

Many people have type 2 diabetes and do not know it. You should find out if you are at risk for diabetes and learn the symptoms. This way you can detect and control it before serious health problems occur.

Risk Factors

Some people have a higher risk of developing diabetes. The disease may run in families, develop from medication use, or be linked to certain lifestyle factors. You should be tested if you have any of these risk factors:

▶ Age 45 or older

▶ Obesity

▶ Family history of diabetes

▶ Ethnic background:
—Native American
—Asian American
—Hispanic
—African American
—Pacific Islander

▶ Previous abnormal glucose screening results

▶ Hypertension

▶ High cholesterol

▶ History of gestational diabetes or a baby weighing more than 9 pounds at birth

Other factors linked to diabetes include polycystic ovary syndrome, long-term medication use (such as steroids), smoking, and heavy alcohol use.

Take the quiz in the box to see if you are at risk for diabetes. If you are at risk, get tested.

Symptoms of Diabetes

Type 1

▶ Extreme thirst or hunger

▶ Weight loss without trying

▶ Feeling tired or weak

▶ Urinating often

▶ Feeling sick to your stomach

Type 2

▶ Any symptoms of type 1 diabetes

▶ Blurred vision

▶ Sores that are slow to heal

▶ Dry, itchy skin

▶ Loss of feeling or tingling in feet

▶ Recurrent infections

▶ Weight gain

▶ Recurrent vaginal or urinary tract infections

▶ Irregular periods

▶ Skin changes

Are You at Risk for Diabetes?

Take this test to see if you are at risk for diabetes. Write in the points next to each statement that is true for you. If a statement is not true, put a zero. Add all the lines for your total score.

1. I am a woman who has had a baby weighing more than 9 pounds at birth.   Yes 1___

2. I have a brother or sister with diabetes.   Yes 1___

3. I have a parent with diabetes.   Yes 1___

4. My weight is equal to or above that listed in the chart.   Yes 5___

5. I am younger than 65 years of age and I get little or no exercise.   Yes 5___

6. I am between 45 and 64 years old.   Yes 5___

7. I am 65 years or older.   Yes 9___

Total___

Scoring 10 or more points

You are at high risk for having diabetes. Only your health care provider can check to see if you have diabetes. See yours soon and find out for sure.

Scoring 3–9 points

You are probably at low risk for having diabetes now. But don't just forget about it. Keep your risk low by losing weight if you are overweight, being active most days, and eating low-fat meals that are high in fruits, vegetables, and whole grains.

American Diabetes Association. Could you have it and not know it? Alexandria, VA: ADA, 1999

At-Risk Weight Chart*

Height (in feet and inches)	Weight (in pounds)
4' 10"	129
4' 11"	133
5' 0"	138
5' 1"	143
5' 2"	147
5' 3"	152
5' 4"	157
5' 5"	162
5' 6"	167
5' 7"	172
5' 8"	177
5' 9"	182
5' 10"	188
5' 11"	193
6' 0"	199
6' 1"	204
6' 2"	210
6' 3"	216
6' 4"	221

*If you weigh the same as or more than the amount listed for your height, you may be at risk for diabetes.

Prevention

To help prevent diabetes, follow a healthy diet and get regular exercise. This also can help keep your weight down—a key part of preventing diabetes. There are steps women can take to help prevent the disease:

▸ Keep your weight in the range that's healthy for you. Many doctors use the body mass index (BMI) chart to assess healthy weight.

▸ Eat a well-balanced diet to help keep your cholesterol, blood glucose, and weight at a healthy level.

▸ Exercise for at least 30 minutes three times a week.

Testing

The purpose of blood glucose testing is to find out whether you have a high level of glucose in your blood. If the blood test shows

If You Have Diabetes

Keeping blood glucose at a normal level in people with diabetes helps reduce the risk of problems. You can stay healthy by:

▶ Reaching and keeping a healthy weight

▶ Eating healthy, low-fat foods

▶ Getting regular exercise

▶ Not smoking

▶ Checking your feet each day. Prevent ingrown toenails, corns, and calluses on your feet to reduce the risk of infection.

▶ Talking to your doctor about pregnancy before you become pregnant

▶ Keeping your blood glucose level close to normal. If glucose cannot be controlled through weight loss, diet, exercise, or medication, insulin therapy may be needed. Insulin can be given by injection, pump, or oral medication.

▶ Asking your doctor about thyroid testing

▶ Getting regular health care. Have your feet, eyes, and kidneys checked by a doctor on a routine basis.

you have a high level of glucose, it may mean you have diabetes. There are three types of tests used to diagnose diabetes:

1. *Fasting plasma glucose*—This is the easiest and most common way to test for diabetes. Before the test, you must fast (not eat or drink anything but water) for at least 8 hours. One sample of blood is obtained.

2. *Random plasma glucose*—Your doctor may screen you when you are not fasting by measuring your glucose levels. If levels are high, a fasting plasma glucose or oral glucose tolerance test will be done to confirm the diagnosis.

3. *Oral glucose tolerance tests*—Before you have this test, you must fast overnight. You will first have a fasting plasma glucose test and then drink a sweet-tasting liquid that contains glucose. Blood samples are taken to measure your blood glucose over several hours.

If your test results are normal, you should be tested again in 3 years. If you are at risk or age 45 and older, you should be tested for diabetes every 3 years. If your test results show you have diabetes, your doctor will talk to you about treatment.

Problems

If diabetes is not controlled, long-term, severe health problems may occur:

▶ Kidney disease that can lead to high blood pressure or kidney failure

▶ Eye problems that can lead to blindness

▶ Nerve damage and blood vessel damage in the feet that can cause pain, numbness, infection, and possibly removal of a foot or toe

▶ High blood cholesterol levels that can lead to stroke and heart disease

▶ Certain infections, such as bladder or kidney infection, yeast infection, and skin infection

▶ Pregnancy complications

▶ Thyroid problems

The best defense against these problems is keeping your blood glucose at a normal level and taking good care of yourself. This can be done with lifestyle changes and taking insulin, if needed.

▶ DIABETES AND PREGNANCY

▶ See also *Diabetes*

Diabetes is of special concern during pregnancy. It can occur in women who are not pregnant, or it can start during pregnancy. The form of diabetes that occurs during pregnancy is called gestational diabetes. Either type of diabetes requires special care during pregnancy.

During pregnancy, the hormones produced by the placenta can change the way insulin works. As a result, gestational diabetes may occur or diabetes that existed before pregnancy may be harder to control.

Gestational diabetes can occur even when no risk factors or symptoms are present. For this reason, many doctors test all pregnant women for diabetes. Gestational diabetes goes away after the baby is born. However, more than half of women who have gestational diabetes will develop diabetes many years later. You should tell your doctor if you have had gestational diabetes.

The risk of diabetes increases with age. Other factors are linked with the condition:

Gestational diabetes affects about 4% of all pregnant women. That's about 135,000 cases in the United States each year, according to the American Diabetes Association.

▶ Obesity

▶ High blood pressure

▶ One or more family members with diabetes

Having these risk factors does not mean you will develop diabetes. It means that the chance is higher.

Effects During Pregnancy

The risk of problems during pregnancy is greatest when diabetes is not well controlled. Some of these problems may increase the chance of a cesarean birth. This is why you need good blood sugar control during pregnancy. Good control of glucose levels, before and during pregnancy, can lower the risks.

If you have diabetes or if you are at risk of developing gestational diabetes, you should understand the problems that may arise:

▸ Birth defects—such as heart defects, kidney problems, and spinal defects—occur more often in babies of women whose diabetes was not well controlled before pregnancy.

▸ Macrosomia (very large baby) occurs when the mother's blood sugar level is high. This allows too much sugar to go to the fetus. It can cause the fetus to grow too large. A baby that is too large can make delivery difficult. For instance, there may be problems delivering the baby's shoulders.

▸ Preeclampsia is high blood pressure during pregnancy. This can pose problems for the mother and the baby. It may require the baby to be delivered early. A woman with a mild form of preeclampsia may need to stay in the hospital so that she and her fetus can be monitored. Severe preeclampsia can lead to seizures.

▸ Hydramnios occurs when there is too much amniotic fluid in the sac surrounding the fetus. This can cause some women discomfort. It may result in preterm labor (labor before 37 weeks of pregnancy) and delivery.

▸ Urinary tract infections can occur without symptoms. If the infection is not treated, it may spread from the bladder to the kidneys and can harm the woman and her fetus.

▸ Respiratory distress syndrome (RDS) can make it harder for the baby to breathe after birth. The risk of RDS is greater in babies of mothers with diabetes.

Testing for Diabetes

The test for diabetes is safe and simple. It is usually done between 24 and 28 weeks of pregnancy. Samples of your blood are taken after you drink a sugar solution. Then the glucose level is measured. A high level suggests that there may be a problem with glucose control. If you have a high level of glucose, you will receive a diagnostic test. This test will diagnose diabetes if you have it.

Many doctors test for diabetes only in women with risk factors. Other doctors find that diabetes is common in the women they care for, so they test all women. In certain groups of people, such as Native Americans, diabetes is so common that some doctors go right to the diagnostic test.

Preparing for Pregnancy

If you have diabetes, preparing for pregnancy can improve your health and that of your future child. Plan to see your doctor before you get pregnant to discuss your care. You should try to have good control over your sugar levels a number of weeks before you become pregnant. Your doctor may suggest changes in your care.

The organs of a fetus begin to develop as soon as you become pregnant, before you may even know you are pregnant. This development can be affected by poorly controlled glucose levels in the weeks before conception or the first few weeks of your pregnancy.

Your doctor will help you monitor your blood glucose levels both before and during your pregnancy. If your glucose levels are high, you may be advised to wait until they are in the normal range before you get pregnant. The normal range for pregnancy may be lower than if you aren't pregnant. It may take several weeks or months to get your blood glucose to a normal level and keep it stable throughout the day. Be patient. This control is vital for the growth of a healthy baby.

Diabetes Control

There are several ways that you can measure your glucose level. All are safe and simple to use on a daily basis. You may need to check your glucose often each day to keep it at a normal level. To be most effective, the results should be kept accurately and reported to your doctor.

Glucose can be controlled with diet and exercise and, in some cases, by taking insulin. You and your doctor will decide together on the best method or mixture of methods for you.

Home Monitoring

Glucose meters or strips can be used to measure glucose levels. Because it is normal for the glucose level to change throughout the day, you may need to check it several times a day. Your doctor will tell you how often to check. Urine tests are not a good way to monitor glucose levels.

Diet

A balanced diet is key in pregnancy. The fetus depends on the food you eat for its growth and nourishment. This is even more important if you have diabetes. Not eating properly can cause glucose levels to change.

The number of calories in your diet will depend on your weight, stage of pregnancy, age, and level of activity. Your doctor may adjust your diet from time to time to improve glucose control or to meet the needs of the growing fetus. Usually the diet consists of small meals and snacks spread throughout the day. A bedtime snack will help keep glucose levels stable during the night.

For a Healthy Pregnancy

Your doctor may want to make some changes to your health care to better control your glucose levels:

▶ *Monitor your glucose levels more often.* You may be asked to check your glucose level more times a day than you have been doing.

▶ *Increase your folic acid.* You may be advised to take more than the recommended 0.4 mg a day of folic acid. Folic acid may help prevent certain birth defects called neural tube defects. It can be taken as a vitamin or can be found in certain foods such as leafy dark-green vegetables, citrus fruits, beans, and bread.

▶ *Change your work and lifestyle.* You may be asked to stop any strenuous work and to stop any habits that could harm the pregnancy.

▶ *Change your diet.* The kinds of food you eat as well as how often a day you eat will affect your glucose levels. Your doctor may make changes in your diet to control your levels.

▶ *Change your medications.* If you're taking certain medications, you may need to switch to others. This may include those bought over the counter.

Changes in Your Diet

During pregnancy, it is vital to eat a balanced diet. Your doctor may make changes in your diet to control glucose levels. For instance, women of medium height and normal weight should eat 2,200–2,400 calories per day. Proteins should make up 12–20% of those calories. Carbohydrates should make up 50–60% of those calories. Fats should account for the remainder of calories. About 25% of the calories should be consumed at breakfast, 30% at lunch, 30% at dinner, and 15% as a bedtime snack. The amount of calories you need is based on your weight before your pregnancy and the body mass index. Ask your doctor for more information how to eat healthy during pregnancy.

Exercise

Moderate exercise is always good. For women with diabetes it is even more important. Regular exercise reduces the amount of insulin needed to keep blood glucose levels normal. The amount of exercise that is right for each woman varies. You and your doctor will decide how much and what type of exercise you need.

Insulin

Some women with diabetes need to use insulin shots to keep their glucose at normal levels. Insulin shots can be safely used during pregnancy to control diabetes.

The amount of insulin needed to control glucose levels throughout the day varies from woman to woman and depends on many factors. Often the insulin dose needs to be changed for good control of glucose levels. Home monitoring of glucose levels helps set the insulin dose.

In many cases, insulin must be taken twice a day or more. Your doctor will tell you about how to use insulin and how many daily shots you'll need. The amounts you need may change during pregnancy.

Some women take pills instead of insulin. The use of pills to control diabetes is not advised during pregnancy. The medicine in such pills may affect the fetus. Women who control their diabetes by taking these pills often need to switch to insulin shots during pregnancy. When insulin is needed to control diabetes during pregnancy, the diet and the insulin dose must be balanced at all times to prevent harmful highs and lows in glucose levels.

Prenatal Care

You play an important role in controlling your diabetes. Prenatal care helps monitor your condition as well as that of the fetus. You may need to see your doctor more often for regular check-ups and tests.

A woman with diabetes often needs to have certain tests done more often in her pregnancy. These tests can help the doctor be aware of any problems and take steps to correct them. Your doctor can answer questions and give you more information about these tests:

- Hemoglobin A_{1C} is a substance in the woman's blood. Its levels may be higher when the woman's glucose level has been too high. Regular checking of hemoglobin A_{1C} can tell the doctor how well the glucose levels have been controlled during the past 2–3 months.

▶ Alpha-fetoprotein (AFP) is a substance made by a growing fetus. In a normal pregnancy, some AFP passes into the amniotic fluid and the mother's blood. Certain birth defects may cause abnormal amounts of AFP in the amniotic fluid and in the woman's blood. Many pregnancies with high maternal AFP levels are normal. If the maternal AFP is abnormal, more tests may be offered.

▶ Ultrasound uses sound waves to create a picture of the fetus. This allows the doctor to check the baby's growth and development.

▶ A kick count is a record of how often you feel your fetus move. A healthy fetus tends to move the same amount each day. You may be asked to keep track of this movement in the latter part of pregnancy and to contact your doctor if the baby is not active. It could mean the need for more tests and sometimes even early delivery of your baby.

▶ Electronic fetal monitoring helps your doctor detect signs of problems the fetus may be having late in pregnancy. Monitors are placed on the woman's abdomen. The heartbeat and activity of the fetus, as well as contractions of the woman's uterus, are then measured and recorded.

▶ Amniocentesis is a procedure used to obtain a small amount of amniotic fluid from the sac that surrounds the fetus. In early pregnancy, this can be done to detect certain birth defects. In late pregnancy, this procedure can help check whether the fetus's lungs are mature. This helps plan when your baby will be delivered. It also helps prevent respiratory distress syndrome (RDS).

A team of health care experts, including a dietician and special nurses, may help your doctor care for you during your pregnancy. Your doctor may consult with them or other doctors from time to time in handling special problems. You may need to stay in the hospital for special care.

Delivery

In most cases, women with diabetes go into labor normally when the time comes. Most women have a normal vaginal delivery. They may require special monitoring of the baby and of glucose levels. If there are problems during pregnancy, labor may need to be induced (brought on) early.

If you have gestational diabetes, your blood sugar level should be checked about 6 weeks after your baby is born. If your blood sugar level is normal at that time, it should be rechecked at least every 3 years.

Postpartum Care

Problems in the Newborn

After birth, your baby may need to spend a number of days in a special care nursery for the care of high-risk newborns. Some problems your baby may have include:

▶ Low glucose levels

▶ Low blood calcium and magnesium levels

▶ An excess of red blood cells

▶ Neonatal jaundice (yellow discoloration of the skin)

▶ Breathing problems (RDS)

These problems are usually not serious. They are all treated fairly easily soon after birth.

Breastfeeding

Women with diabetes can breastfeed their babies in most cases. If you decide to breastfeed, you may need to monitor your glucose levels more often.

Contraception

Good choices for hormonal birth control while you are breastfeeding are the minipill, implants, or injections. These are progestin-only, so they won't affect your milk supply.

Women with diabetes or gestational diabetes need to plan future pregnancies with care. Because you can become pregnant several weeks after childbirth, you should begin using a form of birth control right away. In general, women with diabetes can use most of the available methods. Your doctor can help you make a choice that will be safe and work well.

Glucose Control

If you have been taking insulin during pregnancy, the amount of insulin you use will change after delivery. If you had gestational diabetes, you are more likely to develop diabetes later in life. This is an important part of your medical history. Be sure to tell other doctors you see about it. You also should be tested from time to time for diabetes.

Weight Control

Weight loss during pregnancy is not a good idea—even if you are overweight. You and your doctor should set up a program of diet and exercise for you to follow after delivery. For women with gestational diabetes, diet and exercise may lower the risk of developing diabetes again.

▶ DIAPHRAGM

▶ See also *Barrier Methods of Contraception, Spermicide*

The diaphragm is a form of contraception (birth control). It is a round rubber dome that fits inside the woman's vagina and covers her cervix. It is always used with a spermicidal cream or jelly. Therefore, it acts as both a physical and a chemical barrier. The diaphragm requires a prescription. (The spermicide that is used with it does not.) You will need to see your doctor or nurse if you choose this method.

Diaphragms come in several sizes. You need to be examined to find out which size fits you best. After a type and size of diaphragm is prescribed for you, you will be shown how to insert and remove it. You will also learn how to check that the diaphragm is placed properly. The first time you do this should be in the doctor's office or clinic so that the doctor or nurse can tell you if you are inserting it correctly.

Here are the basic steps to insert a diaphragm. Your doctor or nurse will give you complete instructions.

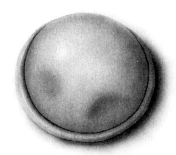

Diaphragm

1. Apply spermicidal cream or jelly around the rim and inside the dome of the diaphragm. The spermicide must be on the side of the diaphragm facing or in contact with the cervix. It also can be put on both sides.

2. Squeeze the rim of the diaphragm between your fingers and insert it into your vagina. When the diaphragm is pushed up as far as it will go, the front part of the rim should be up behind a bone you can feel in front of your pelvis (the pubic bone). Tuck the front rim of the diaphragm up as far as it will comfortably go.

3. Check to see if your cervix is covered. To do this, reach inside and touch your cervix. The cervix feels something like the tip of your nose. If you have trouble finding your cervix, talk with your doctor or nurse about how to place the diaphragm. After the diaphragm is in place, the cervix should be completely covered by the rubber dome.

The diaphragm may be put in place up to 6 hours before you have sex. No matter when you insert the diaphragm, always be sure to use a spermicide. Diaphragms should not be used without this added protection. If you have put in the diaphragm more than 2 hours before having sex, you must insert a fresh supply of spermicide into your vagina just before intercourse. You must also check the position of the diaphragm and add more spermicide before each act of intercourse, no matter how

Of 100 women using diaphragms about 20 will become pregnant during a year of typical use. Of 100 women who use the diaphragm correctly and consistently, about 6 will become pregnant during a year of use.

closely together they occur. To do this, insert the spermicide with an applicator while the diaphragm is still in place. An applicator usually comes with the spermicidal cream or jelly. You can also ask for one when you get your diaphragm.

Do not use any oil-based lubricants such as petroleum jelly when you use a diaphragm. The oil can damage the rubber. Only water-based lubricants can be used safely with a diaphragm.

After sex, the diaphragm must be left in place for about 6 hours. To remove the diaphragm, pull gently on the front rim. Wash it with mild soap and water, rinse the soap off well (soap can harm the rubber and irritate your vagina), dry it, and put it back in its case.

A diaphragm may become discolored over time, but it can still be used unless you notice any holes in the rubber. To check for holes, hold the diaphragm up to the light and stretch the rubber gently between your fingers. Filling the diaphragm with water is another way to check for holes. You should get a new diaphragm about every 2 years.

A properly sized and fitted diaphragm should not cause pain or pressure to either you or your partner during sex. Have your diaphragm checked at your regular exam every year. Also have it rechecked if:

▶ You begin to have trouble with your diaphragm slipping out of place

▶ You have had pelvic surgery or have been pregnant

▶ You have gained or lost a lot of weight

The diaphragm will prevent pregnancy only if you use it correctly each time you have sex. Be sure to use enough spermicidal cream or jelly and check that the diaphragm is placed properly before each act of intercourse.

There may be an increased risk of urinary tract infection with use of the diaphragm. This is an infection of the bladder or the urethra or both. If you get a urinary tract infection, your doctor can give you antibiotics to treat it. If you keep having infections, you may need to use a different size or type of diaphragm. Or, you may want to think about using another type of birth control.

▶ DIARRHEA

Diarrhea, a bowel problem, is having three or more loose bowel movements a day. It may also be accompanied by cramping. Diarrhea is not usually a serious threat to your health, but it can be unpleasant.

Several things can cause diarrhea:

▶ Eating spoiled or improperly handled food

▶ Drinking or eating foods that contain bacteria your body is not used to (for example, when traveling to foreign countries)

▶ Eating or drinking dairy products (if you are lactose intolerant), caffeine, artificial sweeteners, or certain additives

▶ Taking medications, especially antibiotics

Diarrhea can cause dehydration if it continues, so it is important to drink plenty of fluids to replenish those that are lost. If your diarrhea doesn't go away in a few hours, drink electrolyte fluids to replace the lost fluids. Ask your doctor or pharmacist to suggest one. Avoid drinking soda and juices. If diarrhea persists for more than 24 hours or if you also have bloody stools, fever, or severe abdominal pain, see your doctor right away.

Travel Tips

Traveler's diarrhea happens when you eat food or drink water that has bacteria, viruses, or parasites in it. You can take the following precautions to prevent traveler's diarrhea when you go abroad:

▶ Do not drink any tap water, not even when brushing your teeth.

▶ Do not drink unpasteurized milk or dairy products.

▶ Do not use ice made from tap water.

▶ Avoid all raw fruits and vegetables (including lettuce and fruit salad) unless they can be peeled and you peel them yourself.

▶ Do not eat raw or rare meat and fish.

▶ Do not eat meat or shellfish that is not hot when served to you.

▶ Do not eat food from street vendors.

You can safely drink bottled water (if you are the one to break the seal), carbonated soft drinks, and hot drinks like coffee or tea. Depending on where you are going and how long you are staying, your doctor may recommend that you take antibiotics before leaving to protect you from possible infection.

▶ DIETHYLSTILBESTROL

Diethylstilbestrol (DES) is a synthetic (manmade) form of estrogen, a female hormone. Between 1945 and 1971, doctors prescribed DES to help prevent miscarriage in 5 million to 10 million pregnant women. In 1971, doctors were told to stop prescribing DES to expectant mothers because it was found to cause problems in the women and babies exposed to it.

Women who used DES may have a higher risk of breast cancer. These women should be sure to perform a breast self-exam monthly and have mammograms regularly.

It was found that the daughters of women who took DES while pregnant had a higher risk of a cancer called clear cell adenocarcinoma. Certain defects in the vagina, uterus, or cervix were more common. Their periods may be irregular. If they become pregnant, they have an increased risk of miscarriage and preterm births. There is no evidence that children of women whose mothers took DES have a higher risk of birth defects or other problems.

Sons of women who took DES may have defects in their testicles. Doctors still are unsure of all the health problems linked to DES in women and their offspring.

Women who think they may have been exposed to DES before birth should tell their doctor. They should have a complete exam, including:

▶ Pelvic exam

▶ Exam of the rectum, vagina, uterus, cervix, and ovaries

▶ Pap test

▶ Colposcopy (if the results of a Pap test are not normal)

▶ Biopsy (to remove and check any cells that seem abnormal)

▶ Regular breast exams

▶ See also *Miscarriage, Uterine Bleeding*

▶ DILATION AND CURETTAGE

Dilation and curettage (D&C) is a procedure used to diagnose or treat abnormal bleeding from the uterus. It can be used to help detect cancer of the uterus or remove tissue when a miscarriage occurs.

Dilation means to stretch the opening of the cervix to make it wider. Curettage involves removing a sample of the lining of the uterus—endometrium—to be examined later. This may be done with a metal device or with suction.

Reasons

A D&C may be done to assess conditions that could cause abnormal bleeding. It provides a sample of the tissue in the uterus. This sample can be viewed under a microscope to tell whether cells are abnormal. A D&C may be done for a number of reasons.

The Procedure

A D&C can be done in a doctor's office, an outpatient clinic, or a hospital. Your health and the type of anesthesia to be used will play a part in determining where the procedure is performed. The D&C may be done with other procedures such as hysteroscopy, in which a small, lighted telescope is used to view the inside of the uterus. An endometrial biopsy is sometimes performed to obtain similar information about the inside of the uterus. This is an office test and usually does not require stretching or dilating the cervix.

Your doctor may want to start dilating your cervix before surgery. If so, a slender rod (called laminaria) will be inserted into the opening of the cervix. It will be left in several hours.

The rod absorbs water from the cervix. This causes the rod to swell and widen the opening of the cervix.

Before your doctor begins the D&C, you may receive some type of anesthesia. You and your doctor will agree on the type to be used.

With general anesthesia, you will not be awake during the procedure. You will receive medication either through an intravenous (IV) line or a mask.

With local anesthesia, you will be awake. The area around the cervix may be numbed with medication.

During the procedure you will lie on your back and your legs will be placed in stirrups. The doctor will then insert a speculum into your vagina in the same way as for a pelvic exam. The cervix is held in place with a clamp.

The cervix is then slowly opened (dilated). Tissue lining the uterus is removed, either with an instrument called a curette or with suction. The tissue will then be sent to a laboratory for examination.

The D & C Procedure

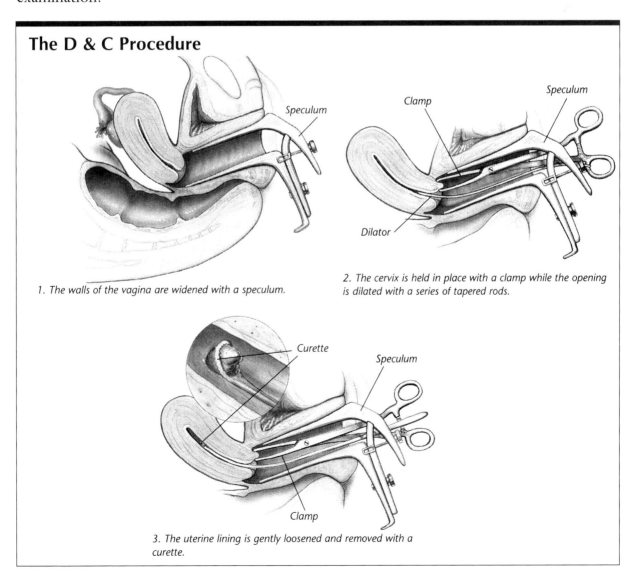

1. The walls of the vagina are widened with a speculum.

2. The cervix is held in place with a clamp while the opening is dilated with a series of tapered rods.

3. The uterine lining is gently loosened and removed with a curette.

Risks

Complications are rare. When they do occur, they include bleeding, infection, or perforation (when the tip of an instrument passes through the wall of the uterus). You should contact your doctor if you have any of the following:

▶ Heavy bleeding from the vagina

▶ Fever

▶ Pain in the abdomen

▶ Foul-smelling discharge from the vagina

Recovery

After the procedure, you will probably be able to go home within a few hours. You will need someone to take you home. You should be able to resume most of your regular activities in 1 or 2 days.

If you had general anesthesia, you may have some nausea and vomiting when you wake up. You may feel groggy and weak for a short while.

During your recovery, you may have:

▶ A sore throat (if a tube was inserted into your windpipe to help you breathe during general anesthesia)

▶ Mild cramping

▶ Spotting or light bleeding

After a D&C, a new lining will build up in the uterus. Your next menstrual period may not occur at the regular time. It may be early or late. It also may be heavier or lighter than normal.

Until your cervix returns to its normal size, bacteria can enter the uterus and cause infection. It is important not to put anything into your vagina after the procedure. Ask your doctor when you can have sexual intercourse or use tampons again.

▶ See also *Alcohol Use* in *Pregnancy, Birth Defects*

▶ DRUGS AND PREGNANCY

It is normal for pregnant women to worry about whether they will give birth to a healthy baby. There are several things you can do to increase the chances that your baby will be born healthy. One of them is to avoid taking drugs while you are pregnant so that your baby can have a good start in life.

Anything you eat, drink, or smoke can affect your fetus. Don't use any drug unless the doctor providing your pregnancy care tells you it's okay. Some prescription drugs can be harmful. If you need help in stopping drug use, you should know that you are not alone and that you can get help.

How Drugs Can Affect Pregnancy

Drug use is widespread. It affects people of all backgrounds. As many as 1 in 10 babies may be exposed to illegal drugs during pregnancy. An even greater number of babies may be exposed to legal drugs, such as alcohol, tobacco, and some prescription medicines. During pregnancy, the use of these drugs can be harmful to the health and growth of your fetus. They have the greatest effect early in pregnancy—so if you are using these drugs you should stop before you get pregnant.

A woman's drug use can affect both her fetus and her newborn. Most drugs cross the placenta—the organ that provides nourishment to the fetus. Some can cause direct toxic (poisonous) effects and drug dependency in the fetus. After birth, some drugs can be passed to the baby through breastfeeding.

How the fetus will react to a certain drug depends on how much of the drug enters the pregnant woman's body, how often the drug is used, and when during pregnancy the drug is used. If drugs are taken together, it can be hard to predict the effects. Sometimes the drugs add to each other's effect.

Drugs can cause problems throughout your pregnancy. For instance, the early part of pregnancy is the most vital for the health of a fetus. This is when the main body systems are forming. Using drugs during this time can cause severe damage. During the last 12 weeks of pregnancy, drug use poses the greatest risk for stunting fetal growth and causing preterm birth.

Drug use may have long-term effects. For instance, using needles that have been used before by others can cause infection. It also can increase the risk of getting hepatitis B virus or human immunodeficiency virus (HIV), the virus that causes acquired immunodeficiency syndrome (AIDS). These viruses then can be passed to the fetus through the placenta.

Alcohol

Alcohol is found in many kinds of drinks. Beer, wine, wine coolers, and liquor all contain alcohol. Alcohol slows down body functions, such as the beating of the heart and breathing. If you are pregnant, alcohol quickly reaches your fetus through your bloodstream. The same level of alcohol that goes through your bloodstream goes through the bloodstream of your fetus.

Women who drink heavily while pregnant have a higher risk of miscarriage than women who don't drink. The more a woman drinks while pregnant, the greater the danger to the fetus. The risk is greatest early in pregnancy.

Do You Have a Drinking Problem?

There are several tests to use to find problem drinking. One is TACE and another is CAGE. See Alcohol in "Women's Wellness."

Accutane

Accutane (isotretinoin) is a prescription drug used to treat severe acne. This drug can cause serious birth defects if taken during a woman's pregnancy. The drug label recommends that any woman of childbearing age who takes Accutane should use two forms of birth control to be sure she does not get pregnant.

Heavy use of alcohol may cause fetal alcohol syndrome. This is the most common cause of mental retardation in babies. Babies can be shorter, weigh less, have heart and face defects, and have poor control over body movements. Hyperactivity can occur. These children are nervous, jittery, and have a poor attention span.

Some of the harmful effects of alcohol for the woman are:

) Vitamin and mineral deficiency

) Damage to the heart, brain, liver, muscles, and digestive system

) Poor muscle control

) Depression

) Higher risk of certain cancers

Is there a safe level of drinking for a pregnant woman? It isn't known how much is harmful. Therefore, the safest course is not to drink alcohol while you are pregnant. This will increase your chances of having a healthy, normal baby.

Smoking

When you smoke before, during, or after birth, you risk not only your own health but that of your baby. Each puff subjects you and the fetus to harmful chemicals such as nicotine, tar, and carbon monoxide. If you or anyone else smokes around the baby after he or she is born, the baby is exposed to the harmful effects of the smoke.

Smoking may make it harder for you to have a normal pregnancy. If you smoke, you are more likely to have:

) An ectopic pregnancy

) A miscarriage

) A stillbirth

) A preterm baby

) Vaginal bleeding

) Problems with the way the placenta attaches to the uterus

) A baby with low birth weight (weighing less than 5½ pounds at birth)

) A baby with sudden infant death syndrome

Prescription Drugs

If you are pregnant or planning to become pregnant, you should discuss the use of any prescription drugs with your doctor. Certain prescription drugs can cause birth defects. These may include drugs used to treat:

) Acne

) Infection

) Epilepsy

) Blood clots

) Breast cancer

If you smoke, you have a higher risk of major disease, including:

▶ Lung cancer

▶ Cancer of the cervix

▶ Bladder cancer

▶ Heart disease

▶ Chronic lung diseases like emphysema and bronchitis

The sooner you quit smoking, the better it will be for both you and your baby. If you stop during the early months of pregnancy, your chance of having a low-birth-weight baby will be close to that of a woman who doesn't smoke. If you can quit while you are pregnant, you can quit for a lifetime.

If you can't quit, cut back to as few cigarettes as possible. Cutting down or stopping smoking at any time while you are pregnant is better than not stopping at all.

Tell your doctor if you need help quitting. If you are a heavy smoker and have not been able to quit or cut down, you may be able to use a nicotine patch to help you quit while you are still pregnant. There are risks to using the patch during pregnancy, but the risk of heavy smoking may be greater.

Cocaine

Cocaine is a highly addictive drug. It can be used by injection with a needle, through the nose (snorting), or by smoking (freebasing).

Cocaine may cause the placenta to detach from the uterus too soon (placental abruption). This can cause bleeding, preterm birth, and fetal death. Women who use cocaine have a 25% higher chance of having a preterm birth. The fetus also may have withdrawal symptoms. Babies born to mothers who use cocaine may:

▶ Grow more slowly

▶ Have smaller heads

▶ Have brain injury

▶ Be irritable and fussy

For the pregnant woman, cocaine use can lead to high blood pressure or sudden death from stroke or heart attack. People who use cocaine can come to depend on it. This can disrupt their home, family, and work life.

For information on treating a drug or alcohol problem, call the Center for Substance Abuse Treatment National Drug and Alcohol Treatment Referral Service at 800-622-HELP. For help to quit smoking, call 800-4-CANCER (800-422-6237).

Marijuana

Marijuana, also called grass or pot, is smoked or eaten. As with cigarettes, your fetus is exposed to the marijuana smoke you inhale. The effects of marijuana use during pregnancy are not well-known. Because marijuana is a drug, it is best not to expose your fetus to it.

Heroin and Other Narcotics

Heroin is smoked or is injected through the veins. Heroin can cause preterm birth or fetal death, addiction in the fetus, and low birth weight. Studies of children of mothers who used heroin showed that some children were smaller, had trouble thinking clearly, and had behavior problems.

Women who use heroin often become addicted to it. They may die from overdose. Sudden withdrawal can harm the woman and the fetus. Methadone often is used to replace heroin in drug treatment centers. This should be used only under a doctor's care.

If you need help kicking a drug habit, talk to your doctor. You also can call 800-COCAINE (800-262-2463) or 800-662-4357 to receive drug and treatment information.

"T's and blues" is the street name for a certain mixture of a prescription narcotic drug and an over-the-counter antihistamine drug. It often is used as a cheap substitute for heroin. Babies of mothers who use T's and blues are more likely to grow more slowly before they are born. They also may have withdrawal symptoms.

PCP and LSD

PCP, or angel dust, often is smoked. It can be eaten, snorted, or injected. Its effects are not always the same. PCP can cause a user to lose touch with what is real. The woman can have flashbacks, seizures, heart attacks, and lung failure that leads to death. Violent acts are common. Use can lead to small babies and babies with poor control of their movements.

LSD, or acid, is taken by mouth. It can cause hallucinations, such as hearing and seeing things when nothing is there. Users may have violent behavior and flashbacks. Use of LSD may lead to birth defects in the baby.

Glues and Solvents

Glues and solvents sometimes are inhaled or sniffed to give a short-term "high" feeling. Glues and solvents can cause light-headedness, dizziness, and even sudden death. They also may cause damage to the liver, kidneys, bone marrow, and brain. The sniffing of these fumes may cause birth defects in the baby like those caused by alcohol.

Amphetamines

Amphetamines, also called uppers or speed, are taken in pill form. They can cause agitation and insomnia. They also cause loss of appetite. Pregnant women who use them may not get enough nutrients for their growing fetus. Users can come to depend on them and can overdose.

Tranquilizers and Sleeping Pills

Tranquilizers and sleeping pills, or downers, are used to produce a calm feeling and relieve stress. If the mother takes these drugs, the newborn can become inactive, have poor muscle tone, and have trouble breathing and feeding. These drugs' effects can last longer in newborns than in adults. For the woman, dependency and overdose can occur.

▶ DYSMENORRHEA

More than half of women who have menstrual periods have some pain for at least 1–2 days each month. Usually, the pain is mild. Sometimes, however, the pain is severe enough to keep them from their normal activities. When the pain is this severe, it is called dysmenorrhea.

Dysmenorrhea is common. Painful periods are the leading cause of women missing work and school.

Causes of Menstrual Pain

The uterus is a muscle, and like all muscles, it contracts and relaxes. This happens throughout the menstrual cycle. During your period, the uterus contracts more strongly. These contractions are caused by prostaglandins—a substance made by the endometrium (the lining of the uterus). Sometimes, when the uterus contracts it produces a cramping pain.

Before your period, the level of prostaglandins in your body increases. Prostaglandin is released when your period starts. As you menstruate, prostaglandin levels decrease. This is why pain tends to lessen after the first few days of your period.

Types of Dysmenorrhea

There are two types of dysmenorrhea. Pain during your period can be classified as either primary or secondary dysmenorrhea.

Primary dysmenorrhea is pain from having a period. Secondary dysmenorrhea is pain during a period that has another cause.

Primary Dysmenorrhea

Primary dysmenorrhea is pelvic pain that is the result of having your period. Women with primary dysmenorrhea may have any of the following symptoms:

▶ Cramps or pain in the lower abdomen or lower back

▶ Pulling feeling in the inner thighs

▶ Diarrhea

▶ Nausea

▶ Vomiting

▶ Headache

▶ Dizziness

Primary dysmenorrhea often begins soon after a girl begins having menstrual periods. As a woman gets older, her periods often become less painful. The pain may lessen after a woman gives birth. Not every woman is the same, however, and some do continue to have pain during their periods. Some cycles may be more painful than others.

Secondary Dysmenorrhea

Secondary dysmenorrhea is menstrual pain that has another cause in addition to menstruation. With secondary dysmenorrhea, pain often begins earlier in the menstrual cycle. It usually lasts longer than normal cramps. For example, it may begin long before your period starts, it may get worse with your period, or it may not go away after your period ends.

Some of the most common causes of secondary dysmenorrhea are:

▶ *Endometriosis*—A condition in which endometrial tissue is found in other areas in the body, such as the ovaries and fallopian tubes. This tissue acts like tissue in the uterus. Endometrial tissue outside the uterus responds to monthly changes in hormones the same way it does inside the uterus. It also breaks down and bleeds. This bleeding can cause pain, especially during your period.

▶ *Fibroids*—Tumors or growths that form on the outside, inside, or in the wall of the uterus. They are not cancerous, but they can cause more pain and heavier bleeding with periods.

▶ *Pelvic inflammatory disease*—An infection of the uterus, fallopian tubes, or ovaries. Most cases develop from sexually transmitted diseases (STDs).

▶ *Intrauterine device (IUD)*— A device placed in the uterus to prevent pregnancy. It can cause pelvic pain and cramping and may make normal menstrual cramps worse.

The intrauterine device may not be the best method of birth control for women with dysmenorrhea. This condition can increase the chance of having problems with an IUD.

Diagnosing Dysmenorrhea

Dysmenorrhea is diagnosed by exams and tests. Some of the tests may need to be done outside the doctor's office. For your doctor to diagnose a cause for dysmenorrhea, you will be asked to describe your history, symptoms, and menstrual cycles. Your doctor will then do a pelvic exam to check for anything abnormal in the reproductive organs. A Pap test, cultures, and blood samples may be taken. An ultrasound exam of the pelvic organs is sometimes done to further check for anything abnormal.

In some cases, the doctor can learn more by looking directly inside your body. This is usually done by laparoscopy. During laparoscopy, the doctor makes a small cut near your navel. A thin lighted scope—a laparoscope—is then inserted into your abdomen. The laparoscope allows the doctor to view the pelvic organs.

Sometimes, the doctor is able to find a cause for the dysmenorrhea. But, often there is no known cause. Based on the results of the tests, you and your doctor will decide which treatment is best for you.

Medications

There are effective ways to treat menstrual pain. Your doctor can prescribe or suggest medications that can help relieve your discomfort.

NSAIDS

NSAIDs (nonsteroidal anti-inflammatory drugs) are drugs that block the production of the prostaglandins that cause menstrual cramps. These drugs also can prevent the other symptoms caused by prostaglandins, such as nausea, diarrhea, and pain. You can buy most NSAIDs, such as ibuprofen or naproxen, over the counter. If these do not relieve your pain, talk to your doctor. He or she may prescribe some stronger medications.

NSAIDs work best when they are taken at the first sign of your period or pain. You usually need to take them only for 1 or 2 days. Do not take more pills than the package recommends. You should avoid taking NSAIDs while drinking alcohol. Women with bleeding disorders, liver damage, stomach disorders, or ulcers should not take NSAIDs.

Finding Relief

Besides medical treatment that your doctor may suggest, there are things you can do on your own to help ease the pain of your menstrual periods:

- **Exercise**—Women who exercise regularly often have less menstrual pain. Aerobic exercise, such as walking, jogging, biking, or swimming, can be helpful.

- **Heat**—A warm bath or a heating pad or hot water bottle on your abdomen can be soothing.

- **Sleep**—Making sure you get enough sleep before and during your period can help you cope with any discomfort.

- **Sex**—Orgasms can relieve menstrual cramps in some women.

- **Relaxation**—Exercises, like meditation and yoga, can help you relax and increase your ability to cope with pain.

Oral Contraceptives

Taking oral contraceptives (birth control pills) also reduces menstrual pain. The birth control pill causes less growth of the endometrium. Less prostaglandin is produced, and there are fewer strong contractions, less flow, and less pain. Birth control pills can be used along with NSAIDs if necessary.

E

▸ EATING DISORDERS

In the United States, 7 million women and girls have eating disorders. Eating disorders are less common in men and boys, but they do occur. The three main types of eating disorders are anorexia nervosa, bulimia nervosa, and binge eating disorder. Eating disorders are serious problems. With proper medical care and counseling, they can be treated.

What Are Eating Disorders?

Eating disorders are not fads and they are not diets. They are serious conditions that can lead to severe health problems—and even death.

A person with an eating disorder is obsessed with food, body weight, and body shape. People with these problems:

▸ Try to manage their weight in ways that are not healthy

▸ Eat too little food or too much food

Eating disorders affect the person as well as her family, friends, and others around her.

Are you worried about your own eating habits or those of someone you know? Call the National Eating Disorders Screening Program at 800-405-9100 to find out where you can get a free screening test.

Who Gets Eating Disorders?

People of all backgrounds and ages can have eating disorders. These problems are most common among women and girls. They most often begin between the ages of 11 and 20.

Eating disorders are complex problems. There is no single cause, but dieting is a common factor. This does not mean that any person who diets has or will have an eating disorder.

People with eating disorders often:

- Have a fear of being fat

- Have a distorted view of their body shape

- Have low self-esteem

- Have depression

- Are very unhappy with their bodies

- Want to be perfect

Eating disorders often arise during stressful times, such as the teenage years. Leaving home or losing a loved one through death or divorce also is stressful.

These disorders often hide other problems. They may be a symptom of family, social, school, or work problems.

Types of Eating Disorders

Anorexia nervosa (also called anorexia), bulimia nervosa (also called bulimia), and binge-eating disorder are the three main types of eating disorders. They often have different warning signs and result in different health problems.

In addition to physical problems, mental and social problems also may result from eating disorders. They can harm a person's family, school, social, and career life.

Anorexia Nervosa

A person with anorexia nervosa diets to extremes because she has a distorted body image—she feels she is too fat. Most girls or women with anorexia have an intense fear of being fat. They want to be thin so badly that they may starve themselves—sometimes to death.

Some women with anorexia do not eat at all or eat very little. Some women with anorexia eat in excess and then purge themselves by vomiting or taking laxatives. They also may exercise to extremes. For many people, anorexia is an addiction, like alcoholism.

People with anorexia often feel shame and guilt. They may become withdrawn. They also may deny that their severe weight loss or dieting is a problem. They may deny that they are underweight. In fact, they do not think they are thin enough.

Anorexia can cause severe and sometimes long-term health problems. These problems may include:

- An irregular heartbeat, which can lead to heart failure and death

- Bone loss, which can lead to osteoporosis

- Low body temperature

Women with anorexia have trouble getting pregnant because they often stop menstruating. They also are at risk of having a baby that's too small or born too early. If they do manage to conceive, these women are more likely to miscarry or to have a cesarean birth.

- Low blood pressure
- Kidney problems
- A slowed metabolism (the body's way of using energy from food)
- Slow reflexes

Treatment in a hospital is needed for many people with anorexia. About 5–10% of people die from problems caused by the disorder. It may lead to a heart attack, a coma, or suicide.

Many people with anorexia also have bulimia at some point. In fact, about half of people with anorexia also have signs of bulimia, or vice versa.

Bulimia Nervosa

People with bulimia nervosa binge (eat large amounts of food in a short time). They then purge the excess calories by:

- Vomiting
- Using laxatives, diuretics (water pills), or emetics (pills that cause vomiting)
- Fasting
- Exercising to extremes

People with bulimia sometimes eat 20,000 calories in a single binge. They often feel out of control and know that their behavior is not normal.

Bulimia is harder than anorexia to detect. This is because the person's weight often is normal or just above normal. The person's weight may quickly go up or down 10 pounds or more because of binges and fasts.

Bulimia can cause severe medical problems such as:

- Dehydration
- Damage to the bowels, liver, and kidney
- Damage to the throat, esophagus, and stomach (caused by self-induced vomiting)
- An irregular heartbeat and sometimes heart failure
- Problems with teeth and gums

Women with bulimia may have a higher rate of miscarriage. They also risk delivering low-birth-weight babies and babies with certain birth defects.

People with bulimia know their eating is out of control, but they are afraid of being fat and of not being able to stop eating. Ridding the body of excess calories may help them feel they have regained control over their bodies.

They often feel very depressed, guilty, and shameful after they binge. They may feel that they must hide the problem from others.

Binge Eating Disorder

Binge eating (also called compulsive eating) may be the most common of the eating disorders. About 2 out of every 100 American adults have this disorder. Slightly more women than men have it.

Binge eating involves eating large amounts of food. In this way, it is like bulimia. Binge eaters do not purge after binging, though. Binge eaters may eat regular meals and snacks throughout the day. Sometimes they may overeat all day rather than binging.

Binge eaters usually become overweight or obese. In fact, up to 40% of obese people may be binge eaters.

Binge eaters often do their binge eating in secret. They then feel depressed, guilty, or shameful.

Anger, sadness, boredom, or anxiety may trigger a binge. Dieting may worsen binge eating in some people.

Signs of Eating Disorders

If you or someone you know has some of the symptoms listed here, seek help. These symptoms may be signs of an eating disorder.

Anorexia Nervosa

- Diets nonstop, even when thin, and refuses to eat except in small portions or wants to eat alone
- Has lost a lot of weight and still thinks they are fat
- Stops having menstrual periods
- Exercises excessively
- Has fine hair growing on the face and arms
- Is losing hair
- Has dry, pale, yellowed skin
- Is withdrawn and irritable

Bulimia Nervosa

- Makes up reasons to go to the bathroom after meals
- Purges by vomiting or abusing laxatives or diuretics
- Is on a strict diet, fasts, or exercises to extremes to lose weight
- Has swelling around the jaw
- Has bloodshot eyes
- Is bloated
- Has problems with teeth and gums
- Is weak and tired
- Has mood swings and seems out of control
- Buys large amounts of food that suddenly disappear

Binge Eating Disorder

- Weight goes up and down
- Is obese
- Eats a large amount of food in a short time
- Eats quickly
- Diets often
- Is withdrawn socially and often eats alone
- Becomes depressed, irritated, and disgusted after overeating

The causes of binge eating are not known. As many as half of all people with this problem have a history of depression. Many binge eaters have trouble keeping other areas of their lives under control.

Binge eating may cause severe medical problems, such as:

- High blood pressure
- High cholesterol levels (which can cause the arteries to harden and can cause heart disease and heart attacks)
- Gall bladder disease
- Diabetes
- Certain types of cancer

Getting Help

There is treatment for eating disorders. The first step to overcoming an eating disorder is to know that a problem exists and that help is needed. Family and friends can help the person become aware of the problem. Eating disorders may be diagnosed by a doctor or other health care worker.

People with eating disorders may become angry or defensive when someone tries to help, or they may be relieved that someone wants to help. Be sensitive to the person's feelings. Let her know that you care about her well-being.

Treatment often involves a doctor's care or going into the hospital. Medication also may be used to help treat the disorder as well as the health problems caused by it. Treatment also includes either single, family, or group counseling.

Ask for help if you believe that you, a family member, or a friend has an eating disorder. Not all doctors are trained to treat eating disorders. They can refer you to someone who can help. You also may want to contact local self-help and support groups that help people with eating disorders.

▶ ECTOPIC PREGNANCY

Sometimes the fertilized egg doesn't reach the uterus. It begins to grow in the fallopian tube or, rarely, attaches to an ovary or other organs in the stomach. This is called an ectopic pregnancy. Because it is outside the uterus, an ectopic pregnancy cannot grow as it should and must be treated. About 1 in 60 pregnancies is ectopic.

Almost all ectopic pregnancies occur in the fallopian tube. Because the tube is so narrow and its wall is so thin, the pregnancy

Ectopic Pregnancy

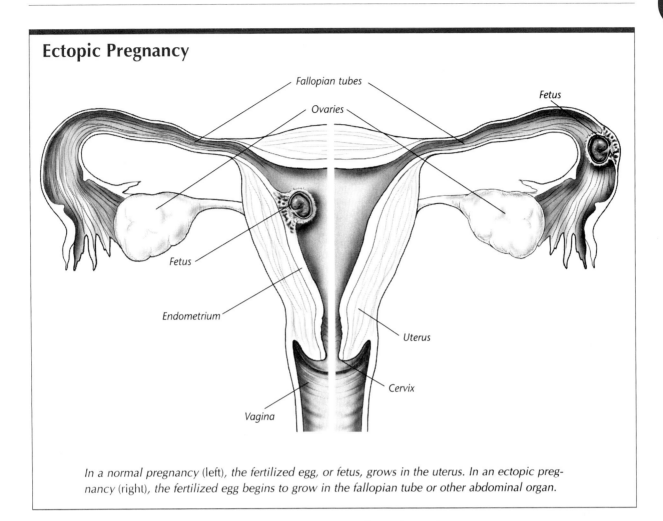

In a normal pregnancy (left), the fertilized egg, or fetus, grows in the uterus. In an ectopic pregnancy (right), the fertilized egg begins to grow in the fallopian tube or other abdominal organ.

can grow to only about the size of a walnut before the tube bursts. This can occur any time in the first 3 months of pregnancy. Because the tube may burst and cause major bleeding, ectopic pregnancy must be treated promptly once it is found.

Women who have abnormal fallopian tubes are at higher risk for ectopic pregnancy. These abnormalities may be present in women who have had:

- Pelvic inflammatory disease or salpingitis

- Previous ectopic pregnancy

- Infertility

- Pelvic or abdominal surgery (for instance, appendectomy)

- Endometriosis

Symptoms and Diagnosis

Ectopic pregnancies can be hard to diagnose. Some women may have no symptoms at all and may not even know that they are pregnant. The symptoms of ectopic pregnancy sometimes include the symptoms of pregnancy, such as tender breasts or upset stomach. Other symptoms may include:

▶ *Vaginal bleeding.* Bleeding will be unlike your normal menstrual bleeding. Bleeding may be lighter or heavier than is normal.

▶ *Abdominal pain.* This can be sudden and sharp and ache without relief or seem to come and go. It often occurs on one side of the stomach.

▶ *Shoulder pain.* Blood from the ruptured fallopian tube area can build up in the stomach under the diaphragm (the area between your chest and stomach). This causes pain that is felt in the shoulder.

▶ *Weakness, dizziness, or fainting*

Because an ectopic pregnancy can occur without warning, you should call your doctor right away about any pain or bleeding. Call even if you do not think there really is a problem.

If your doctor suspects that you may have an ectopic pregnancy, he or she may give you a pelvic exam, perform blood tests, or give you an ultrasound exam. The results may not be clear right away, and these tests may need to be done again. Surgery may be needed to be certain of the presence of an ectopic pregnancy. Your doctor may perform a laparoscopy, in which a slender, light-transmitting telescope is inserted through a small opening in your stomach. This test is done in an operating room with general anesthesia. It allows the doctor to see inside your body. A dilation and curettage (D&C) is another option. It may be performed to check for signs of an early miscarriage.

If your doctor suspects that you have an ectopic pregnancy that has ruptured, it is an emergency. You will need to have surgery right away.

Treatment

If your doctor thinks you have an ectopic pregnancy, he or she will decide on the best treatment based on your medical condition and your future plans for pregnancy.

Sometimes, if the pregnancy is small and the tube is not ruptured, the pregnancy can be lifted out through a hole made in the tube during a laparoscopy. A bit of pregnancy tissue may remain after the procedure. Blood testing over a few weeks may be needed after the treatment to check for this.

A laparotomy—in which a larger incision is made in the stomach—may be needed if the pregnancy is large or the blood loss is thought to be life threatening. During laparotomy, the

A woman who has an ectopic pregnancy may be treated with the drug methotrexate, which allows the body to absorb the pregnancy tissue and may save the fallopian tube. This treatment is most effective early in the pregnancy. If the tube has become stretched or it has ruptured and started bleeding, all or part of the fallopian tube may have to be removed.

pregnancy may be lifted out through an opening in the tube or some or all of the tube may be removed.

Sometimes medications can be prescribed to stop the growth of the pregnancy tissue and permit the body to absorb it over time. These medications are used only when the pregnancy is small, the tube has not ruptured, and there is no bleeding. Not all medical centers provide this type of treatment. Careful follow-up over time is needed.

If your tube bursts, you will have bleeding inside the stomach. The bleeding may be heavy. Bleeding needs to be stopped promptly, and emergency surgery is needed. If little damage has been done to the tube, the doctor may try to repair it. But in many cases, a ruptured tube must be removed.

If the tubes have been left in place, there is a fairly good chance that you can have a normal pregnancy in the future. Once you have had an ectopic pregnancy, though, you are at higher risk for having another one.

▶ EMERGENCY CONTRACEPTION

▶ See also *Birth Control, Birth Control Pills*

Emergency contraception is used to prevent pregnancy after having sex without birth control or after a birth control method used has failed. It is a good option for women who have had unprotected sex.

When Can Emergency Contraception Be Used?

Emergency contraception can be used if you have unprotected sex and don't want to get pregnant. It should not be used instead of birth control on a routine basis—regular use of a birth control method (such as condoms or birth control pills) is most effective. You may need emergency contraception if:

▶ You didn't use any birth control

▶ You had sex when you didn't plan to

▶ A condom broke or slipped off

▶ Birth control was not used correctly

▶ You were forced to have sex (rape)

There are many more reasons why someone has unprotected sex. No matter the reason, emergency contraception may be a good choice to prevent you from getting pregnant.

If you need emergency contraception but cannot contact your physician or do not have an advance prescription for it, you can call the toll-free, 24-hour hotline (888-NOT-2-LATE). It provides the names and numbers of five health care providers near you who prescribe emergency contraception.

Doctor's offices, family planning clinics, and hospital emergency rooms can prescribe emergency contraception pills. They can be bought at a drug store with a prescription.

Call your doctor's office right away if you have had unprotected sex. Be sure to tell him or her you need treatment without delay. In some cases, your doctor can call in a prescription for you to your local drug store. Emergency contraception pills must be started within 72 hours of having unprotected sex.

You may want to talk to your doctor about giving you an advance prescription for emergency contraception pills. This way, you will have it on hand if you need it.

Types of Emergency Contraception

The most commonly used method of emergency contraception is pills. The intrauterine device (IUD) also can be used for emergency contraception.

There are two types of emergency contraceptive pills. One type is combined oral contraceptives—birth control pills that contain the hormones estrogen and progestin. The other type uses only one of the hormones—progestin.

Both types of pills work the same way. Both are given in a higher dose than that used normally for birth control. The higher doses of these pills prevent pregnancy because they disrupt the normal hormone patterns in the menstrual cycle.

The emergency contraception pills may be prescribed to you in three forms:

1. A combination of regular birth control pills (contains estrogen and progestin)

2. A prepared kit with a pregnancy test and four pills (contains estrogen and progestin)

3. A package with two pills (contains progestin only)

The Intrauterine Device

The intrauterine device (IUD) is another type of emergency contraception. The IUD must be inserted within 5–7 days of having unprotected sex. A benefit of the IUD is that it can be left in for long-term use. The intrauterine device may be a good choice if you cannot take birth control pills. The IUD is not a good choice for someone who is at risk for STDs.

The kit with the pregnancy test and four pills also contains detailed instructions. You should read them first. Then, take the pregnancy test to confirm you are not pregnant from a previous time you had sex.

If the pregnancy test results are positive, do not take the pills. Emergency contraception will not work if you are pregnant. Talk to your doctor. If the test results are negative, take the pills as directed to prevent pregnancy.

How to Take the Pills

For the pills to work, timing is everything. The sooner you start them, the better. The pills are given in two doses. To prevent pregnancy, the first dose of birth control pills must be taken by mouth within 72 hours of having unprotected sex. A second dose is taken 12 hours after the first dose. The number of pills in the dose depends on the brand of pill used.

After taking emergency contraceptive pills, you may have some nausea and vomiting. The progestin-only pills cause less nausea and vomiting. Any nausea and vomiting will go away in about 1 or 2 days. Your doctor may give you an anti-nausea medicine to take 1 hour before you take the birth control pills.

If you vomit within 1 hour of taking either dose, let your doctor know right away. You may need to repeat that dose.

Other side effects may include:

◗ Abdominal pain and cramps

◗ Tender breasts

◗ Headache

◗ Feeling dizzy

Any side effects will go away within a few days. Also, your next period may not be regular—it may be early or late or light or heavy.

Follow-Up Care

If you use emergency contraceptive pills within 72 hours of unprotected sex, your chance of getting pregnant is greatly reduced. But, there is still a chance you could become pregnant. It is not as effective as using birth control on a regular basis. Ask your doctor about a method of birth control that you can use regularly.

If you have sex after you use emergency contraceptive pills, you should use a backup method such as a condom, spermicide, cervical cap, sponge, or diaphragm until you get your period. If you were taking birth control pills before, you should keep taking the pills and use a backup method. If you have not had a period within 21 days of taking the pills, you should see your doctor for a pregnancy test.

Keep in mind that emergency contraception does not prevent sexually transmitted diseases (STDs). Your doctor may suggest that you be tested for STDs. There are steps you can take to protect yourself, such as using a condom every time you have sex.

ENDOMETRIAL CANCER

Cancer of the endometrium—the lining of the uterus—occurs most often in women between the ages of 60 and 75, although it can occur at other ages. The warning signs of endometrial cancer include abnormal bleeding or discharge between periods, prolonged and heavy bleeding during periods, and, most importantly, any bleeding after menopause.

Your risk is higher if you:

- Have a history of irregular periods
- Started your period before age 12
- Have had fertility problems
- Have not had children
- Had a late menopause
- Are obese
- Have diabetes
- Have high blood pressure

Cancer of the endometrium is the most common gynecologic malignancy in the United States. It has occurred more often over the past 50 years because of the longer life expectancy of women, improved methods of diagnosis, and an increased frequency of certain conditions believed to cause the problem.

Cancer of the endometrium is more common in women who take estrogen therapy without a progestin hormone after menopause. Women who take birth control pills appear to have a lower risk.

To detect endometrial cancer, your doctor may perform certain tests, such as:

- Endometrial biopsy
- Ultrasound
- Dilation and curettage (D&C)
- Hysteroscopy

If cancer of the endometrium is found, surgery will be done to decide the stage of the disease and how it should be treated. Staging helps your doctor decide what treatment has the best chance for success. The chance for a cure decreases as the cancer becomes more advanced.

To treat endometrial cancer, most patients have both hysterectomy (removal of the uterus) and salpingo-oophorectomy (removal of the ovaries and fallopian tubes). Tissue from lymph nodes in the pelvic region may be tested to find out if the cancer has spread. Some cases of endometrial cancer may also require radiation therapy after surgery.

If tests show that the cancer has spread or come back after surgery or radiation, your doctor may advise more drug therapy. Chemotherapy may be used to treat endometrial cancer that has spread to other organs.

▶ ENDOMETRIAL HYPERPLASIA

▶ See also *Polycystic Ovary Syndrome, Uterine Bleeding*

Endometrial hyperplasia is a condition that occurs when the lining of the uterus (endometrium) grows too much. It is a benign (not cancer) condition. However, in some cases it can lead to cancer of the uterus. If you are having problems with your menstrual periods or any vaginal bleeding after menopause, your doctor may want to test you for endometrial hyperplasia. He or she will suggest treatment if this condition is found.

What Is the Endometrium?

The endometrium is the lining of the uterus. This lining grows and thickens every month to prepare the uterus for pregnancy. If pregnancy does not occur, the lining is shed during the menstrual period.

The female hormones—estrogen and progesterone—control the changes in the uterine lining. If these hormones are at the correct levels, the lining sheds and a woman has regular, normal menstrual cycles.

Estrogen builds up the uterine lining. Progesterone maintains and controls this growth. If an egg is not fertilized, hormone levels decrease. This decrease triggers the menstrual period.

What Is Endometrial Hyperplasia?

If estrogen is too high or progesterone is too low, the endometrium may grow too thick and cause abnormal bleeding. This is called endometrial hyperplasia.

In some cases of endometrial hyperplasia, the cells of the lining become abnormal. When this occurs, endometrial hyperplasia can lead to cancer of the uterus. This is called atypical hyperplasia.

Who Is at Risk?

Endometrial hyperplasia is more likely to occur in women who:

▶ Have abnormal bleeding.

▶ Are in the years around menopause.

▶ Skip menstrual periods often or have no periods at all

▶ Have polycystic ovary syndrome.

▶ Take estrogen without progesterone to replace the estrogen their body is no longer making and to relieve symptoms of menopause.

▶ Are overweight. (They may make too much estrogen and not enough progesterone.)

Tests

If you have abnormal bleeding along with any of the other risk factors, you may need to be tested for endometrial hyperplasia. One or more tests may be required.

Ultrasound

Your doctor may suggest you have an ultrasound exam. For this test, a device is placed in your vagina. Fluid may be placed in your uterus. Ultrasound uses sound waves to make a picture of the uterine lining. If the lining looks thicker than normal, you will need more tests.

Biopsy

Endometrial hyperplasia also can be found with a biopsy of the endometrium. Endometrial biopsy is a simple office procedure. Your doctor puts a slender device inside the uterus to take a sample of cells. (You will feel some cramping during the test.) The cells will be sent to a lab and checked under a microscope.

The results of this test will let your doctor know if you have endometrial hyperplasia. Endometrial biopsy results also can help detect if cancer of the uterus is present or if the condition is likely to lead to cancer. If your endometrial biopsy results are abnormal, your doctor may want to do other tests to check the rest of your uterus for cancer.

Dilation and Curettage

For dilation and curettage (D&C), the opening of the uterus is stretched open (dilated). A special device is used to gently loosen the uterine lining. This tissue then is studied in the lab to check for cancer.

Hysteroscopy

For hysteroscopy, your doctor inserts a slender, telescope-like device into the uterus to look for areas that might be thick or swollen. He or she then removes cells from these areas and sends the sample to a lab for testing.

Treatment

In most cases, endometrial hyperplasia can be treated with medication that is a form of the hormone progesterone. This hormone is given to work against the estrogen. Taking progesterone when you have gone some time without a period can prevent the lining of the uterus from growing too much. It often will cause your period to begin.

You may have to take progesterone pills for a number of months. In some cases, you may get progesterone shots. Your

Hysteroscopy is minor surgery that may be done in a doctor's office or operating room with local, regional, or general anesthesia. In some cases, little or no anesthesia is needed. The procedure poses little risk for most women. Hysteroscopy may be used for diagnosis, treatment, or both.

doctor will find a form of progesterone and a dose that is right for you. After treatment, another endometrial biopsy may be done to find out if the medication worked. If medications do not work, your doctor may suggest surgery to remove the uterus (hysterectomy). Hysterectomy may be an option if you have completed your family and your biopsy showed cells that could become cancer.

Prevention of Endometrial Hyperplasia

Women can take steps to help prevent endometrial hyperplasia. If you are overweight, losing weight may help. Also, your doctor may suggest taking certain hormones.

Women who take estrogen after menopause also need to take a form of progesterone to reduce the risk of endometrial hyperplasia and cancer of the uterus. If you don't have regular periods and you have a uterus, your doctor may suggest that you take a form of progesterone to help prevent the lining of the uterus from growing too much.

Birth control pills (oral contraceptives) contain estrogen along with a form of progesterone. They may help protect against endometrial hyperplasia in women who don't have regular periods.

▶ ENDOMETRIOSIS

▶ See also *Dysmenorrhea, Infertility, Pelvic Pain*

The lining of the uterus is called the endometrium. Sometimes, tissue similar to that which normally lines the uterus grows elsewhere in the body. When this happens it is called endometriosis.

Endometriosis can cause pain, especially during the menstrual period. For some women, the pain is mild. For others, it can be severe. Endometriosis may also cause infertility.

What Is Endometriosis?

In endometriosis, tissue similar to the endometrium is found in other areas in the body and acts like tissue in the uterus. Endometrial tissue may attach to organs in the pelvis or to the peritoneum. It may also be found in other parts of the body, although this is very rare. It most often appears in places within the pelvis, including the:

▶ Ovaries

▶ Fallopian tubes

▶ Outside of the uterus

▶ Cul-de-sac (the space behind the uterus)

Although the pregnancy rates for women with endometriosis are lower than those of women without endometriosis, most women with endometriosis do not have fertility problems.

▶ Bowel

▶ Bladder

▶ Rectum

Endometrial tissue outside the uterus responds to monthly changes in hormones the same way it does inside the uterus. It also breaks down and bleeds. This bleeding can cause pain, especially during your period. The breakdown and bleeding of this tissue each month can cause scar tissue, called adhesions. Sometimes adhesions bind organs together. Adhesions can also cause pain. If blood is trapped in the ovary because of adhesions, it can form an endometrioma (a type of cyst).

No one is certain of the cause of endometriosis. One theory is that blood sometimes backs up and carries tissue from inside the uterus into the fallopian tubes during your period. The tissue then travels out of the tubes and attaches to other places. Another theory is that endometrial cells are transported through blood and lymph vessels.

About 7% of women of childbearing age in the United States have endometriosis. It is most common in women in their 30s and 40s, but it can occur anytime in women who menstruate. Endometriosis occurs more often in women who have never had children. Women whose mothers, sisters, or daughters have had endometriosis are more likely to have it.

The symptoms of endometriosis often get worse over time. It will progress in more than half of women who are not treated and in 20% of women who are treated. Treatment may help keep the condition from getting worse.

Symptoms

Symptoms of endometriosis include pelvic pain. Such pain may occur with intercourse, during bowel movements or urination, or just before a menstrual cycle. Endometriosis may also cause spotting or infertility.

Although these symptoms may be a sign of endometriosis, they could also be signs of other problems. If you have any of these symptoms, see your doctor.

The amount of pain does not tell you how severe your condition is. For example, some women with slight pain may have a severe case, whereas others who have a lot of pain may have a mild case.

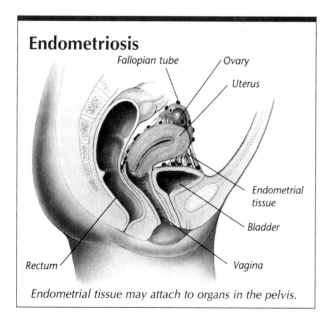

Endometriosis

Fallopian tube *Ovary*

Uterus

Endometrial tissue

Bladder

Rectum *Vagina*

Endometrial tissue may attach to organs in the pelvis.

Some women with endometriosis have no symptoms. In fact, they may first find out that they have endometriosis if they are unable to get pregnant. Endometriosis is found in about one third of infertile women.

Women often find that symptoms are relieved while they are pregnant. In fact, many of the products used to relieve endometriosis are based on the hormonal effects of pregnancy.

Diagnosis

Your doctor may suspect something is abnormal while performing a pelvic exam. The only way to confirm a diagnosis of endometriosis is to look directly inside the body. This is usually done by laparoscopy. Laparoscopy is often done with general anesthesia. The doctor makes a small cut near your navel. A thin lighted scope—a laparoscope—is then inserted into your abdomen. The laparoscope allows the doctor to view the pelvic organs. The doctor can then better tell the extent of the endometriosis.

Endometriosis can also be treated with laparoscopy. If endometrial tissue is found during the laparoscopy, your doctor may decide to remove it right away, if possible.

Sometimes a small amount of tissue is removed during the procedure. This is called a biopsy. Studying the tissue in a laboratory helps confirm the diagnosis.

Women with a first-degree relative (mother or sister) who have had endometriosis have almost 10 times the risk of developing endometriosis.

Treatment

Treatment for endometriosis depends on your symptoms and whether you want to have children. It may be treated with medication, surgery, or both. Although symptoms of endometriosis may come back, therapy can relieve pain for a time.

Medications

Hormones may be used to relieve pain. The hormones may help slow the growth of the endometrial tissue. The most commonly prescribed hormones include oral contraceptives, gonadotropin-releasing hormone (GnRH) agonists, progestin, and danazol. Not all women, however, get pain relief from medications. Medication does not reduce adhesions or scar tissue, which may be the cause of pain.

These medications are not for all women. As with most medications, there are some side effects linked to hormone treatment. Some women, however, may find the relief of pain is worth the discomfort of the side effects.

Oral contraceptives. Birth control pills are often prescribed for symptoms of endometriosis. The hormone in them helps keep the menstrual period regular, lighter, and shorter and can relieve pain. There is no evidence that birth control pills shrink endometriosis or increase fertility. Your doctor may prescribe the pill in a way that prevents you from having periods.

GnRH agonists. GnRH is a hormone that helps control the menstrual cycle. GnRH agonists are drugs that are similar to human GnRH but are many times more potent than the natural substance. GnRH agonists lower estrogen levels by turning off the ovaries. This produces a temporary condition similar to menopause.

GnRH agonists can be given as a shot, an implant, or nasal spray. Usually, patches of endometriosis shrink and pain is relieved. GnRH may help relieve pain during sex. Women taking GnRH may have hot flushes (hot flashes), headaches, and vaginal dryness.

Treatment with GnRH usually lasts up to 6 months. After stopping GnRH, you will have periods again in about 6–10 weeks. Symptoms of endometriosis will recur in at least half of women who take GnRH, especially if symptoms are severe.

Progestin. The hormone progestin is also used to shrink patches of endometriosis. Progestin works against the effects of estrogen on the tissue. You will no longer have a menstrual period when taking progestin. Progestin is taken as a pill or injection.

Danazol. Danazol is a synthetic hormone that shrinks endometrial tissue. It is taken as a pill and stops the menstrual cycle. You will no longer have a period while taking danazol.

Danazol works very well to decrease pelvic pain and pain during sexual intercourse. Symptoms of endometriosis usually return in about 6 weeks after you stop taking the medication. The side effects of danazol may include weight gain, acne, deepening of the voice, and hair growth.

Danazol treatment is not for everyone. Women who have liver, kidney, or heart problems cannot take danazol.

Surgery

Surgery may be performed to remove endometriosis and the scarred tissue around it. Healthy ovaries and normal fallopian tubes are left alone as often as possible to increase the chances of pregnancy later.

Until recently, surgery for endometriosis was always done by laparotomy. This surgery is a more extensive procedure than laparoscopy. Now, surgery is most often done by laparoscopy. Laparoscopy has many benefits over open surgery. It requires a shorter hospital stay, a smaller incision, and shorter recovery time.

Not all conditions can be handled with laparoscopy. Sometimes laparotomy may still be needed. Ask your doctor what to expect.

Surgery is often successful, both for treating pain and infertility, but symptoms may return. Many patients are treated with both surgery and medications to reduce recurrence. About one third of women who have had surgery will need more surgery within 5 years. When pain is severe and doesn't go away after therapy, your doctor may suggest that you have your uterus, fallopian tubes, and ovaries removed. This is major surgery. After this procedure, a woman will no longer have periods or be able to get pregnant.

Coping

In addition to seeking further treatment, women with pain from endometriosis often find that it helps to make a few lifestyle changes. These changes include exercise, following a healthy diet, and practicing relaxation techniques. Feeling fit may make it easier to handle stress, which makes it easier to cope with pain.

It may also help to talk with other women who are coping with endometriosis. Ask your doctor or nurse to recommend a support group in your area.

▶ EPISIOTOMY

An episiotomy is a small cut made into the perineum (the region between the vagina and the anus) to widen the vaginal opening for delivery of a baby. It is one of the most common operations in the United States. This procedure is sometimes necessary because when your baby's head appears at the opening of the vagina, the tissue of the vagina becomes very thin and tightly stretched. Sometimes it is hard for the baby's head to fit through without tearing the woman's skin and muscles.

The doctor also may do an episiotomy if he or she needs to get the baby out quickly. The area is numbed with a local anesthetic before the cut is made, so you shouldn't feel a thing. (An episiotomy will hurt as it heals, though.)

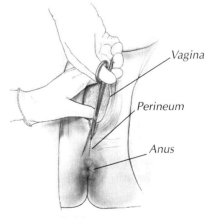

Vagina

Perineum

Anus

Episiotomy

EXERCISE DURING PREGNANCY

Regular exercise builds bones and muscles, gives you energy, and keeps you healthy. It is just as important when you are pregnant. Exercise helps you look and feel better during a time when your body is changing.

Benefits of Exercise

You're tired. You're gaining weight. You may not feel your best. Although these symptoms are normal during pregnancy, there is a way to find relief. Becoming active and exercising on most, if not all, days of the week can benefit your health in many ways:

▶ Helps reduce backaches, constipation, bloating, and swelling

▶ Gives you energy

▶ Improves your mood

▶ Improves your posture

▶ Promotes muscle tone, strength, and endurance

▶ Helps you sleep better

Regular activity also helps keep you fit during pregnancy and may improve your ability to cope with the pain of labor. This will make it easier for you to get back in shape after the baby is born. You should not, however, exercise to lose weight while you are pregnant.

The type of exercise you can safely do depends on your health and fitness level. Pregnancy is not a good time to take up a new sport. If you were active before getting pregnant, though, you should be able to keep it up, within reason.

Changes in Your Body

Pregnancy causes many changes in your body. Some of these changes will affect your ability to exercise.

Joints

The hormones produced during pregnancy cause the ligaments that support your joints to become relaxed. This makes the joints more mobile and more at risk of injury. Avoid jerky, bouncy, or high-impact motions that can increase your risk of injury.

Balance

Remember that during pregnancy you are carrying extra pounds—as much as 20–30 pounds at the end of pregnancy.

The extra weight in the front of your body shifts your center of gravity and places stress on joints and muscles, especially those in the pelvis and lower back. This can make you less stable, cause back pain, and make you more likely to lose your balance and fall, especially in later pregnancy.

Heart Rate

The extra weight you are carrying will make your body work harder than before you were pregnant. Exercise increases the flow of oxygen and blood to the muscles being worked and away from other parts of your body. So, it's important not to overdo it.

Try to exercise moderately so you don't get tired quickly. If you are unable to talk normally while exercising, your activity is too strenuous.

A pregnant woman should listen to her body's signals when she exercises. Even mild to moderate exercise should allow her to retain her pre-pregnancy level of fitness.

Getting Started

Before beginning your exercise program, talk with your doctor to make sure you do not have any health conditions that may limit your activity. Ask about any specific exercises or sports that interest you. Your doctor can offer advice about what type of exercise routine is best for you.

Women with one of the following conditions may be advised by their doctor not to exercise during pregnancy:

- Pregnancy-induced hypertension (high blood pressure)
- Symptoms or history of preterm labor (early contractions)
- Vaginal bleeding
- Premature rupture of membranes

Pregnant women with certain other medical conditions, such as preexisting high blood pressure, heart disease, and lung disease, will be advised by their doctor when and if exercise is appropriate.

Choosing Safe Exercises

Most forms of exercise are safe during pregnancy. But, some types of exercise involve positions and movements that may be uncomfortable, tiring, or harmful for pregnant women. For instance, after 20 weeks of pregnancy, women should not do exercises that require them to lie flat on their back because it may be more difficult for the blood to circulate.

Walking is considered the best exercise for anyone. Brisk walking gives a good total body workout and is easy on the joints and muscles. Other good activities for pregnant women include swimming and stationary biking.

Your Routine

Exercise during pregnancy is most practical during the first 24 weeks. During the last 3 months, it can be difficult to do many exercises that once seemed easy. This is normal.

If it has been some time since you've exercised, it is a good idea to start slowly. Begin with as little as 5 minutes a day and add 5 more minutes a week until you can stay active for 30 minutes a day.

Always begin each exercise session with a warm-up period for 5–10 minutes. This is light activity, such as slow walking, that prepares your muscles for activity. During the warm-up, stretch your muscles to avoid stiffness and soreness. Hold each stretch for at least 10–20 seconds—do not bounce.

After exercising, cool down by slowly reducing your activity. This allows your heart rate to return to normal levels. Cooling down for 5–10 minutes and stretching again also helps you to avoid sore muscles. Hold each stretch for 20–30 seconds—don't bounce.

Things to Watch

The changes your body is going through can make certain positions and activities risky for you and your baby. While exercising, try to avoid activities that call for jumping, jarring motions, or quick changes in direction that may strain your joints and cause injury.

There are some risks from becoming overheated during pregnancy. This may cause loss of fluids and lead to dehydration and problems during pregnancy. Overheating in the first 8 weeks of pregnancy may be a contributing factor to the development of birth defects. Exercising does not cause miscarriage.

When you exercise, follow these general guidelines for a safe and healthy exercise program:

Wear the right shoes for your sport. There are shoes made just for walking, running, aerobics, and tennis, for instance. Also, be sure the shoes have plenty of padding and give your feet good support.

▶ After 20 weeks of pregnancy, avoid doing any exercises on your back.

▶ Avoid brisk exercise in hot, humid weather or when you are sick with a fever.

▶ Wear comfortable clothing that will help you to remain cool.

▶ Wear a bra that fits well and gives lots of support to help protect your breasts.

▶ Drink plenty of water to help keep you from overheating and dehydrating.

▶ Make sure you consume the extra 300 calories a day you need during pregnancy.

While you exercise, pay attention to your body. Do not exercise to the point that you are exhausted. Be aware of the warning signs that you may be exercising too strenuously. If you notice any of these symptoms, stop exercising and call your doctor.

After the Baby Is Born

Having a baby and taking care of a newborn is hard work. It will take a while to regain your strength after the strain of pregnancy and birth. Taking care of yourself physically and allowing your body time to recover is important. If you had a cesarean delivery, a difficult birth, or complications, your recovery time may be longer. Check with your doctor before starting or resuming an exercise program.

Walking is a good way to get back into exercising. Brisk walks several times a week will prepare you for more strenuous exercise when you feel up to it. Walking has the added advantage of getting both you and the baby out of the house for exercise and fresh air. As you feel stronger, consider more vigorous exercise.

You will want to pick an exercise program that meets your own needs. Your doctor, nurse, or community center can help. There are also special postpartum exercise classes that you can join.

Warning Signs

Stop exercising and call your doctor if you get any of these symptoms:

- Pain
- Vaginal bleeding
- Dizziness or faintness
- Increased shortness of breath
- Rapid heartbeat
- Difficulty walking
- Uterine contractions and chest pain
- Fluid leaking from the vagina

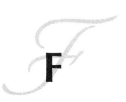

▶ FETAL MONITORING

Labor and delivery can be the most stressful times of a pregnancy for both mother and baby. Problems may arise at any point that need attention. Because of this, the heart rate of the baby is monitored during labor to check its well-being. Certain changes in the heart rate of the baby can signal a problem, so every woman gets some form of monitoring while she is in labor. Most babies will have changes in their heart rate some time during labor and delivery. Fetal monitoring cannot prevent a problem from occurring, but it can alert your doctor or nurse to warning signs. No form of fetal monitoring is perfect,

Women who are monitored electronically often are asked to spend their labor in bed. This helps keep the monitor in place.

but techniques have improved over the years, and today more is known about what can happen to the baby during labor.

Types of Fetal Monitoring

There are two methods of fetal heart rate monitoring. One method, called auscultation, involves listening to your baby's heartbeat at certain times. The other method, electronic fetal monitoring, uses equipment to record the heart rate on an ongoing basis. At the same time, the contractions of the uterus are measured. This can be done by feeling the abdomen or by using electronic equipment.

Auscultation and electronic fetal monitoring are both good ways to measure your baby's responses to labor and delivery. The choice of which method is used depends on:

▶ How your labor is progressing

▶ Your chance of problems

▶ Your doctor's judgment

▶ Availability of equipment

▶ Number of nurses and doctors at your hospital

Fetal heart monitoring will be done at different times depending on your stage of labor and if you are at risk for problems. You may be monitored as often as every 5 minutes or every 30 minutes, or it may be done continuously.

Auscultation

There are two ways of listening to the baby's heartbeat with auscultation:

1. A special device like a stethoscope, called a fetoscope, is placed in your doctor's or nurse's ears with the open end pressed on your abdomen. This device allows your baby's heartbeat to be heard clearly.

2. A Doppler ultrasound is a small, hand-held device that is pressed against your abdomen. It uses sound waves that are reflected from your baby to create a signal of the heartbeat that can be heard.

Your doctor or nurse will monitor the heart rate of the baby before, during, and just after a contraction. This is done to tell how the baby is reacting to the contraction.

Electronic Fetal Monitoring

Electronic fetal monitoring uses electronic equipment to measure the response of the baby's heart rate to contractions of the uterus.

It provides an ongoing record that can be read by the doctor or nurse. Electronic fetal monitoring is either external or internal.

External monitoring requires that two small devices be placed on the mother's abdomen. One device uses ultrasound to detect the fetal heart rate. The other measures the length of uterine contractions and the time between them. Two types of tests can provide reliable information on the fetus's health and can give early warning if the fetus is in trouble:

1. *Nonstress test:* This test measures the way a fetus responds to its own body movements. Normally, the fetal heart rate increases when the fetus moves. Each fetal movement felt by the mother or noted by the doctor or nurse is marked on a paper recording of the fetal heart rate.

2. ***Contraction stress test:*** This test measures how the fetus may react to the stress of labor. It is often used if the nonstress test shows no change in fetal heart rate in response to fetal movement. In the contraction test, mild contractions of the mother's uterus are brought on with a drug called oxytocin or by having the mother stimulate her nipples. The fetus's heart rate in response to the contractions is then recorded.

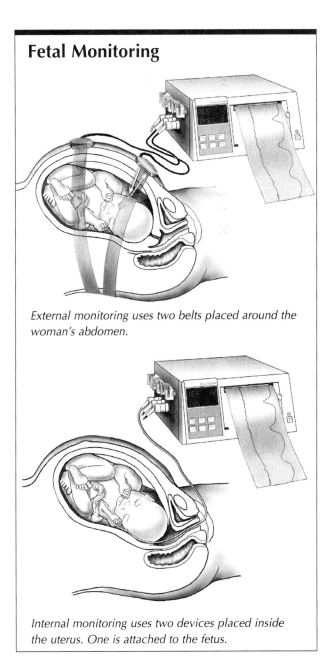

Fetal Monitoring

External monitoring uses two belts placed around the woman's abdomen.

Internal monitoring uses two devices placed inside the uterus. One is attached to the fetus.

Internal monitoring can be used only after the membranes of the amniotic sac have ruptured (that is, after "your water breaks"). A small device called a fetal scalp electrode is inserted through the vagina and attached to your baby's scalp. This device records the heart rate. At the same time, a thin tube called a catheter may be inserted through the vagina into your uterus. The tube measures the strength of contractions. You may feel some discomfort when the tube is inserted. Once it is inserted, though, there is little or no discomfort.

With either external or internal monitoring, information about the mother and the baby is sent to a small machine. The information is recorded on a long strip of paper that is read by your doctor or nurse. You may need to stay in bed during both types of monitoring, but you can move around and find a comfortable position.

What Do Abnormal Patterns Mean?

An average fetal heart rate varies between 110 and 160 beats per minute. This is much faster than your own heart rate, which is about 60–100 beats per minute.

Changes in the fetal heart rate that occur along with contractions form a pattern. Certain changes in this pattern may suggest a problem. One such problem could be that the umbilical cord, which connects the mother and baby, is being squeezed.

If there is an abnormal fetal heart rate pattern, you may be:

▶ Asked to change positions

▶ Given oxygen through a mask

▶ Given intravenous fluids

▶ Given medication to decrease the strength of contractions and relax the uterus

▶ Given fluids into the uterus

Abnormal fetal heart rate patterns do not always mean there is a serious problem, nor do they point to the exact problem. Other tests may be used to get a better idea of what is happening with your baby. Electronic monitoring may be done if abnormal patterns are found with auscultation. If the baby's heart rate patterns don't improve, your doctor may decide to speed the delivery of your baby.

Risks

There are no known risks with auscultation or with external electronic monitoring. With internal electronic monitoring, there is a small risk of infection.

Women who have a high risk for problems during labor and delivery will most likely have electronic fetal monitoring. In women who are high risk or whose babies show an abnormal heart rate pattern with electronic fetal monitoring, the delivery of the baby is more likely to be by cesarean birth or with special instruments (forceps).

Other Forms of Monitoring

There are a number of tests that can help the doctor check on the health of the baby. These tests often are begun at around 40–41 weeks of pregnancy. You can do some tests on your own at home. Some are done in the doctor's office, and others are done in the hospital:

▶ A kick count is a record of how often you feel your baby move. Healthy babies tend to move about the same amount each day. Your doctor will want to know about any sudden decrease in movement right away. More tests may be needed to see if the baby should be delivered soon.

▶ Electronic fetal monitoring records the baby's heart rate as the baby moves or the mother's uterus contracts. Two tests that can provide this information are the nonstress test and the contraction stress test.

▶ Ultrasound can show the position and size of the baby and placenta. It can show the baby's heartbeat, breathing, and body movements. It also can be used to measure the amount of amniotic fluid.

▶ A biophysical profile uses electronic fetal monitoring and ultrasound results to assess the level of amniotic fluid, tone, movement, heartbeat, and breathing.

If you have passed your due date, your doctor may discuss inducing labor.

▶ FIBROCYSTIC BREAST CHANGES

▶ See also *Breast Cancer, Breast Problems, Breast Self-Exam* in *"Women's Wellness,"* *Mammography*

Fibrocystic breast changes cause lumpy, tender breasts. These changes most often occur near the time of your period. Fibrocystic breast changes do not mean that you have a disease or that you are more likely to have cancer. However, a lump should be checked to see if it is solid or a cyst (a small sac filled with fluid).

Changes in Your Breast

Your breasts respond to changes in levels of the hormones progesterone and estrogen. These hormone levels change during your monthly menstrual cycle. They also change during pregnancy and menopause. You also may notice changes if you take hormones, such as oral contraceptives or hormone replacement therapy (HRT). Hormones cause a change in the amount of fluid in the breast. This may make fibrous areas in the breast more painful.

Many women have fibrocystic changes in their breasts. These changes are most common during childbearing years. They also can occur after menopause in women taking HRT.

Fibrocystic breast changes can cause lumps, thickened tissue, and swelling. Pain in your breasts can occur at any time of your cycle. The breast lumps may become larger or more tender near the time of your period, though.

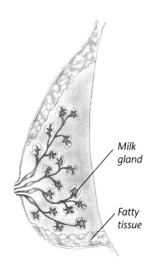

Normal breast

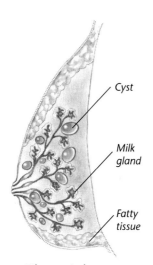

Fibrocystic breast

Symptoms include sharp, burning, itching, or aching pain in the breast. One breast may hurt more than the other. Any nipple discharge should be checked by your doctor. A clear, white, creamy, or green discharge from the nipple may occur off and on. Bloody (red) discharge should be checked right away.

Fibrocystic breast changes are benign (not cancer). If you have fibrocystic breast changes, you should become aware of the shape and location of all of the lumps you have. This will help you detect any changes.

Fibrocystic breast changes may make a breast exam harder to do. You should have regular exams to help detect any problems.

Detection

Breast changes can be found through a physical exam of the breast by:

▶ Breast self-exam

▶ Partner exam

▶ Health professional exam

All women should do a breast self-exam. If you have fibrocystic breast changes, it is even more important to check your breasts each month. That is because the changes in your breast may hide other problems. Knowing what is normal for your breasts will help you detect any changes that may signal a problem. Doing the exam helps you know what is normal for your breast and makes it easier to find an odd or new lump.

If you find a lump, it should be checked by your doctor to see if it is solid or a cyst. A cyst is a small, fluid-filled cavity that can be almost any size. Cysts are benign in most cases. Lumps that are cancer often appear in only one breast. Benign lumps often appear in both breasts in an even pattern. Signs of concern include:

▶ New lumps

▶ A lump that grows in size

▶ A distinct lump rather than a lumpy area

▶ A change in breast size

Other Tests

You or your doctor cannot tell a benign mass from cancer just by touching it. Your doctor may request a diagnostic mammogram, ultrasound, or biopsy to rule out cancer. Often, more than one of these tests will be used. Your doctor may refer you to a surgeon for the biopsy. You may be asked to return in 2–6 months for a checkup.

If a cyst is found, your doctor may suggest you have a fine-needle aspiration or needle biopsy. This draws fluid out of the cyst with a needle attached to a syringe. If the fluid is clear and the cyst goes away, it is likely that no more tests will be needed. If no fluid is obtained, further tests need to be done.

Relief of Symptoms

Most fibrocystic changes do not cause problems and do not require treatment. Some things may worsen the discomfort caused by fibrocystic breast changes. Although fibrocystic breasts are hard to treat, there are a few things you can try for relief:

▶ Avoid caffeine (coffee, tea, cola, and chocolate) for a few months. This works in many women.

▶ Take over-the-counter pain relief. Nonsteroidal antiinflammatory drugs (NSAIDs) are the most helpful.

▶ Reduce the amount of fluid you retain by not eating foods with a lot of salt, especially the week before your period.

Your doctor may suggest treatment to change your hormone patterns if the symptoms do not improve.

What Can I Do?

To find changes early, do a breast self-exam once a month. The best time to do it is about a week after your period begins, when breast swelling has gone down. Avoid things that may cause your condition to worsen. Have a mammogram once every 1–2 years from age 40 to 50. After age 50, have a mammogram once a year.

Things to Tell Your Doctor if You Find a Lump

Discuss your answers to these questions with your doctor:

▶ Have you had any previous breast problems?

▶ Have you had a breast biopsy in the past? When and where?

▶ Do you have any family history of breast cancer? Who and when?

▶ What was the date of your last period?

▶ What medications are you taking?

▶ When did you find the lump?

▶ What size is the lump? Has it gotten smaller or larger?

▶ How does the lump feel?

▶ Where is the lump?

▶ Do you have any nipple discharge? If so, what color is it?

▶ FOLIC ACID

▶ See also *Birth Defects, Genetic Disorders, Nutrition During Pregnancy*

Folic acid (vitamin B_9) is an important part of a healthy diet, especially during pregnancy. The U.S. Public Health Service has recommended that all reproductive-aged women take 0.4 mg of folic acid daily. Taking this amount each day will help

Folic acid may have benefits for pregnant and nonpregnant women of all ages. Scientists are now studying folic acid as a prevention for heart disease.

reduce the risk of neural tube defects in your children if you become pregnant. It can be taken as a vitamin or can be found in certain foods such as leafy, dark-green vegetables; citrus fruits; beans; and bread and cereals.

Women who have had a previous pregnancy that involved a neural tube defect have a higher risk of it recurring in a future pregnancy and should take 10 times more folic acid than the amount recommended routinely. Such women should take 4 mg daily for 1 month before pregnancy and during the first 3 months of pregnancy. These women should take folic acid alone, not as a part of a multivitamin preparation. To get enough folic acid from multivitamins, a woman would be getting an overdose of the other vitamins.

▶ See also *Vacuum Extraction*

▶ FORCEPS

Most of the time a woman goes through labor with no problems. Sometimes, when it's time to push, though, she may bear down for hours without making much progress. Other times, the baby's heartbeat may become slow or erratic. Still other times, the baby's position makes delivery harder. Also, a woman may become too tired to push.

In such cases, a doctor may need to help delivery along by using forceps. Forceps look like two large spoons. Forceps are inserted into the vagina. Next, the doctor places the forceps around the baby's cheeks and jaw (the fat there provides a nice cushion). Then the doctor uses the forceps to help the mother push the baby's head out of the birth canal.

In most cases, using forceps to help delivery causes no major problems. Still, this method of delivery can bruise the baby's head or tear the vagina or cervix.

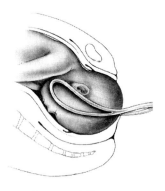

Forceps delivery

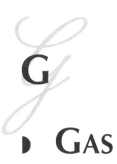

▶ GAS

Foods that are hard to digest can remain in the large intestine and cause gas. Gas affects many women who are lactose intolerant or who have trouble digesting beans or vegetables such as cabbage or broccoli. Your body may get used to these foods if you eat them regularly.

There are things you can do to prevent gas:

▶ Figure out which foods give you gas and eliminate them from your diet.

▶ Try over-the-counter remedies that help reduce gas.

▶ GENETIC DISORDERS

▶ See also *Birth Defects*

Problems in the genes or chromosomes of the fetus are called genetic disorders. They may be inherited—that is, they are passed from parent to child—or they may occur on their own.

Some genetic disorders are more likely if you have a certain ethnic background or if you have a family history of a disorder. Counseling can help predict your risk and testing may find the disorder.

What Is Genetics?

Genetics is the study of how traits—such as blood type—are passed from parent to child through genes and chromosomes. Each cell in your body has pairs of genes and chromosomes. They control your physical makeup.

Normally, a man's sperm and a woman's egg have 23 chromosomes each. All other cells in the body have 46. When an egg is fertilized by a sperm, 23 chromosomes from the mother and 23 chromosomes from the father join to form the 46 chromosomes of the cell that will become the fetus.

One pair of these chromosomes—one each from the sperm and the egg—is the sex chromosomes. There are two types of

DNA

Cells are the basic building blocks of the body. Inside each cell is a nucleus. Inside each nucleus are the chromosomes. All cells in the body have 46 chromosomes, except for the eggs and sperm, which have 23 each. The chromosomes are made up of DNA (deoxyribonucleic acid) molecules. The DNA molecule is double stranded. The two strands are in the shape of a double helix that resembles a spiral stair. The double strands are connected at what are called base pairs. Each chromosome contains anywhere from 50 million to 250 million base pairs, depending on the size of the chromosome. There are about 3 billion base pairs of DNA in the human body. DNA contains the genetic code for the entire body.

A gene is a segment of a DNA molecule that is coded to pass along a specific characteristic. In humans, there are about 50,000–100,000 genes. Each one has a specific position on the chromosome and a specific function.

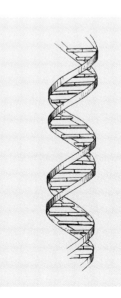

Preimplantation Genetic Diagnosis

Preimplantation genetic diagnosis (PGD) is sometimes used as a way to test embryos for genetic disorders before they are implanted in the uterus. Only the embryos that show no disorders are used. Not all genetic disorders can be found this way, though PGD allows couples with genetic disorders to decrease the risk of having a child who has the same problem. This technique is offered only in a few centers and raises some ethical issues.

If both parents are carriers of a recessive disorder, there is a 25% chance that a boy or girl will be affected, a 50% chance that a child will be a carrier, and a 25% chance that the child will not carry the gene.

sex chromosomes: X and Y. A normal sperm has either an X or a Y chromosome. A normal egg always has an X chromosome.

The sex chromosome in the sperm determines the sex of the child. If a sperm with a Y chromosome joins with an egg, the fetus is male (XY). If the sperm has an X chromosome, the fetus is female (XX).

Each chromosome carries many genes. Genes also come in pairs. Half of a fetus's genes come from the mother. The other half come from the father. Some traits, such as blood type, are controlled by a single gene pair. Other traits—including skin color, hair color, and height—are the result of many pairs of genes working together.

A gene or a genetic disorder is either dominant or recessive. If one gene in a pair is dominant, the trait it carries cancels out the trait carried by the recessive gene. For a recessive trait to appear, the gene that carries it must be inherited from both parents.

Types and Causes of Disorders

Genetic disorders may be caused by problems with either genes or chromosomes. Some disorders may be caused by a mix of factors (multifactorial). The actual cause of these multifactorial disorders is unknown. They can run in families or can occur on their own with no family history. Some dominant disorders can be found by testing, and others cannot. Also, some dominant disorders can be treated and are not serious.

Dominant Disorders

Just one gene from either parent can cause a dominant gene disorder. If a parent has the gene, each of his or her children has a 1-in-2 (50%) chance of inheriting the disorder.

Recessive Disorders

A pair of genes—one from each parent—causes recessive disorders. In these cases, both genes are abnormal.

Each person carries a few recessive genes. Most of the time, these genes are canceled out by dominant genes. If you have a recessive gene for a certain disorder, you are a carrier. Although you may show no signs of the disorder yourself, you still can pass it on to your children.

If both you and your partner are carriers for the same recessive disorder, each of your children has a 1-in-4 (25%) chance of having the disorder. If one of you has the disorder and the other doesn't (and isn't a carrier), your children always will be carriers. Some recessive disorders are more common in certain ethnic groups.

X-Linked Disorders

Disorders that are caused by genes on the X chromosome are called X-linked or sex-linked disorders. In most X-linked disorders, the abnormal gene is recessive.

A woman may carry this gene but not have the disorder. That's because the normal gene on her other X chromosome cancels out the abnormal gene. A male child who inherits the X chromosome with the abnormal gene, however, may get the disorder. That's because he doesn't have another X chromosome with a normal gene to cancel that one out (he has a Y chromosome). Color blindness is a common X-linked trait.

If you're a carrier for an X-linked disorder and the father of the baby isn't, there is a 1-in-2 (50%) chance a son will have the disorder and a 50% chance a daughter will be a carrier. Very rarely, a daughter has an X-linked recessive disorder. In this case, her father has the disease and her mother is a carrier.

Chromosomal Disorders

Genetic disorders also may be caused by problems with the fetus's chromosomes. Most are caused by an error that occurred when the egg and sperm were forming. Extra, missing, or incomplete chromosomes often cause severe health problems. Most children with chromosomal disorders have physical defects and below-average intelligence.

The older you are, the greater your risk of having a child with a chromosomal disorder (Table 16). If you're age 35, for instance, the chance is about 1 in 192 (less than 1%). If you're age 40, it's about 1 in 66 (1.5%).

Who Is at Risk?

When you are planning to become pregnant or when you start prenatal care, your doctor may give you a list of questions like the ones in the box "Risk Factors for Genetic Disorders." If you answer "yes" to any of them, you may be at increased risk for having a baby with a genetic disorder. Sometimes genetic disorders occur even when there is no history of problems in the family.

Table 16. The Risk of Having a Baby with a Chromosomal Disorder at Birth

Mother's Age at Delivery	Risk of Down Syndrome	Risk of Any Chromosomal Disorder
20	1/1,667	1/526
25	1/1,250	1/476
30	1/952	1/385
35	1/378	1/192
40	1/106	1/66
41	1/82	1/53
42	1/63	1/42
43	1/49	1/33
44	1/38	1/26
45	1/30	1/21

Modified from Hook EB, Cross PK, Schreinemachers DM. Chromosomal abnormality rates at amniocentesis and in live-born infants. JAMA 1983; 249:2034–2038 (ages 33–49); Hook EB. Rates of chromosome abnormalities at different maternal ages. Obstet Gynecol 1981;58:282–285

Risk Factors for Genetic Disorders

▶ Will you be age 35 or older when your baby is due?

▶ If you or your partner is of Mediterranean or Asian descent, do either of you or anyone in your families have thalassemia?

▶ Is there a family history of congenital heart defects?

▶ Is there a family history of Down syndrome?

▶ Have you ever had a child with Down syndrome?

▶ If you or your partner are of eastern European Jewish or French Canadian descent, is there a family history of Tay–Sachs disease?

▶ If you or your partner are of eastern European Jewish descent, is there a family history of Canavan disease?

▶ If you or your partner are African American, is there a family history of sickle cell disease or trait?

▶ Is there a family history of hemophilia?

▶ Is there a family history of muscular dystrophy?

▶ Is there a family history of cystic fibrosis?

▶ Is there a family history of Huntington disease?

▶ Is anyone in your or your partner's family mentally retarded?

▶ If so, was that person tested for fragile X syndrome?

▶ Do you, your partner, anyone in your families, or any of your children have any other genetic diseases, chromosomal disorders, or birth defects?

▶ Do you have a metabolic disorder such as diabetes or phenylketonuria?

▶ Have you had more than two miscarriages in a row?

▶ Have you ever had a baby who was stillborn?

Genetic Counseling

If you are at risk for having a baby with a disorder, genetic counseling can help you decide whether to:

▶ Take tests to find out if you and your partner are carriers

▶ Become pregnant

▶ Have prenatal testing to see if your fetus has a problem

A genetic counselor is someone with special training in genetics. He or she can:

▶ Give you an idea of the risk you face

▶ Tell you about the types of genetic disorders and how they affect babies born with them

▶ Help you weigh your options

▶ Discuss any concerns you have

Your genetic counselor will ask you and your partner for a detailed family history. If a family member has a problem, the counselor may ask to see that person's medical records. He or she also may refer you or your partner for physical exams, blood tests, or prenatal tests. Using all the information he or she can gather, the counselor will try to figure out the risk of your baby having a problem and explain it to you.

Testing

Whether to have genetic testing is up to you and your partner. Some couples would rather not know if they're at risk for a problem. However, finding out has benefits before and during pregnancy.

Before You Become Pregnant

If you have carrier testing before trying to conceive, the results can help you decide whether to become pregnant. If you learn that you have a strong chance of having a child with a genetic defect, you may want to explore other options for starting a family.

Carrier testing or genetic testing can give you information that will help other family members. Siblings and other relatives who may want to have children of their own can benefit from the knowledge that your family has the gene for a certain disorder.

During Pregnancy

Testing can help you prepare for the birth of a child with special needs. You can learn about the disorder, line up special medical care for your baby, and seek out others for support.

Genetic testing done during pregnancy can help you decide whether to continue your pregnancy. If you find out your baby has a severe problem, you have the chance to think about not continuing the pregnancy and trying again.

Many parents with risk factors can have a baby who's just fine. Testing may spare you from spending the months before your child's birth in a state of fear.

There are other issues to think about as well. Testing:

▶ May involve testing of other family members

▶ Will reveal the father of the baby

▶ May be costly

▶ May not be covered by health insurance

Types of Tests

Some genetic tests are offered to all pregnant women. These are called screening tests. Others may be offered if your medical history, family history, or physical exam show you may be at risk. These are called diagnostic tests.

It may take a while to receive the results of some genetic tests. This time is stressful. You may need to make choices and think about your options. Your doctor can help you do this.

Human Genome Project

The Human Genome Project is an international effort to map the entire human genome. Scientists are trying to pinpoint each gene's place on a chromosome and the role it serves. By knowing the role and placement of each gene, scientists can better understand how it affects the body in both health and disease.

For many genetic disorders, there is no test. Most tests focus on a single disorder and will not find any other problems.

Screening Tests

Screening tests are done even when a woman has no symptoms or known risk factors. A positive screening test often is followed by further tests to confirm the results. Screening tests include:

▶ Blood tests of the parents

▶ Ultrasound exam

Diagnostic Tests

Diagnostic tests usually are offered after a screening test raises concerns. If a woman is already at an increased risk of having a baby with a disorder, she may be offered a diagnostic test first. Diagnostic tests include:

▶ Amniocentesis

▶ Chorionic villus sampling

▶ Fetal blood sampling

▶ Detailed ultrasound exam

▶ See also *Chlamydia, Condoms, Pelvic Inflammatory Disease, Sexually Transmitted Diseases*

▶ GONORRHEA

One of the most common sexually transmitted diseases (STDs) in both women and men is gonorrhea. This infection is passed from person to person through sex. It often occurs with another STD called chlamydia. About 25–40% of women with gonorrhea have chlamydia at the same time. The factors that place a person at risk for both are the same. They also infect the same sites in a woman's reproductive tract. For these reasons, the two are often diagnosed and treated together.

Gonorrhea can cause serious health problems if it is not treated. These problems include pelvic infection. If a pelvic infection is not treated, it can damage the fallopian tubes and make ectopic pregnancy more likely. A woman who has had a severe infection may not be able to become pregnant. She may also have problems during pregnancy or after birth that pose risks to herself and her baby.

What Is Gonorrhea?

Gonorrhea infects about 1 million people each year in the United States. In the past 20 years, the rate of this infection has declined. It is still high, though, in some groups. For example, it may be increasing in teenagers.

In both women and men, gonorrhea can occur without symptoms. As many as half of all women who get this disease have no symptoms in the early stages. Men are more likely to have symptoms, but they, too, may have no symptoms in the early stages. If your partner has symptoms, you should avoid having sex.

The most common site of infection in women is the cervix (opening of the uterus). Untreated, gonorrhea can spread upward into the uterus and fallopian tubes. The rectum can also become infected, either through anal sex or from the spread of the infection from a woman's vagina. The urethra (the opening through which urine is passed) is also a common site of infection. Gonorrhea also can infect the mouth and throat of a person who has oral sex with an infected partner.

Health Risks

If not treated, gonorrhea can pose serious, long-term risks to your health. The sooner this disease is found and treated, the lower the chance that serious problems will develop.

Pelvic Inflammatory Disease

Gonorrhea can cause pelvic inflammatory disease (PID) if it is not treated. PID is an infection of the uterus, fallopian tubes, and other structures inside a woman's pelvis. It is the most common serious infection in women aged 16–25 years.

PID almost always results from an untreated infection that spreads upward into the pelvic area. It is the most common and the most serious complication of gonorrhea. It is also the most common preventable cause of infertility in the United States. It can lead to long-term pelvic pain.

Problems During Pregnancy

Gonorrhea can cause problems for a pregnant woman and her baby, both during pregnancy and after birth. Gonorrhea increases the risks of preterm birth (birth before 37 weeks of pregnancy) and premature rupture of membranes (in which the sac that surrounds the fetus breaks before labor begins). A newborn can also become seriously ill if he or she gets gonorrhea from the mother. Gonorrhea can also result in a miscarriage.

Symptoms of Gonorrhea

Many women and men with gonorrhea have few or no symptoms when they are first infected. When they do occur, symptoms may appear anywhere from 2 days to 3 weeks after contact with an infected partner. The most common symptoms in women include:

▶ A yellowish vaginal discharge

▶ Painful or frequent urination

▶ Burning or itching in the vaginal area

▶ Redness, swelling, or soreness of the vulva

▶ Pain in the pelvis or abdomen during sex

▶ Abnormal vaginal bleeding

The most common symptoms in men include:

▶ Discharge form the penis

▶ Pain and burning during urination

In both women and men, a gonorrhea infection in the rectum can cause discharge, itching around the anus, and pain during bowel movements. A woman or man whose throat is infected may also have a sore throat.

None of these symptoms in either sex is a sure sign of gonorrhea. Any of them, though, should prompt you to see your doctor.

Gonorrhea can be passed to the fetus before birth. A baby born to a woman with gonorrhea may develop an eye infection that can lead to blindness. For this reason, babies are treated with an eye medicine soon after birth, whether or not the mother has gonorrhea.

Because of the risks posed to both mother and baby by this infection, tests for gonorrhea are offered to pregnant women who are at risk for this disease. Some states require that all pregnant women be tested for certain STDs. There is less risk to the baby when the mother is treated for gonorrhea during pregnancy.

Risk Factors

Like other STDs, gonorrhea is passed on by sexual contact. The risk of getting this infection is high if you have sex—vaginal, anal, or oral—with someone who is infected.

Anyone who has sex can get this disease. But the risk is higher in young women and those who:

▶ Have more than one sexual partner

▶ Have sex with someone who has or has had more than one partner

▶ Began sexual activity at an early age

▶ Have other types of STDs, either now or in the past

▶ Have had gonorrhea before

▶ Use illegal drugs

Diagnosis

If you have any of the risk factors described here, or if you think you may have been exposed to someone with this infection, contact your doctor to get tested. Lab tests can be done to find out whether or not you have gonorrhea.

It is possible to have more than one STD at the same time. Your chances of having another STD are higher if you have gonorrhea. The same factors that place you at risk for this infection also increase your risk of having other STDs. For this reason, your doctor may also test you for other STDs, such as chlamydia, genital herpes, syphilis, or human immunodeficiency virus (HIV) infection.

Because the most common site of gonorrhea in women is the cervix, diagnosis is usually done by a pelvic exam and culture of the cervix. During the exam, your doctor will look at your cervix and any discharge. A sample of cells will then be taken from the cervix. These cells will be tested. Other sites that may be cultured are the rectum, urethra, and throat.

Using a condom the correct way every time you have sex is a very effective way to prevent most STDs. For more information about STDs and condom use, visit www.acog.org or call the CDC National STD hotline at 800-227-8922.

Treatment

Gonorrhea can be treated. Antibiotics that act against this infection can be taken by mouth or injected into a muscle. Treatment may last for up to 7 days.

For treatment to work, it's important to follow these guidelines:

▶ *Finish all of your medicine.* Even if your symptoms go away before you finish all the medicine your doctor prescribes, you can still be infected. If you stop taking the medicine, the infection may progress silently. Remember, many women have these infections with no symptoms at all.

▶ *Your sexual partner should also be tested and treated.* If your partner is infected and does not get treatment, the disease can be passed back to you.

▶ *Don't have sex until you are fully cured.* Gonorrhea can be passed to your sexual partner while you are being treated. If this happens, you may end up passing the infection back and forth, and you could be reinfected. After you and your partner have completed treatment, you can resume having sex.

Females aged 15–19 years have the highest rates of gonorrhea in the United States. About 50% of women with gonorrhea have no symptoms. Without early screening and treatment, 10–40% of women with gonorrhea will develop pelvic inflammatory disease.

Prevention

Even if you have already had gonorrhea, there are things you can do to keep from getting it again. These safeguards can also help protect against other STDs:

▶ Limit your sexual partners.

▶ Know your partner.

▶ Use a condom.

▶ Use a spermicide containing nonoxynol 9.

▶ If you think you may be at risk, get tested.

▶ GROUP B STREPTOCOCCUS AND PREGNANCY

Group B streptococcus (GBS) is a type of bacteria that can be found in up to 40% of pregnant women. A woman with GBS can pass it on to her fetus when she is pregnant or to her baby during delivery or after birth. Most babies who get GBS from their mothers do not have any problems. A few, though, will become sick. This can cause major health problems or even threaten their lives.

What Is GBS?

GBS is one of the many bacteria that do not usually cause serious illness. It may be found in the digestive, urinary, and reproductive tracts. In women, it is most often found in the vagina and rectum.

A person who has the bacteria but shows no symptoms is said to be colonized. If the bacteria grow and cause symptoms, infection has occurred. GBS is different from group A streptococcus, which is the bacteria that causes "strep throat." GBS is not a sexually transmitted disease (STD).

Being colonized with GBS usually does not pose any danger to a woman's health, and, in most cases, a woman will not need to be treated. If a woman is pregnant, however, she can pass GBS to her fetus. It can also be passed to the baby after birth. For this reason, a woman may be tested or treated during pregnancy or labor even if she doesn't have symptoms.

Effects on the Baby

Because many women are colonized with GBS, infection can occur during pregnancy or delivery. If the bacteria is passed from a woman to her baby, the baby may develop GBS infection. This happens to only 1 or 2 of every 100 babies whose mothers have GBS. Babies who do become infected may have early or late infections.

Early Infections

Early infections occur within the first 7 days after birth. Most occur within the first 6 hours. In most newborns with early infection, GBS is passed to them by their mother during labor and delivery.

Late Infections

Late infections occur after the first 7 days of life. About half of late infections are passed from the mother to the baby during birth. The other half result from other sources of infection, such as contact with other people who are GBS carriers.

Both early and late infection can be serious. They can cause inflammation of the baby's blood, lungs, brain, or spinal cord. Both early and late infections can lead to death of the newborn in about 5% of infected babies.

Testing for GBS

Tests are available to detect GBS and provide rapid results. These tests are of limited use because they work best with high levels of bacteria and not as well with low levels. Cultures are better tests for GBS.

During the 1990s, efforts were made to prevent the spread of GBS disease to newborns. Thanks to these efforts, from 1993 to 1998 the occurrence of the disease during the first week of life declined by 65%.

With cultures, samples are taken from the mother's vagina, perineum, and rectum during pregnancy. These samples are then grown in a special substance. A urine sample may also be used for cultures. It may take up to 2 days to get the results. If your culture is positive for GBS, you should receive antibiotics during your labor to help prevent GBS from being passed to your baby.

The usefulness of cultures is limited in early pregnancy. Cultures done at 35–37 weeks of pregnancy have a better chance of accurately telling whether GBS is present and might be passed to the baby during delivery. However, a culture cannot always detect women who will be colonized at the time of delivery. For this reason, your doctor may decide not to use cultures to test for GBS. Rather, he or she may decide to treat you based on whether you have a risk factor for GBS infection.

> ## Risk Factors for GBS
>
> ▶ Labor that begins before 37 weeks of pregnancy (preterm labor)
>
> ▶ Breaking of the amniotic sac before 37 weeks of pregnancy (preterm premature rupture of membranes)
>
> ▶ More than 18 hours have passed since the amniotic sac broke (prolonged rupture of membranes)
>
> ▶ Prior baby with GBS infection
>
> ▶ Fever during labor

Treatment

There are two ways to reduce the risk of GBS infection in the baby. One way is to treat all mothers who test positive for GBS with antibiotics during labor. Another way is treat those who have risk factors for GBS.

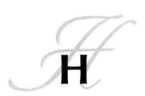

▶ HEADACHE

Everyone has had a headache at some time or another. Most headaches are minor and can be treated with over-the-counter pain relievers. However, an estimated 45 million Americans have chronic headaches—headaches serious enough to interfere with daily life.

Types of Headaches

Tension

The most common type of headache is a tension headache. Tension headaches usually create a steady squeezing or pressing

To help prevent tension headaches, maintain good posture to prevent the muscle cramps that sometimes cause the problem. Also, regular aerobic exercise (such as walking, biking, or jogging) may help prevent tension headaches.

pain on both sides of the head. It feels as if a band is being tightened around your head.

Tension headaches can occur occasionally or they can be chronic. They can last from 30 minutes to several days. They often occur upon waking.

Migraine

Migraine headaches affect 18% of women and 6% of men in the United States. Although many people believe they suffer from migraine headaches, most headaches that people get are not migraine.

Migraine is a severe throbbing pain on one or both sides of the head. It may occur with other symptoms, such as nausea and sensitivity to light and noise. Migraine headaches occur occasionally—once or twice a week, or sometimes every few years. They do not typically happen every day.

There are two types of migraine headaches—"migraine with aura" and "migraine without aura." An aura is a symptom that usually occurs 10–30 minutes before a migraine headache. During an aura, the person may see lines or flashing lights. They may temporarily lose vision or have speech problems or tingling in the face or hands. People who have migraines without aura may have symptoms that include mood changes, fatigue, diarrhea, increased urination, and nausea.

Cluster

Cluster headaches affect only a small percentage of people. The cause of cluster headaches is not known. This is the only type of headache that is more common in men than women.

Cluster headaches are described as a very severe, nonthrobbing pain felt behind one eye. They usually occur periodically over several weeks or months. The pain can lasts up to 3 hours.

Headache Triggers

Limiting stress, avoiding triggers, and getting regular exercise can help keep headaches under control. If your headaches persist, become severe, or differ from what is normal for you, see a doctor.

You may notice that certain factors trigger your headache. Some known headache triggers include:

- *Diet*—Alcoholic beverages, caffeine, and foods that contain certain substances

- *Eating and sleeping patterns*—Fasting or skipping meals, getting too much or too little sleep, or becoming dehydrated (not drinking enough water)

- *Emotions*—Stress, anxiety, excitement, or anger

▶ *Medications*—Medications such as those to treat chest pain (angina) and high blood pressure

▶ *Environment*—Things in your workplace and home, including bright lights; noise; eyestrain; and inhaling fumes from substances, such as gasoline, insecticides, or cleaning agents

For women, one main trigger is a change in the body's level of hormones. Many women notice that headaches occur around their menstrual periods or during pregnancy. Using oral contraceptives (birth control pills)—which alter the level of hormones in the body—can also bring on headaches.

Headaches can also be caused by sinus or dental problems. A sinus headache can arise from an allergy or a cold.

Controlling the Pain

Keeping track of your headaches in a "headache diary" can help you pinpoint what causes them. For 1 or 2 months, write down the times you have a headache and any events that could have triggered it, such as meals, noise, or your menstrual cycle. Look for patterns when your headaches occur.

Once you know what triggers your headaches, it may be easier to prevent them. Most headaches can be controlled by making a few lifestyle changes:

▶ *Exercise*—Exercising releases your body's endorphins, its natural painkilling agent. Regular exercise also relieves stress and helps you sleep better.

▶ *Avoid eyestrain*—Have your eyesight checked regularly.

▶ *Avoid food triggers*—Be aware of what foods cause your headaches and remove them from your diet.

▶ *Relax*—Try relaxation techniques that help reduce stress, such as massage, biofeedback, and meditation.

▶ *Keep your routine*—Avoid changes in the number of meals you eat or hours you sleep.

▶ *Drink plenty of water*—Drink at least 8 glasses of water a day to prevent dehydration.

Food Triggers

Some foods contain substances that are known to trigger a headache.

Tyramine, a natural chemical, can be found in:

▶ Chocolate

▶ Yogurt

▶ Sour cream

▶ Aged cheese

▶ Red wine

Nitrites, a preservative, can be found in:

▶ Smoked fish

▶ Bologna

▶ Sausage

▶ Hot dogs

Monosodium glutamate (MSG), an additive, can be found in:

▶ Chinese food

▶ Processed or frozen foods

When to See a Doctor

Most headaches do not require medical attention. Some headaches, however, can be a sign of a more serious problem, such as high blood pressure. It is rare for a headache to be caused by a brain tumor. Be aware of the symptoms that may signal a problem, and call your doctor if you experience any of them.

If you visit your doctor for treatment of headaches, diagnosing the cause of your headache is the first step. He or she may ask detailed questions about your headaches, such as:

▶ How often do you have headaches?

▶ Where is the pain?

▶ How long do the headaches last?

▶ When did you start having headaches?

Your doctor may also obtain a history of your health, including questions about any past head injuries and about your use of medications. Special tests or a referral to a specialist may be recommended. This information will help your doctor determine what type of treatment is necessary.

Treatment

Most tension headaches can be relieved with over-the-counter pain relievers, such as aspirin, acetaminophen, or ibuprofen. However, avoid taking these medications daily or almost every day.

Heavy use of pain relievers may hamper the body's own system for fighting pain. This can lead to a condition known as "rebound headache." When pain relievers are overused, they no longer ease the pain, which leads to the use of more medication. Rebound headaches can usually be relieved by stopping the use of the medication all at once—or "cold turkey." Although a withdrawal headache may occur for 2 or 3 days, most people notice fewer headaches within 2 weeks.

Migraine headaches can sometimes be relieved with ice packs or by putting pressure on the temple on the painful side of the head. For mild migraine headaches, aspirin or acetaminophen may give some relief. If the over-the-counter medications do not work, your doctor may prescribe stronger medications. If you have two or three migraine headaches per month, your doctor may suggest medications to help prevent them.

Warning Signs

If your headache is more severe than usual and you have any of the following symptoms, see your doctor right away—it could be a signal of a more serious problem:

▶ Stiff neck along with high fever

▶ Confusion, dizziness, weakness

▶ Convulsions

▶ HEART DISEASE

▶ See also *Cholesterol, Diabetes, High Blood Pressure*

Many women are not aware of their risk of heart disease. In the United States, heart disease is the leading killer of women older than age 40. More than 233,000 women die of heart attacks each year. By comparison, about 43,000 women die from breast cancer each year.

There are a number of factors that can raise your risk of heart disease. Many of the risks can be lessened by lifestyle changes.

The Heart and Its Function

All the cells in your body need oxygen to function normally. Your cardiovascular system (the heart and blood vessels) carries oxygen in the blood throughout the body. There are different types of blood vessels:

▶ Arteries carry oxygen-rich blood from the heart to the body.

▶ Veins carry blood back from the body to the heart.

Causes of Heart Disease

The vessels that supply blood to the heart are called the coronary arteries. The most common cause of heart disease is coronary artery disease. This is a narrowing of blood vessels to the heart by the buildup of plaque. Plaque is a fatty substance that forms in the arteries when too much cholesterol is present. Over the years, plaque causes the arteries to harden and narrow. This is called atherosclerosis.

Atherosclerosis begins in young adulthood, but it may be decades before symptoms of heart disease appear. It puts you at risk for angina (pain in the chest) and heart attack.

There are two forms of cholesterol, one that helps prevent heart disease—HDL (high-density lipoprotein) "good" cholesterol—and one that is harmful—LDL (low-density lipoprotein) "bad" cholesterol. HDL carries cholesterol out of the blood vessels to the liver, where it

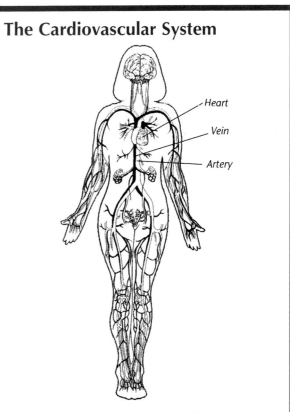

The Cardiovascular System

Heart

Vein

Artery

The heart pumps blood rich in oxygen through the arteries (light blood vessels) to the body. Veins (dark blood vessels) carry blood back from the body to the heart.

is broken down to be passed from the body. LDL tends to stay in the body and build up on artery walls, forming plaque, and making it harder for blood to move through the arteries. HDL clears the arteries, while LDL clogs them.

When the blood vessels narrow, the supply of oxygen to the heart may be cut off. This can lead to a heart attack, in which the heart tissues are damaged. A sign that the heart may not be getting enough oxygen may be chest pain. However, not everyone will have this symptom.

Sometimes the signs that a heart attack may be starting are hard to detect. The box lists the warning signs of a heart attack. If you have any of these symptoms, don't wait. Call an ambulance.

Risks

Some factors that increase your risk of heart disease cannot be changed. You should, however, be aware of them when assessing your own health. One such factor is family history—having a parent, grandparent, or sibling who has had a heart attack. Age is another factor—as you get older, your risk increases.

Other risks of heart disease are related to a person's lifestyle. These risks can be reduced by making a few lifestyle changes. The box gives tips on what you can do to have a healthy heart.

High Cholesterol

High levels of cholesterol increase your risk of atherosclerosis. Levels more than 240 mg/dL are considered high.

It is important to monitor your level of cholesterol. Your goal should be to keep HDL cholesterol high (more than 60 mg/dL) and LDL cholesterol low (less than 130 mg/dL). Women with risk factors for heart disease should be tested every 1–2 years. Risk factors include family history of high cholesterol and heart disease. Women without risk factors should be tested every 5 years beginning at age 45.

If your cholesterol level is high, take steps to reduce it by eating foods low in fat and cholesterol and by exercising. If your doctor has prescribed a medication to lower your cholesterol, take it as directed.

High Blood Pressure

When arteries are narrowed by plaque, blood pressure increases. Untreated high blood pressure (or hypertension) is a major risk for heart disease.

Warning Signs of a Heart Attack

Many heart attacks in women go unnoticed because women's symptoms are sometimes different from men's. Most men, for example, develop a crushing pain in the chest. Although some women also have chest pain, others have nausea as their first symptom along with chest pain. Know the warning signs of a heart attack:

▶ Sudden, intense pressure or pain in the chest

▶ Shortness of breath

▶ Chest pain that spreads to the shoulders, neck, or arms

▶ Feelings of light-headedness, fainting, sweating, or nausea

If any of these symptoms last more than 5 minutes, you could be having a heart attack. Call an ambulance and go to the hospital. While you're waiting, take an aspirin, lie down, and breathe slowly. This may help limit the damage to your heart muscle.

The only way to check for high blood pressure is to have it measured with an inflatable cuff that is wrapped around your arm. A blood pressure reading has two numbers separated by a slash, the systolic pressure and diastolic pressure. A reading of more than 140/90 is considered high and requires attention.

Controlling high blood pressure will lower your risk of heart disease. Getting regular exercise and maintaining a healthy weight can help. If these steps don't keep your blood pressure in the normal range, medication may be necessary.

> **For a Healthy Heart**
>
> Follow this prescription for a healthy heart:
>
> ▶ Eat a well-balanced diet that is low in fat.
> ▶ Have your blood pressure checked regularly.
> ▶ Don't smoke.
> ▶ Exercise at least three times a week.
> ▶ Monitor your cholesterol levels.

Lack of Exercise

Lack of exercise can raise your risk of heart disease. Exercise can help control high blood pressure, obesity, and high cholesterol, all of which increase your chances of getting heart disease.

It is important to get active and stay active. Regular exercise can help you lose weight and keep it off, which is also healthier for your heart. The best exercise to strengthen your heart is aerobic exercise, such as brisk walking, dancing, jogging, or climbing the stairs. You should exercise about 30 minutes every day.

Obesity

Obesity (being more than 30% above your ideal weight) increases your risk of heart disease, diabetes, and high blood pressure. Women with fat around their abdomen (apple-shaped) are at higher risk for heart disease than women who gain extra pounds around their hips and thighs (pear-shaped).

Maintaining a healthy weight can lower your risk of health problems. If you need help, talk with your doctor about a diet and exercise program that is right for you.

In 1988, not one state in the United States had an obesity rate higher than 15% of the population. By 1998, all but 10 states had reached or topped that mark. Almost a quarter (22%) of Americans are obese.

Diabetes

Diabetes increases a woman's chances of developing heart problems. Diabetes is a condition that causes high levels of glucose (sugar) in the blood. Women who have diabetes often have other risk factors for heart disease, such as high blood pressure, high cholesterol, and obesity.

Cigarette Smoking

Smoking doubles the risk of heart disease in women. Women older than age 35 who smoke and use oral contraceptives (birth control pills) are at an even higher risk for heart attack. Women who stop smoking decrease their risk for heart disease to that of a nonsmoker in 5–10 years.

Especially for Women

The female hormone estrogen helps protect the heart and arteries against cholesterol that clogs blood vessels. It keeps arteries open and increases HDL cholesterol, resulting in less plaque. After menopause, a woman's level of estrogen decreases and she loses this benefit. Women who are menopausal can take hormone replacement therapy (HRT) to replace the estrogen their body is no longer making.

By age 65, women without estrogen have the same heart attack rate as men. HRT may reduce a woman's risk of heart disease by as much as 50%. Discuss the benefits of HRT with your doctor to see if it is right for you.

Many women also take aspirin, which has been found to help prevent heart attacks in men because of its blood-thinning qualities. More research is needed to know if this is also true for women.

▶ HEARTBURN

About 60 million American adults have heartburn at least once a month. Heartburn is a symptom of something called gastroesophageal reflux disease (GERD). With GERD, the valve that connects the esophagus (throat) with the stomach is weak and does not keep acid and food from flowing backwards. Heartburn happens when acidic juices from the stomach splash upwards. Heartburn's burning and pressure may last as long as 2 hours. It is often worse after eating, lying down, or bending over.

Heartburn feels like a burning chest pain behind the breastbone. The feeling can extend to the throat and neck. It may seem like food is coming back into the mouth and you may notice an acid or bitter taste.

Tips for preventing and treating heartburn and GERD include:

▶ Avoid foods that irritate the stomach lining or affect the pressure in the lower esophagus. These include fried and fatty foods, peppermint, chocolate, alcohol, coffee, citrus fruits and juices, and tomato products.

▶ Lose weight.

▶ Stop smoking.

▶ Elevate the head of the bed 6 inches. You can put blocks under the legs or use a foam wedge.

▶ Avoid lying down 2–3 hours after eating.

Although heartburn is a very common digestive problem in the United States, it is rarely life-threatening. It may, however, limit daily activities. Once the causes are found and treatment begins, most people find relief.

Heartburn pain is sometimes mistaken for a heart attack. A way to tell the two conditions apart is with heart disease, exercise makes the pain worse and rest relieves it. Heartburn is usually not affected by exercise.

Most of the time, taking an antacid can treat bouts of heartburn very well. These are sold over the counter in pharmacies and many grocery stores. If you need antacids for more than 3 weeks, see your doctor. Taking antacids for too long can cause side effects. People with chronic GERD and heartburn can sometimes benefit from other drugs that reduce acid in the stomach.

HEMORRHOIDS

Hemorrhoids are swollen blood vessels in and around the anus and lower rectum that stretch under pressure. They can become painful, itchy, and irritated, especially by straining to have bowel movements. Hemorrhoids may be caused by:

- Being overweight
- Pregnancy
- Standing or sitting for long periods
- Straining during physical labor
- Constipation

The symptoms of hemorrhoids can be relieved with ice packs to reduce swelling and by applying hemorrhoidal cream or suppositories to the affected area. Witch hazel also may help relieve symptoms. Increasing fiber and fluids in your diet is an important factor in preventing hemorrhoids. In more severe cases, surgery may be needed to remove troubling hemorrhoids.

HEPATITIS VIRUS

See also *Hepatitis B Virus*

Hepatitis is a virus that attacks and damages the liver. This infection makes your liver swell and prevents it from working as it should. The most common types of hepatitis are hepatitis A, hepatitis B, and hepatitis C. Although these forms of hepatitis differ in many ways, they all have certain things in common.

How It Is Spread

Hepatitis A is spread when a person eats food or drinks water infected with stool that contains the virus. Some people are at high risk for hepatitis A virus. You should be vaccinated if you have one or more of these risk factors:

▶ Live with someone who has the disease

▶ Work in a daycare center or have children in daycare

▶ Are a man who has sex with men

▶ Travel to other countries

Hepatitis B and hepatitis C are spread through blood and body fluids, such as sharing needles or having unprotected sex with someone who is infected. It also may be passed from a mother to a baby during birth. If you had an organ transplant or blood transfusion before 1992, you might have hepatitis C. Before 1992, there was no way to check blood for the virus.

Symptoms and Diagnosis

Symptoms for each type of hepatitis are about the same. You may be tired, lose your appetite, or feel like you have the flu, with nausea, fever, diarrhea, and pain in the stomach, muscles, or joints. Some people get dark-yellow urine, light-colored stools, and yellowish eyes and skin. Many people often have no symptoms at all.

If you have these symptoms or have been exposed to hepatitis, see your doctor. Your blood will be tested for a special protein, called an antigen, that is found in blood infected with the virus. In some cases, a tiny piece of your liver will be removed with a needle to check for abnormal cells. This is called a biopsy.

Treatment

Most people with hepatitis A get well on their own after a few weeks. You may need to rest in bed for a few days or even weeks. Your doctor may give you medicine to treat your symptoms. You should not drink alcohol until you are well again.

Some people with hepatitis B or C have chronic infections that never go away. Often these people do not feel sick. Yet they may get liver damage known as cirrhosis. They also have a higher risk of liver cancer.

Prevention

The best way to avoid getting hepatitis A or B is to get the vaccine. A vaccine is a type of medicine you are given, often as a

For more information on hepatitis, contact:

Hepatitis Foundation
   International
30 Sunrise Terrace
Cedar Grove, NJ 07009-1423
Phone: 800-891-0707
Web Address: www.hepfi.org

shot, to keep you from getting a certain type of disease, such as hepatitis. The hepatitis virus vaccine triggers the body's immune system to make antibodies, proteins found in the blood produced in reaction to foreign substances such as bacteria or viruses. These antibodies then fight off the virus when you are exposed to it. The vaccine will not help people who are already infected. Your doctor may also give you gamma globulin, which contain antibodies to the virus. This will protect you against the virus until the vaccine triggers your body to make its own antibodies. There is no vaccine to prevent hepatitis C.

Other steps for preventing hepatitis A:

▶ Wash your hands after using the toilet and before fixing food or eating.

▶ Wear gloves if you have to touch other people's stool. Wash your hands when you are finished.

▶ Drink bottled water when you are in another country. Do not use ice cubes or wash fruits and vegetables in tap water.

Other steps for preventing hepatitis B and C:

▶ Don't share drug needles with anyone.

▶ Wear gloves if you have to touch anyone's blood.

▶ Don't use an infected person's toothbrush, razor, or anything that could have blood on it.

▶ If you get a tattoo or body piercing, make sure the tools are clean.

▶ Use a condom when you have sex.

A new combined hepatitis A and B vaccine is being studied to see if it is more effective than the current vaccine method. The new vaccine takes less time than the current method. It may be most useful for travelers, who often need the vaccine quickly.

▶ HEPATITIS B VIRUS

Hepatitis B is a serious infection of the liver caused by the hepatitis B virus. Each year, about 300,000 people in the United States get infected with the hepatitis B virus. The disease can be fatal. About 5,000 deaths a year are due to liver diseases caused by the virus.

What Is Hepatitis B?

Hepatitis B is a type of hepatitis virus that attacks and damages the liver—an organ located at the upper-right side of the abdomen. The liver cleanses the body of waste. It breaks down and filters out any harmful substances that you consume. The liver also makes bile, which helps you to digest food.

There are over 1 million carriers of hepatitis B virus in the United States. Children are at especially high risk. About 90% of babies who become infected with the virus at birth, and up to 50% of children who are infected before they reach 5 years of age, become chronic carriers.

Infection with hepatitis B can damage the liver over time and lead to cirrhosis of the liver. With this condition, cells of the liver die and are replaced by scar tissue. Over time, the liver stops working. Hepatitis B is also the most common cause of liver cancer.

A person may be infected with the hepatitis B virus and not know it—sometimes the virus does not cause any symptoms. When symptoms do occur, they may include:

▶ Jaundice (yellowing of the skin and eyes)

▶ Extreme fatigue

▶ Loss of appetite

▶ Nausea

▶ Headache

▶ Stomachache

▶ Muscle aches

In most adults, the infection clears up completely in a few weeks. Most adults then become immune to the virus—that is, they will not get it again. They can no longer pass the virus to others.

However, in about 5–10% of infected adults (and in many children younger than age 5), the infection never clears up completely. This is known as chronic infection. These people keep the virus for the rest of their lives and are known as carriers. They may not always have symptoms. About 1 million people in the United States are carriers of the hepatitis B virus. All carriers can pass the virus to others.

Testing for the Virus

A blood test can show whether someone has been infected with hepatitis B virus. For the test, a small sample of blood is taken and tested for a special protein, called an antigen, which is found in blood infected with the virus.

If your test result is negative, it means you had not been infected with the virus at the time the test was done. If your test result is positive, it means you have been infected with the virus and can infect others, including your baby if you are pregnant. Your doctor will want to do more tests to learn whether your liver is still healthy. A positive test result means that your children, your sexual partner(s), and others living in your household are at risk of infection. They should be told about testing and vaccination and decide whether to have them done.

If you are pregnant, you should be tested for the virus. The test should be done early enough in pregnancy to allow time to prepare treatment for the baby and test family members if your test result is positive.

How Is It Spread?

Hepatitis B is spread by direct contact with the body fluids (blood, semen, vaginal fluids) of an infected person. This can happen during sexual intercourse, while sharing needles used to inject ("shoot") drugs, and during delivery of a baby. Hepatitis B can also be spread if you live with an infected person and share household items that may transmit body fluids, like toothbrushes or razors.

Hepatitis B cannot be spread by casual contact with people and objects. Casual contact includes shaking hands, sharing food or drink, or coughing and sneezing.

Who Is at Risk?

Anyone can get hepatitis B virus. Your risk is higher if you:

▶ Inject illegal drugs, such as crack or heroin

▶ Have had a sexually transmitted disease

▶ Have had multiple sexual partners

▶ Are a health care or public safety worker

▶ Live with someone who is infected with the virus

▶ Have worked or lived in a home for the disabled

▶ Have been on dialysis or worked in a dialysis unit

▶ Have received treatment (clotting factors) for a bleeding disorder

Other groups at risk include homosexual or bisexual men and sexual partners of infected men. The risk of infection is also high in Asian and Inuit populations. Infection is more likely if you or your sexual partner have a tattoo or have served time in prison.

The hepatitis B vaccine is safe for use during pregnancy. There is no risk of getting hepatitis or other diseases, such as AIDS, from the vaccine.

If any of these risk factors apply to you or your partner, ask your doctor about being tested and about ways to protect against the infection.

A simple blood test can show whether you are infected with the hepatitis B virus and can pass it to others. If you test positive, it is important for you to take certain steps to avoid passing the infection to others:

▶ Do not donate blood or plasma or arrange to be an organ donor.

▶ Do not share toothbrushes or razors or other objects that could be in touch with blood.

▶ Tell sex partners—past and present—and the people who live with you.

Most infants who receive the hepatitis B vaccine have no side effects. Some may have minor problems, such as redness or tenderness where the shot was given. Serious problems are rare.

Prevention

There is no cure for hepatitis B. It is best to take steps to prevent it. You can help prevent it by avoiding the risky habits that can pass the virus.

The best protection against hepatitis B, however, is a vaccine. The vaccine triggers your body's immune system to fight off the virus when you are exposed to it. It is usually given in three doses: the first dose is followed by a second dose in 1 month and a third dose in 6 months. The vaccine is recommended for:

▶ All babies, children, and adolescents aged 18 years and younger

▶ Anyone at high risk

Some doctors suggest that all teenagers should get the vaccine to protect themselves and any children they may have later. If you are a teenager and are at high risk, you should get the vaccine.

People who have been recently exposed to the virus and are not vaccinated are usually given the vaccine along with a shot of hepatitis B immune globulin. Hepatitis B immune globulin (HBIG) contains antibodies to the virus. It gives temporary protection (about 3–6 months) against hepatitis B.

There are also lifestyle changes you can make to lower your risk of getting the virus:

▶ Use a latex condom during sex.

▶ Practice "safer" sex (know your partner's sexual history and have only one sexual partner).

▶ If you are injecting drugs, get help and try to stop—if you can't stop, do not share needles.

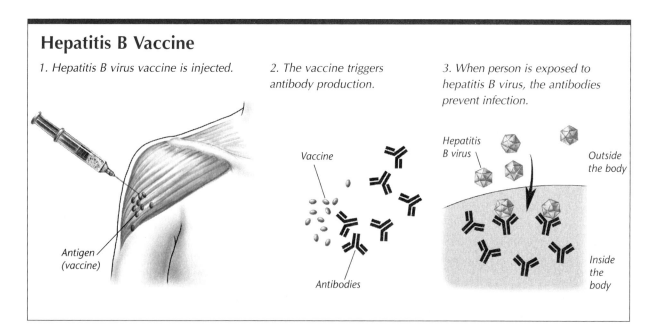

Hepatitis B Vaccine

1. Hepatitis B virus vaccine is injected.

2. The vaccine triggers antibody production.

3. When person is exposed to hepatitis B virus, the antibodies prevent infection.

Antigen (vaccine)

Vaccine

Antibodies

Hepatitis B virus

Outside the body

Inside the body

Effects During Pregnancy

Infection with hepatitis B virus is a special problem for pregnant women. About 1 in every 500–1,000 pregnant women has hepatitis when she gives birth. More pregnant women may be infected but not show any signs.

When a pregnant woman is infected with hepatitis B virus, there is a chance she may infect her fetus. Whether the baby will get the virus depends on when infection occurred. If it was early in pregnancy, the chances are less than 10% that the baby will get the virus. If it was late in pregnancy, there is up to a 90% chance the baby will be infected.

Hepatitis may be severe in babies. It can threaten their lives. Even babies who appear well may be at risk for serious health problems.

Infected newborns have a high risk (up to 90%) of becoming carriers. They, too, can pass the virus to others. When they become adults, these carriers have a 25% risk of dying of cirrhosis or liver cancer.

All infants should get the hepatitis B virus vaccine. If you are pregnant and have the virus, your baby will receive HBIG soon after birth. Your baby also will receive the first dose of the vaccine. Two more doses of the vaccine will be given later—one at 1 month and one at 6 months of age. This plan is 95% effective in protecting babies from becoming hepatitis B virus carriers.

If you had a negative test result, your baby should get the first dose of vaccine before you leave the hospital. If it cannot be given by then, it should be given within 2 months of birth. Check with the baby's doctor to find out when the second and third doses should be given.

If you were not tested, your baby should get the first dose of vaccine and you then should be tested. The rest of your baby's treatment depends on whether you are positive or negative.

▶ HERPES

Genital herpes is a viral infection spread through sexual contact. It affects 1 in 5 adults in the United States—about 50 million people.

What Is Genital Herpes?

Genital herpes is a sexually transmitted disease (STD). It is spread through close contact, most often during sexual activity.

Genital herpes is probably best known for the sores and blisters it causes. These sores appear around the genitals or lips. The place where the sores appear is the original site where the

Do You Know?

The herpes virus belongs to the same group of viruses that include the herpes zoster or varicella zoster that causes chickenpox in children and shingles in adults.

virus entered your body. In most cases, genital herpes is spread through direct contact with these sores.

How Infection Occurs

The herpes virus passes through a break in your skin. It also can enter the moist membranes of the penis, vagina, urinary opening, cervix, or anus.

Once the virus gets into your body, it infects healthy cells. Your body's natural defense system then begins to fight the virus. This causes sores, blisters, and swelling.

Besides the sex organs, genital herpes can affect the tongue, mouth, eyes, gums, lips, fingers, and other parts of the body. During oral sex, herpes can be passed from a cold sore around the mouth to the partner's genitals or vice versa. You can even infect yourself if you touch a sore and then rub or scratch another part of your body, especially your eyes.

The herpes virus can survive for a few hours outside the body. There is no proof it can be picked up from toilet seats, hot tubs, or other objects.

Symptoms

Many people infected with herpes have no symptoms. When symptoms do occur, they vary with each person. Some people have painful attacks with many sores. Others have only mild symptoms.

If you get symptoms, they will appear about 2–10 days after the herpes virus enters your body. At this time, you may feel like you have the flu. You may get swollen glands, fever, chills, muscle aches, fatigue, and nausea. You also may get sores. Sores appear as small, fluid-filled blisters on the genitals, buttocks, or other areas. The sores often are grouped in clusters. Stinging or burning when you urinate also is common.

The first bout with genital herpes may last as long as 3 weeks. During this time, lesions break open and "weep." Over a period of days, the sores become crusted and then heal without leaving scars.

If lesions recur, you may feel burning, itching, or tingling near where the virus first entered your body. You also may feel pain in your lower back, buttocks, thighs, or knees. These symptoms are called a prodrome. A few hours later, sores will appear. In recurrent infections there is usually no fever and

If You Have a Herpes Outbreak

The following tips may help relieve some discomfort of herpes:

- Keep the lesions clean and dry.

- Use a hair dryer on the low setting to dry sores that are very sensitive or hard to reach.

- Wear loose-fitting cotton underclothes and avoid pantyhose. Nylon and other synthetics hold in heat and moisture, which may slow the healing process.

- Take aspirin or acetaminophen to relieve the pain.

no swelling in the genital area. Sores heal more quickly—within 3–7 days in most cases.

See your doctor right away if you have symptoms of genital herpes. Similar symptoms may be caused by other infections, so your doctor should confirm the diagnosis.

Diagnosis

One way your doctor can diagnose herpes is to examine the genitals. There are also a number of tests to detect infection. The most accurate way is to obtain a sample from the sore and see if the virus grows in a special fluid. Test results may take about 1 week. A positive result confirms the diagnosis, but a negative result does not rule it out.

Because the test for herpes has a high rate of false negative results (60–70%), the infection usually is diagnosed by examining a lesion.

Treatment

There is no cure for genital herpes. However, there are oral medications to help control the course of the disease. Medication can shorten the length of an outbreak and help reduce discomfort.

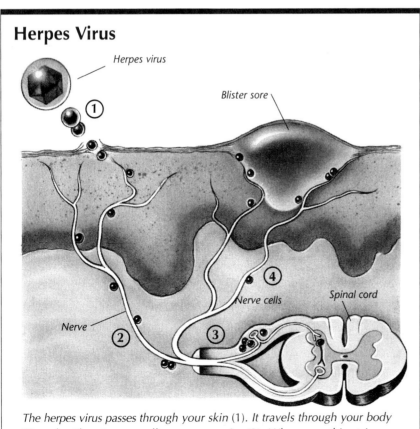

Herpes Virus

The herpes virus passes through your skin (1). It travels through your body (2) and settles at nerve cells near your spine (3). When something triggers a new bout of herpes, the virus leaves its resting place and travels along the nerve, back to the surface of the skin (4).

If you have repeat outbreaks, taking medication on a daily basis can greatly reduce the attacks. In many cases, it can prevent attacks completely. Ask your doctor whether this type of treatment is right for you.

Most people can tell when they are having an outbreak. Learning what to do during an outbreak can also help reduce discomfort that goes with it.

Avoiding Recurrence

Although some people with herpes report that their outbreaks are triggered by stress, illness, or having a menstrual period, outbreaks often are not predictable. In some cases, outbreaks may be connected to exposure to sunlight.

Although herpes sores heal in days or weeks, herpes does not leave your body. The virus travels to nerve cells near your spine. It stays there until some event triggers a new bout. Then the viruses leave their resting place and travel along the nerves, back to where they first entered the body. This causes new blisters to occur.

No one is sure why some people have recurrences of herpes. One trigger seems to be stress—both emotional and physical. Outbreaks may recur when you are under pressure, or they may recur when your resistance is lowered by a cold or flu. Keep your body strong—get plenty of rest, eat a balanced diet, and learn to cope with stress.

About 90% of people with herpes have repeat bouts. How often these bouts occur varies greatly from person to person. Some people have only one or two outbreaks a year. Others have as many as five to eight. Fortunately, most recurrent infections are milder than the first.

Spread Prevention

If you or your partner have oral or genital herpes, avoid sex from the time of prodromal symptoms until a few days after the scabs have gone away. Not having sex doesn't mean you can't kiss, hug, or cuddle. Just be sure that lesions and their secretions do not touch the other person's skin. Wash your hands with soap and water after any possible contact with lesions. This will keep you from reinfecting yourself or passing the virus to someone else.

Using a condom may not protect against herpes. Although the virus does not cross through the condom, lesions not covered by the condom can cause infection. Using a condom will help protect you from other STDs, though.

Genital Herpes and Pregnancy

If you are pregnant and have herpes, tell your doctor. During pregnancy, there are increased risks to the baby, especially if it's the mother's first outbreak.

Most newborns become infected while they are being born through the mother's infected birth canal. If you have sores at the time of delivery, your doctor may suggest a cesarean birth. Cesarean birth may reduce the chance the baby will come in contact with the virus.

A cesarean delivery takes place through a surgical cut in the abdomen, where the tissue is not infected with the virus. However, a baby can be infected without passing through the vagina. The infection can occur if the amniotic sac (fluid-filled sac in which the baby grows) has broken a few hours before birth.

▶ HIGH BLOOD PRESSURE

▶ See also *Cholesterol, Diabetes, Heart Disease, High Blood Pressure During Pregnancy*

High blood pressure (or hypertension) has long been called a "silent killer" because it often causes no symptoms. After age 50, high blood pressure is more common in women than men. Untreated, high blood pressure can lead to other serious health conditions, such as heart disease, stroke, and kidney disease.

What Is Blood Pressure?

Blood pressure is vital for the body's circulatory system—the heart, arteries, and veins—to function. It is created in part by the steady beating of the heart. Each time the heart contracts, or squeezes, it pumps blood into the arteries. The arteries carry the blood to the body's organs. The veins return it to the heart.

Small arteries, called arterioles, also affect blood pressure. These blood vessels are lined with a layer of muscle. When the blood pressure is normal, this muscle is relaxed and the arteri-

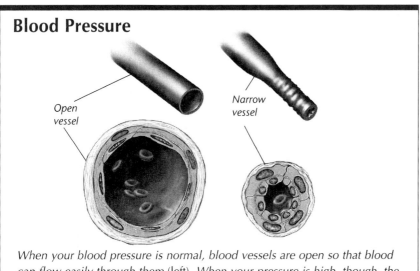

Blood Pressure

Open vessel

Narrow vessel

When your blood pressure is normal, blood vessels are open so that blood can flow easily through them (left). When your pressure is high, though, the vessels are narrow (right). This makes it harder for the blood to flow.

oles are dilated (open) so that blood can flow through them easily. However, if a signal is sent to increase the blood pressure, the muscle layer tightens and the arterioles narrow. This makes it harder for the blood to flow. The pressure then increases in the arteries.

Imagine that an arteriole is the nozzle on a hose. When the nozzle is open, the water can escape, so the pressure in the hose is normal. When it is closed, the water is trapped. The pressure in the hose increases, but less water comes out.

Blood pressure is checked with a stethoscope and a device made of a pressure gauge and a cuff that inflates. A blood pressure reading has two numbers. Each number is separated by a slash: 110/80, for instance. (You may hear this referred to as "110 over 80.")

The first number is the pressure in the arteries when the heart contracts. This is called the systolic pressure. The second number is the pressure in the arteries when the heart relaxes between contractions. This is the diastolic pressure.

Blood pressure can go up and down throughout the day. Blood pressure that is consistently more than 140/90 (read as "140 over 90") is considered hypertension. The box shows how your doctor classifies your blood pressure reading as normal or high.

Every woman should have her blood pressure checked yearly—the test is simple and painless. To measure your blood pressure, an inflatable cuff that is pumped with air is wrapped around your upper arm. Your pressure reading is taken while the cuff is squeezing your arm.

How High Blood Pressure Affects Your Body

High blood pressure can have a number of causes and often runs in families. People with high blood pressure often have no symptoms and feel fine. Long before high blood pressure causes symptoms, however, it can damage vital organs in your body. If it is not treated, high blood pressure can lead to very serious health problems.

The Blood Vessels

Long-term high blood pressure can damage blood vessels. The buildup of plaque also can lead to a narrowing of blood vessels. Plaque is a fatty substance that forms in the arteries when too much cholesterol is present. Over the years, plaque causes the arteries to narrow and harden. This is called atherosclerosis. The combination of atherosclerosis and high blood pressure sets the stage for stroke and heart attack.

How High Is Too High?

The chart below shows different blood pressure readings and how they are classified for adults aged 18 and older. Find your systolic and diastolic pressure readings to see whether your blood pressure is normal.

Category	Systolic (mm Hg)	Diastolic (mm Hg)
Optimal	Less than 120	Less than 80
Normal	Less than 130	Less than 85
High normal	130–139	85–89
Hypertension	More than 140	More than 90

Joint National Committee on the Prevention, Detection, Evaluation, and Treatment of High Blood Pressure. Sixth Report of the Joint National Committee on the Prevention, Detection, Evaluation, and Treatment of High Blood Pressure (JNC VI). Bethesda, Maryland: National Heart, Lung, and Blood Institute, 1997

The Heart

As blood pressure increases, the heart has to work harder to deliver oxygen to the tissues. Over time, the heart enlarges and may have trouble doing its work. This can lead to heart failure.

Your Blood Pressure Reading		
110 = systolic =	pressure in the arteries when heart contracts
80 = diastolic =	pressure in the arteries when heart relaxes

The Brain

High blood pressure can cause a blood vessel to the brain to burst and lead to stroke. Brain cells in that part of the brain may die. A stroke that continues for a few minutes can cause permanent brain damage or death. Depending on the part of the brain affected, signals from the brain to the body can be disrupted and can affect speech, movement, and other bodily functions.

The Kidneys

The kidneys filter the blood to remove waste from your body. The blood vessels in the kidneys can be easily damaged by high blood pressure. When the kidneys are not working normally, their ability to control salt and water balance in the body is disrupted. This can lead to kidney failure.

The Eyes

High blood pressure can also narrow the blood vessels in the eyes. This can cause your vision to become worse and may even lead to blindness.

Risks for High Blood Pressure

Lifestyle habits can increase your risk for high blood pressure. Women who are overweight, are not physically active, smoke cigarettes, or drink large amounts of alcohol are more at risk. Diet and stress also play a role.

There are factors, however, that increase the risk for high blood pressure that are not related to lifestyle habits and cannot be changed:

▶ *Age*—Blood pressure increases with age, and high blood pressure occurs most often among women older than 40.

▶ *Race*—High blood pressure is more common in African Americans than in any other racial group.

▶ *Family history*—High blood pressure tends to run in families.

▶ *Medical conditions*—Certain diseases, such as diabetes and kidney disease, can be linked to high blood pressure.

"White coat hypertension" occurs when your blood pressure increases in your doctor's office, but not at other times. Most of the time, this diagnosis is not thought to be a health risk.

Managing High Blood Pressure

You can lessen your risk of high blood pressure and its long-term effects by adopting a healthy lifestyle. The following methods may help decrease your blood pressure:

▶ *Lose weight*—If you are overweight, losing weight is the single most effective way to reduce your blood pressure. Even as little as a 5-pound weight loss can make a difference.

▶ *Exercise regularly*—Daily exercise decreases your blood pressure. You can benefit from doing moderate aerobic exercise, such as brisk walking, swimming, or bicycling, for at least 30 minutes a day.

▶ *Quit smoking*—Cigarette smoking is a major risk for high blood pressure and heart disease. When you quit smoking, the benefits begin right away.

▶ *Limit alcohol drinking*—Heavy alcohol drinking (more than two drinks a day) is linked to an increase in blood pressure.

▶ *Cut back on salt*—Heavy salt (sodium) consumption can increase blood pressure in some people. Some people with high blood pressure are "salt sensitive"—their blood pressure increases when on a high-salt diet and decreases when on a low-salt diet.

▶ *Change your diet*—If your high blood pressure is linked to atherosclerosis, a low cholesterol diet may be helpful.

▶ *Relieve stress*—Stress that is not managed or relieved can affect your health. Relaxation techniques, exercise, or getting professional counseling can help you cope with stress.

Medical Treatment

Your doctor may prescribe medications to decrease your high blood pressure. He or she will discuss with you which ones are best for your condition.

Medications to treat high blood pressure can have side effects. If you think you are having any side effects, talk to your doctor—it's possible that you can try different therapy. Do not stop taking your medication—this could cause your blood pressure to increase to a very high level. It is important to continue taking your medication even when you are feeling healthy.

About 50 million Americans have high blood pressure, but about a third do not know it. Of those that do know they have it, only 27% have it under control.

HIGH BLOOD PRESSURE DURING PREGNANCY

See also *High Blood Pressure*

Blood pressure is the pressure in the vessels that carry blood through the body. Normal levels are key to good health. When pressure becomes too high, it is known as hypertension. This can pose health risks at any time. It is even more of a risk during pregnancy.

High blood pressure can be present before a woman becomes pregnant. It also can first appear when a woman is pregnant. If it is not treated, it can cause severe problems for both mother and baby. If you are pregnant and have any of the risk factors that may lead to high blood pressure, you may need special care.

Blood Pressure

Blood pressure changes from person to person. It changes often during the day. It can increase if you are excited or if you exercise. Most often, it decreases when you are resting. These short-term changes in blood pressure are normal. It is only when a person's blood pressure stays high for some time that it may signal a problem.

In most nonpregnant women, readings less than 130/80 are normal. If you are pregnant and your systolic pressure is 140 or the diastolic pressure is 90, it is too high.

Because of the normal ups and downs in blood pressure, if you have one high reading, another reading may be taken again later to see if it is your normal level. Your normal blood pressure can be an average of a number of readings taken at rest.

A single reading of high blood pressure is not enough to confirm the diagnosis of high blood pressure. Whether you use a home monitor or a monitor in a drug store or grocery store, be sure to confirm your results with your doctor.

Types of High Blood Pressure

When high blood pressure has been present for some time before pregnancy, it is known as chronic hypertension. This condition remains during pregnancy and after the birth of the baby. When high blood pressure occurs for the first time during pregnancy, it is known as pregnancy-induced hypertension (PIH).

Both types can pose a risk during pregnancy. If high blood pressure is controlled, the risks are reduced.

Chronic Hypertension

If it is not treated, chronic hypertension can lead to health problems such as heart failure or stroke. Women with chronic hypertension who took medication to control their blood pressure before they were pregnant often can keep on taking it during pregnancy under their doctor's care. If you take medication to control your blood pressure, ask your doctor if it is safe to use during pregnancy.

Pregnancy-Induced Hypertension

Pregnancy-induced hypertension, sometimes called preeclampsia, may occur some time after the 20th week of pregnancy. It goes away soon after the baby is born. With PIH, high blood pressure and other problems are present. Women with chronic hypertension are at increased risk of developing PIH.

Pregnant women should be aware of the symptoms of PIH. They are not always easy to detect. A pregnant woman could have PIH for weeks and not know it. The serious risks of high blood pressure in pregnancy can be decreased if it is found and treated early. The only way to detect PIH is to measure the blood pressure regularly.

Effects on Pregnancy

In a healthy pregnancy, the fetus receives from the mother all of the nutrients and oxygen it needs for normal growth. This happens when the correct amount of the mother's blood flows through the placenta and the nutrients and oxygen pass through the umbilical cord to the baby.

When a woman has high blood pressure in pregnancy, it may cause less blood to flow to the placenta. This means that the fetus receives less of the oxygen and nutrients it needs. This causes the growth of the fetus to slow. Thus, the growth and health of the fetus may be checked using ultrasound and electronic fetal monitoring.

When PIH is mild, blood pressure increases only slightly. If the mother's blood pressure is kept under control, she most likely will have a healthy baby. During pregnancy, high blood pressure that is mild will not harm the mother in most cases.

When PIH becomes more severe, other conditions can develop and affect the mother:

▶ Her organs—such as the kidneys, liver, brain, and eyes—can become damaged.

▶ Her heart may be weakened.

▶ Her urine tests may show that there is protein in her urine.

▶ She may have swelling (edema) of her hands and face. (It is normal for pregnant women to have some swelling of the feet. In women who have high blood pressure, though, this can be a sign of severe PIH.)

▶ She may develop HELLP syndrome (Hemolysis, Elevated Liver enzymes, and Low Platelets).

▶ In extreme cases, she may have seizures. This is sometimes called eclampsia.

If PIH is not treated, it can be life-threatening for the mother and baby. The baby may be born too small. In severe cases, the baby may die. Severe PIH may require early delivery, even if the baby is not fully grown. A baby born before 37 weeks of pregnancy may have problems breathing because its lungs may not be fully developed.

Risk Factors

Most women with PIH have never had high blood pressure. Doctors do not know why some women get PIH. They do know that some women are at a higher risk than others. The risk of developing PIH is higher in women who:

▶ Have a history of chronic hypertension or PIH

▶ Are pregnant for the first time

▶ Are older than age 40

▶ Are carrying more than one fetus

▶ Have certain medical conditions such as diabetes or kidney disease

Pregnancy-induced hypertension occurs more often in women with a family history of the condition. It also occurs more often in African-American women. If you are at high risk for PIH, talk with your doctor about what might be best for you.

Prenatal Care

If a woman knows she has high blood pressure before or during pregnancy—or if she knows she may be at risk—there are steps she and her doctor can take to reduce the chance of severe effects to herself or her baby. For this reason, the best thing a woman can do is to see her doctor before pregnancy and get regular prenatal care.

Warning Signs of Pregnancy-Induced Hypertension

If you notice any of these symptoms, you should call your doctor right away:

▶ A sudden weight gain of more than about 1 pound a day

▶ Swelling (edema) of the face and hands

▶ Severe or constant headaches

▶ Blurred vision or spots in front of the eyes

▶ Pain in the upper right part of the abdomen

What You Can Do

Until more is known about what causes PIH, the best approach is to prevent it from becoming too severe. If you have chronic high blood pressure or are at risk for PIH, follow these steps to help make your pregnancy safer:

Before pregnancy:

▶ If you have high blood pressure, work with your doctor so that you can get it under control.

▶ Take medication as prescribed.

▶ Lose weight through diet and exercise, if needed.

▶ Check with your doctor to see if your blood pressure medication is safe to use during pregnancy.

During pregnancy:

▶ See your doctor regularly, starting as soon as you can, so that changes in your blood pressure and weight can be found as soon as they occur.

▶ If you have high blood pressure, kidney disease, or any other risk factors, be sure to tell your doctor early in pregnancy.

▶ If you develop any of the warning signs of PIH, tell your doctor right away.

▶ Check your blood pressure and weight at home, if your doctor suggests you do so.

▶ Tell your doctor about all the medications you are taking, including over-the-counter products.

At each prenatal visit, a woman's weight and blood pressure are taken. This helps detect any changes that might have occurred. Once the doctor is aware that a woman's blood pressure is high or that she is at risk for PIH, she may be checked more often. A urine sample also is tested for protein in the urine. Its presence is a sign of PIH.

If high blood pressure occurs, it can be watched closely and treated. This may prevent other problems. The type of treatment depends on whether the high blood pressure is mild or severe and how long a woman has been pregnant.

Treatment of Mild PIH

When blood pressure increases slightly and the woman is not near the end of her pregnancy, bed rest may help control the pressure. Bed rest may be at home or in the hospital. If the blood pressure does not increase to dangerous levels, pregnancy will be allowed to continue until labor begins naturally.

Treatment of Severe PIH

Although most symptoms of PIH can be controlled, the only real cure for PIH is having the baby. The decision to deliver the baby depends on both the risks to the mother and whether the risk to the baby is greater in the mother's uterus or in a special nursery. The delivery may occur naturally or labor may be induced (brought on). Sometimes a cesarean birth is needed.

Before deciding to deliver your baby early, your doctor may wait to see if your condition improves. During labor you may be given medication to help prevent seizures or lower your blood pressure.

▶ See also *Polycystic Ovary Syndrome*

▶ HIRSUTISM

Hirsutism is excessive hair growth. Some women grow coarse hair on the face, chest, belly, back, upper arms, or upper legs in a pattern like that of men.

Some women naturally have more hair than others. Some ethnic or racial groups tend to grow dark hair on the upper lip, face, or body. Although these women may feel their hair growth is heavy, it is normal for them.

Hirsutism arises when the level of male hormones in a woman's body is too high. All women produce male and female hormones. These hormones can get out of balance for several reasons:

▶ *Polycystic ovarian syndrome (PCOS).* In this disorder, cysts grow on the ovaries and produce large amounts of male hormones. Women with PCOS may have irregular periods, as well.

▶ *Ovarian or adrenal tumors.* Tumors that grow on the ovaries or adrenal glands can sometimes cause hirsutism and male-like balding.

▶ *Late-onset adrenal hyperplasia.* This inherited disorder causes the adrenal glands to produce increased amounts of male hormones.

▶ *Insulin resistance syndrome.* Women with this syndrome produce too much insulin (a hormone that decreases the levels of sugar in the blood), which causes the ovaries to produce too much male hormone.

▶ *Medicines.* Some drugs used to treat illness have the same traits as male hormones. They may cause hair growth and acne.

Women who think they have hirsutism should see a doctor. Early treatment brings the best results. Blood tests, ultrasound, or special X-rays may be done to find the reason for excess hair growth. Then, depending on the cause, drugs may be given to block or reduce male hormones. In the case of cysts or tumors, surgery may be needed. After treatment, unwanted hair growth may slow down or go away completely.

Unwanted hair that remains after treatment—or has no medical cause—can be removed. Plucking, waxing, shaving, and depilatory agents remove hair for a while. Bleaching creams can lighten hair so it's not as easy to see. The only long-term method of hair removal is electrolysis. In electrolysis, an electric current is sent through a fine needle into the hair root to kill it. It is a slow, costly process, but works well when done by a trained technician.

Your doctor may prescribe a drug to decrease excess hair growth. However, the drug often takes 3–6 months to work and will only reduce the amount of new hair growth. It is unlikely to change the amount of hair you already have.

▶ HORMONE IMPLANTS

▶ See also *Birth Control*

Implants are a form of hormonal birth control. With hormonal birth control, a woman takes hormones like those her body makes naturally. These hormones prevent ovulation. Implants are match-size, soft plastic tubes that are placed just under the skin of the upper arm. This is done through a small cut (inci-

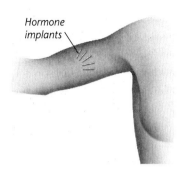

Hormone implants

sion) after the woman is given an injection of local anesthesia. After the tubes are inserted, you don't need to do anything else to prevent pregnancy. Implants provide birth control for up to 5 years. They can be removed when a woman wishes to stop using them or can be replaced with new implants after 5 years. They are removed by making another small cut at or near the original site. Removal of the implants may be more difficult than insertion and takes slightly longer.

The hormones in implants may make your periods irregular. You may spot at any time in your cycle.

▶ See also *Birth Control*

▶ HORMONE INJECTIONS

Hormone injections are a type of birth control. With hormonal birth control, a woman takes hormones to prevent ovulation. When there is no egg to be fertilized, pregnancy cannot occur.

There are two types of hormone injections available. One type of injection provides birth control for 1 month, so a woman needs 12 injections each year. Other injections provide birth control for 3 months, so a woman needs only four injections each year. During the time that the injection is effective, you don't have to do anything else to prevent pregnancy. Hormonal injections are very effective. You may have irregular periods.

▶ See also *Menopause* in *"Women's Bodies," Osteoporosis, Selective Estrogen Receptor Modulators*

▶ HORMONE REPLACEMENT THERAPY

Hormones are chemicals that control when and how certain organs work. They are made by glands in the body. In women, the hormone estrogen plays a key role in the reproductive system. Changes in the level of estrogen lead to menstrual periods each month. Estrogen also affects a woman's bones and the health of her heart and blood vessels.

At menopause, a woman's body makes less estrogen and she stops having menstrual periods. This is a natural stage in a woman's life. The lack of estrogen can bring on symptoms such as hot flushes (a sudden feeling of heat that spreads over the body) and vaginal dryness. It can also increase the risk of heart disease and osteoporosis (bone loss). Because of this, many women take hormone replacement therapy to restore estrogen after menopause.

Your Body's Estrogen

Estrogen is made mainly by the ovaries—two glands on either side of the uterus. The ovaries make estrogen from puberty until menopause.

The amount of estrogen produced by the ovaries slowly decreases as a woman ages. At some point, the ovaries stop making enough estrogen to thicken the uterine lining. This is when the menstrual periods stop. The average age of a woman's last menstrual period is 51, but the normal range is from ages 45 to 55.

If a woman's ovaries are removed during surgery, her estrogen level will decrease. The decrease will be a sudden, rather than a slow, decline, which will bring on symptoms of menopause.

The hormones estrogen and progesterone can be replaced after menopause. Women who have a uterus need to take both hormones, and those who have had their uterus removed can take just estrogen.

Benefits of Hormone Therapy

Hormone replacement therapy can relieve the symptoms of low estrogen—hot flushes and vaginal dryness. However, the major benefits of therapy are that it prevents osteoporosis and protects against heart disease—problems that can have long-term effects on your life and health. The decision to begin hormone replacement therapy depends on your:

) Medical history

) Symptoms

) Risk of bone loss and cardiovascular disease

Relief from Hot Flushes

About 75% of all women going through menopause have hot flushes (hot flashes). Hot flushes may occur a few times a month or several times a day, depending on the woman. Hot flushes can happen anytime—day or night. When they occur at night, they can disrupt your sleep. Estrogen causes them to go away.

Protection from Cardiovascular Disease

Cardiovascular disease, which causes heart attack and stroke, is more likely after menopause. It occurs when the blood vessels leading to the heart and brain become narrowed. Cardiovascular disease is the leading cause of death in women in the United States. Once the ovaries stop making estrogen, a woman's risk of cardiovascular disease increases over time to equal that of a man's.

Hormone replacement therapy (HRT) was first developed to treat symptoms of menopause, such as hot flushes, vaginal dryness, and pain during intercourse. It became clear over time that HRT also can prevent certain chronic illnesses.

Women who use hormone replacement therapy may reduce their risk of heart disease. Hormone replacement therapy decreases the "bad" low-density lipoprotein (LDL) cholesterol in the bloodstream that can build up inside the blood vessels. At the same time, estrogen increases the "good" high-density lipoprotein (HDL) cholesterol that removes LDL cholesterol from the bloodstream. Estrogen, therefore, helps to keep arteries clear.

Protection from Osteoporosis

Osteoporosis is another result of low estrogen levels in women. Estrogen helps protect against bone loss. After menopause, a woman's bones slowly lose strength and become more fragile. As a result, older women are more likely to break bones. The hip, wrist, and spine are most often affected.

Hormone replacement therapy is a good way to slow bone loss after menopause. Estrogen preserves bone and works with other hormones to increase bone mass. Estrogen helps bones absorb calcium, which gives them strength.

Relief from Dryness

When estrogen levels decrease, the walls of the vagina may become thin and dry. These changes can cause pain during sex and lead to infection. Taking estrogen can relieve dryness.

Tissues in the urinary tract also change with age. Some women may need to urinate more often. Women may be more prone to getting urinary tract infections after menopause. Hormone replacement therapy restores the elasticity of these tissues and can help to prevent various urinary tract problems.

Other Benefits

Some studies have shown that estrogen has a positive effect on mood and short-term memory in women. Estrogen may also protect against Alzheimer's disease, which is a brain disease that causes early senility. This disease is more common in women than men.

Concerns and Risks

Like most treatments, hormone replacement therapy is not free of risk. Using estrogen alone causes the lining of the uterus to grow and can increase the risk of endometrial cancer. To reduce this risk, your doctor may also prescribe another hormone called progestin (a synthetic hormone that acts like progesterone). The progestin keeps the lining of the uterus from growing too much. The drawback of using a progestin is that monthly bleeding may resume. Although bleeding may occur for only a short time, many women don't want to have menstrual cycles at all and, therefore, find this side effect of progestin bothersome.

An ongoing study called the Women's Health Initiative, which began in 1993, is a group of clinical trials and observational studies that involves more than 164,000 postmenopausal women across the United States. New and current treatments, including hormone replacement therapy, are being tested to see if they prevent problems such as heart disease, cancers of the breast, fractures due to osteoporosis, and memory loss.

An issue of great concern to women is whether hormone replacement therapy increases the risk of breast cancer. There have been many studies of this issue, with most showing no increase in risk. A report by the American Cancer Society of 422,000 postmenopausal women followed for 9 years reported that the use of hormone replacement therapy was linked to a significantly decreased risk of fatal breast cancer. Although this is reassuring, a definite conclusion cannot yet be made. If there is an increased risk of hormone replacement therapy increasing breast cancer, the increase appears to be small—especially compared with the risks of disease that estrogen prevents.

With or without hormone replacement therapy, there are things you can do to remain healthy. Eating a balanced diet (rich in calcium and low in fat), getting enough exercise, and avoiding alcohol and tobacco can help reduce the rate of bone loss and protect against heart disease.

Treatment

Hormone replacement therapy can be given by pills or patches. It can also be given as a cream for vaginal dryness, but this form usually does not relieve other symptoms.

Your doctor may prescribe one of several types of therapy:

▶ *Cyclic therapy:* This is the most common therapy prescribed. Estrogen is taken throughout the cycle and progestin is added for certain days in the month. The exact times can vary. You may have some bleeding if you are not taking hormones on certain days.

▶ *Continuous cyclic therapy:* Estrogen is taken every day in cycles of 4 weeks. The progestin is added only during the first 2 weeks. During the time when the estrogen is taken alone, you may have some bleeding.

▶ *Continuous-combined therapy:* Estrogen and a progestin are taken every day. It is common to have irregular bleeding the first few months, but within 1 year, most women stop all bleeding.

▶ *Transdermal patch:* Instead of taking pills, you place a patch usually on your abdomen or thigh. The estrogen passes from the patch, through the skin, and into the body.

Most women who have not had a hysterectomy receive estrogen and a progestin. The amount of each hormone needed to prevent low-estrogen symptoms varies from person to person. Changes in the dose may be needed. If you take hormones to guard against osteoporosis and heart disease, life-long treatment is needed. The protection is lost if you stop taking replacement hormones.

Other Medications

Sometimes, your doctor may prescribe other medications to manage or protect against various diseases. For example, to build strong bones and prevent osteoporosis your doctor may prescribe alendronate or raloxifene. Women who already have thin bones, or who have had a fracture, may be asked to use alendronate, raloxifene, or calcitonin. For women with severe hot flushes, the hormone androgen may be given along with estrogen. A medication called calcitonin works against osteoporosis. Calcitonin is given by injection or as a nasal spray. Other medications used to build strong bones are etidronate and alendronate.

When taking hormone replacement therapy or other medications, you should follow your doctor's advice carefully and get regular checkups. If you have any unexpected vaginal bleeding, tell your doctor right away. Follow-up visits will include a blood pressure check, breast and pelvic exams, and a Pap test. An endometrial biopsy may also be done, especially if you are not taking a progestin.

> See also *Condoms, Human Immunodeficiency Virus Infection and Pregnancy*

▶ HUMAN IMMUNODEFICIENCY VIRUS INFECTION

The human immunodeficiency virus (HIV) causes acquired immunodeficiency syndrome (AIDS). Many people think AIDS is a disease that affects only homosexual men and intravenous (IV) drug users. This is not true. The rate of HIV infection is increasing most rapidly among heterosexual women. HIV infection has become the third leading cause of death among women 25–44 years old. As a woman, you should know how HIV infection can affect you.

HIV and AIDS

How Infection Occurs

The virus enters the bloodstream by way of body fluids—in most cases, blood or semen. Once in the blood, the virus invades and kills cells of the immune system. These cells are white blood cells called CD4 cells. When these cells are destroyed, the body is less able to fight disease. The number of white blood cells often decreases in patients with advanced HIV infection.

How Infection Is Spread

HIV infection is spread through contact with the body fluids of an infected person. This can happen during sex or by sharing needles used to inject drugs. An infected woman who is preg-

The number of CD4 cells may remain normal for many years as the immune system tries to fight the virus. During this time, disease symptoms, such as weight loss, lack of energy, frequent fevers and sweats, and persistent skin rashes, are uncommon.

nant can pass the virus to her baby. Women with HIV who breastfeed also can pass the virus to their babies. Once someone is infected, he or she always will carry the virus and can pass it to others.

People may become infected with HIV if they are exposed to infected blood or blood transfusions during a medical procedure. This was not known until 1985, so persons who received blood transfusions before then could have been infected this way. All donor blood in the United States is now screened for diseases such as HIV. The risk of getting infected this way is very low.

People also may become infected if they are exposed to infected blood by accident. For instance, some health care workers have become infected from contact with their patients' blood.

HIV cannot be spread by casual contact with people and objects. The virus cannot get through skin that is not broken.

Effects of HIV

A person who has been infected with HIV does not get sick with AIDS right away. The virus breaks down the immune system over time. Shortly after infection, some people have a brief illness like the flu. As the immune system becomes weaker, people infected with HIV may have weight loss, fatigue, and fever.

The infection is called AIDS when a person has certain conditions or symptoms that result from a weakened immune system. It also is called AIDS when the number of a person's CD4 cells drops below a certain level.

Over time, HIV infection results in severe illness. The body is left open to harmful infections and certain types of cancer. Such conditions attack the body when the immune system is weak. Sometimes these conditions can be treated. They often come back after treatment, though.

It may be months or years before HIV becomes AIDS. On average, it takes about 11 years from the time of infection to develop AIDS. In some cases, though, it takes much less time. Because symptoms do not appear right away, a person may not know that he or she is infected with HIV. Someone who looks healthy can carry the virus for years without knowing it and can pass it to others.

There is no vaccine to prevent HIV infection, and there is no cure for AIDS. There are some medications that fight HIV-related infections and help protect the immune system.

What Doesn't Spread HIV

You should know the ways that HIV cannot be spread, or in which there is no known risk. HIV has *not* been shown to spread through:

▶ Hugging, kissing, or touching

▶ Coughing or sneezing

▶ Being exposed to another person's tears or sweat

▶ Giving blood

▶ Sharing food or drink

▶ Touching objects such as bedsheets, towels, toilet seats, telephones, and door knobs

▶ Using swimming pools, hot tubs, steam baths, or saunas

HIV Transmission in Women

Most women get the HIV virus by using IV drugs or having sex with men who use such drugs. Heterosexual activity has increased as a way of passing the virus to women.

During sex, the virus is spread more easily from men to women than from women to men. The risk of spreading HIV from woman to woman during sex is not known, but it is thought to be low.

Testing for HIV

A simple blood test can tell you whether you have been infected with HIV. It looks for HIV antibodies in the blood. This test is not an AIDS test. It does not tell you if you have AIDS or if you will get sick.

Who Should Be Tested

Women who are of childbearing age should think about being tested for HIV. All pregnant women should be tested for HIV as part of their prenatal care—even if they don't think they may be infected. It's a good idea to have counseling after getting the results.

What the Results Mean

A positive test result means that you are infected with HIV and can pass the virus on to others. You will need to get special health care and take measures to protect others.

A negative test result means that HIV antibodies were not found in your blood. In most cases, antibodies show up in the test within 6–12 weeks after a person is infected. Sometimes it may take longer. For this reason, you may want to take a second test after about 6 months to be sure to get an accurate result. Even if your test results are negative, you should still protect yourself by stopping any behavior that could pose a risk.

Protecting Yourself and Others

The number of people in the United States who are infected with HIV is growing. There are things you can do to lower your chances of getting or spreading the virus.

Use a Condom

The best way to help prevent the spread of HIV infection during sex is by using latex condoms. Latex condoms also can help prevent the spread of other sexually transmitted diseases (STDs), such as gonorrhea, syphilis, and chlamydia. Condoms made from natural skin or lambskin do not stop infection. Condoms don't offer complete protection against HIV infection. When used properly, though, they can reduce the chances

In people who are not infected with HIV, CD4 counts range from 500 to 1,500 CD4 cells per cubic millimeter of blood. People who are infected with HIV routinely have their CD4 counts measured as a way to know how many of these cells are available to help fight infection.

that one partner will infect the other. For best protection, condoms should be worn every time you have sex.

Practice Safer Sex

The safest practice of all is to not have sex. However, "safer" sex means sexual practices that reduce the risk of HIV transmission. There are aspects of safer sex you should know about.

▶ *Know your partner.* Keep in mind that it's not just your own behavior that can put you at risk, it's your partner's too. Ask about your partner's sexual history and whether he or she has ever used IV drugs. There is no way of knowing for sure if someone has HIV infection. You and your partner may want to be tested before you begin having sex.

▶ *Limit sexual partners.* The chances of getting infected with HIV increase with each sexual partner you have. The safest kind of relationship is one in which neither partner has had sex with anyone else.

▶ *Avoid risky sex practices.* The riskiest sex is vaginal or anal sex without a condom. Anal sex is the most common way HIV is spread sexually. Anal sex poses the most risk because it is more likely to tear or break the skin. This makes it easier for HIV (from an infected partner) to enter the bloodstream.

Hugging, kissing, massage, and fondling are all thought to be safer sex. Mutual masturbation also poses less risk.

Don't Use Drugs

Injecting ("shooting") drugs greatly increases your chances of HIV infection. If you are using IV drugs, get help and try to stop. If you can't stop, do not share needles. If you share needles, the HIV-infected blood left in the needles after injecting can get into you or your partner. Make sure that the needle is clean. Needles should be cleaned after every use with both laundry bleach and water.

Concerns for HIV-Positive Women

Women who are HIV positive have special health concerns. These include birth control, certain conditions, as well as pregnancy and childbirth.

If You Are Infected

A positive HIV test result means that you are infected with the virus. You should take certain steps to avoid passing the infection to others:

▶ Tell sex partners—past and present.

▶ Don't share needles to inject drugs; if you have, tell the person.

▶ Practice safer sex.

▶ Never donate or sell your blood or plasma or arrange to be an organ donor.

▶ Do not share toothbrushes, razors, or other objects that could have blood on them.

▶ Be sure to tell every health care provider who treats you, including your dentist, that you are HIV-positive.

▶ Avoid getting pregnant because your baby will be at risk. However, if you are pregnant, talk to your doctor about special care for you and your newborn.

Women and HIV

Did you know that:

▶ Women account for about 47% of people living with HIV and AIDS.

▶ Between 107,000 and 150,000 women in the United States are living with HIV infection.

▶ During 1999, over 5 million new HIV infections occurred world-wide—about 15,000 infections each day.

▶ In 1998, almost 40,000 new HIV infections occurred in the United States. About 30% of these cases were women.

▶ Mother-to-child transmission is responsible for 90% of HIV-infections in infants and children.

Birth Control

An HIV-infected woman can avoid pregnancy by using effective birth control. If she becomes pregnant, the fetus is at risk of infection. If you are infected and using birth control to prevent pregnancy, your partner still should use latex condoms during sex to avoid getting the virus from you.

Certain Conditions

A woman infected with HIV is more likely to get yeast infections and pelvic inflammatory disease—an inflammation of the reproductive organs. Normally, these conditions are easy to treat. In an HIV-infected woman, though, the conditions may resist treatment. They also may be more severe and recur more often.

If you are infected with HIV, you will need to be tested for other STDs. You should be vaccinated against hepatitis B, influenza, and pneumonia if you are not immune to these diseases. Women who are HIV infected should have a Pap test at least once a year.

▶ See also *Human Immunodeficiency Virus*

▶ HUMAN IMMUNODEFICIENCY VIRUS INFECTION AND PREGNANCY

Human immunodeficiency virus (HIV) causes acquired immunodeficiency syndrome (AIDS). Because there is no cure for AIDS, infection with HIV is a serious health threat to all people. HIV infection has increased among women of childbearing age. It affects women in all walks of life. If you are pregnant and have the HIV infection, it can harm your baby. However, there are steps you can take to help protect your baby from getting infected. This is why all pregnant women should be tested for HIV.

Passing HIV to Your Baby

Almost 2 out of every 1,000 pregnant women are infected with HIV. A woman can pass the infection to her baby as early as her 8th week of pregnancy. Mothers can pass HIV infection to their babies during pregnancy, labor, and delivery. Breastfeeding is another way a mother can pass HIV to her baby. HIV infection during pregnancy causes almost all cases of HIV infection in children.

During pregnancy, a woman can prevent passing HIV to her baby by taking medication. For this reason, all women should be tested for HIV during pregnancy so they can be treated if they test positive. Once the baby is born, a woman with HIV can help prevent her baby from being infected with HIV by not breastfeeding.

HIV Testing

There are blood tests that can show if you have been infected with HIV. As part of prenatal care, all pregnant women should have an HIV test. It is vital for both you and your doctor to know your HIV status. If you have concerns about this test, talk to your doctor. If you test positive, a counselor will talk to you about treatment options.

For more information about HIV and AIDS, call the National AIDS Hotline at 800-342-2437.

Testing

There are several types of HIV tests. The most common test—called the ELISA—searches for HIV antibodies in your blood. If this test is positive, another test called the Western blot is used to confirm the results. These tests do not tell you if have AIDS or if you will get sick. They only tell you if you are carrying the virus.

Your Test Results

If your results are negative, it means the HIV antibodies were not found in your blood. It takes the body some time to make enough antibodies to be detected by the test. If you were infected recently, your test results could be negative even if you are infected. For this reason, you may want to take a follow-up test in 6 months to ensure results remain negative. A woman may need a second test if she is at high risk for infection.

If your test results are negative, be aware of things you can do to prevent getting infected with HIV or sexually transmitted diseases (STDs). If you test positive for having HIV antibodies, you are infected with the HIV virus. You can pass the infection to your baby and to others. You will need special health care.

Treatment

Pregnant women infected with HIV need to have their health checked closely. If you are HIV positive, you should report all symptoms to your doctor so that he or she can ensure you get proper care. You will be tested for other infections, such as STDs. Your doctor may prescribe medications to help prevent other infections.

Treatment with special medications during pregnancy may help prevent the infection from being passed from the mother to her baby. Without treatment, about 25% of babies (1 out of 4) born to women infected with HIV will get the virus. With medication, that number drops to less than 8%, or about 1 out of 12. For some women, cesarean birth may be recommended.

▶ See also *Cervical Disorders, Sexually Transmitted Diseases, Vulvar Disorders*

▶ HUMAN PAPILLOMAVIRUS INFECTION

Human papillomavirus (HPV) is a virus that causes warts. HPV is one of the most common sexually transmitted diseases (STDs). An estimated 24 million people in the United States are infected with HPV.

What Is HPV?

HPV is a virus. Like all viruses, it needs to infect cells in order to live. The virus enters a cell, then it directs the cell to make copies of itself and to infect other healthy cells.

Over time, the cells infected with the virus die. When this happens, they are shed from the body just as skin cells are shed. The virus is shed along with the dead cells. When the virus is shed, it can be passed to another person who also can become infected.

The virus is spread from person to person during vaginal, anal, or oral sex. Contact with the genitals, mouth, or rectum can transmit HPV. The virus also can be found in semen.

There are many types of HPV. Some types tend to infect cells in the genital areas of a man or woman, while other types infect other parts of the body.

HPV can cause warts. Warts that grow in the genital area are called condyloma acuminata. These growths may appear on the outside or inside of the vagina or penis and can spread to nearby skin. They can be pink, red, flesh-colored, or brown. Sometimes they grow in groups and look like cauliflower. Although the warts may go away over time, the virus may remain in the body.

Some types of HPV are associated with cancer of the cervix. The Pap test can detect changes in the cervix that may be an early sign of cancer. This is why it's important to have a regular exam that includes a Pap test.

In some cases, the virus causes changes that cannot be seen by the naked eye. Signs of HPV can appear on a Pap test done as part of a regular exam. If your doctor finds these changes, further testing may be done.

About 25 types of HPV can infect the genital area. These types are split into "high-risk" and "low-risk" groups based on whether they are associated with cancer of the cervix. Cancer of the cervix affects about 4,500 women each year.

Treatment

The warts caused by HPV can be treated. Although warts may go away on their own, the virus can remain. If warts do not go away or if they recur, they may need treatment. The type of treatment depends on where the warts are on your body. Warts can be treated with medication applied to the area or surgery to remove them.

If you have a lot of warts, or very large ones, your doctor may recommend that they be removed with surgery. Although all these treatments destroy the warts, the virus may still be in nearby tissue. It can produce new growths weeks or even months after the old ones are gone. You may then need more treatment. Over time, though, the warts usually go away either with treatment or on their own.

HPV Infection and Pregnancy

Most of the time, HPV does not create problems during pregnancy. Rarely, a baby may get warts during birth, but they may not appear until later. Most warts caused by HPV can be treated during pregnancy.

Your doctor may prefer to treat you after you have your baby. In that case, you will be checked closely throughout your pregnancy.

Warts can grow in number and size when a woman is pregnant. Very rarely, warts can grow so big they narrow or block the birth canal. If this occurs, a cesarean birth is needed. In a cesarean birth, the baby is born through a surgical cut made in the mother's abdomen and uterus.

Scientists have identified more than 60 types of HPV. Some types of the virus cause common skin warts. About one third of HPV types are spread through sexual contact and live only in genital tissue.

Prevention

There is no vaccine to protect against HPV, and there is no cure for it. The best way to prevent being infected with HPV is to lower your risk:

▶ Limit your number of sexual partners—the more partners you have, the greater your risk.

▶ Use condoms when you have vaginal, anal, or oral sex—the virus may be found in semen even if no warts are present.

If You Have HPV

If you have HPV, you also need to take steps to protect your health and prevent spreading the disease to someone else:

▶ Tell your doctor if there are new warts. You may need treatment for weeks or months until all signs are gone.

▶ Ask your doctor if you should be tested for other STDs.

▶ *See also Endometriosis, Pelvic Pain, Pelvic Support Problems, Uterine Bleeding, Uterine Cancer, Uterine Fibroids*

▶ HYSTERECTOMY

Hysterectomy —the removal of the uterus—is one of the most common types of surgery performed in women. A hysterectomy is one way of treating problems affecting the uterus. Because it is major surgery, your doctor may suggest trying other treatments before hysterectomy. For severe conditions—and those that have not responded to other treatment—a hysterectomy may be the best choice. The choice depends to some extent on the effect of the condition, and the surgery, on your life. You should be fully informed of all options before you decide.

Conditions Affecting the Uterus

Hysterectomy may be performed to treat conditions that can affect the uterus. Some are benign (not cancer), and others are cancer. Some have symptoms that cause discomfort, while others can threaten your life.

Your condition may be treated with medicine or various types of surgery, including hysterectomy. The choice of treatment depends on the nature and extent of your condition as well as personal factors. These factors include your plans to have children in the future, the amount of discomfort you are having, and other options available. Other forms of treatment often are tried first. If they don't work, hysterectomy may be considered. Following are some of the conditions for which hysterectomy may be performed:

▶ Uterine fibroids

▶ Uterine bleeding

▶ Uterine cancer

▶ Pelvic support problems

▶ Endometriosis

▶ Pelvic pain

About Hysterectomy

There are three types of hysterectomy:

1. Partial (or subtotal), in which the upper part of the uterus is removed but the cervix is left in place

2. Complete (or total), in which the entire uterus, including the cervix, is removed

3. Radical, in which the entire uterus, lymph nodes, and support structures around the uterus are removed. This is done when the cancer is extensive.

The ovaries and fallopian tubes may be removed at the same time. This is called a salpingo-oophorectomy.

The uterus may be removed through a cut in the abdomen or through the vagina. The method used depends on the reason for the surgery and the findings of a pelvic exam. During a vaginal hysterectomy, some doctors use a laparoscope to help them see

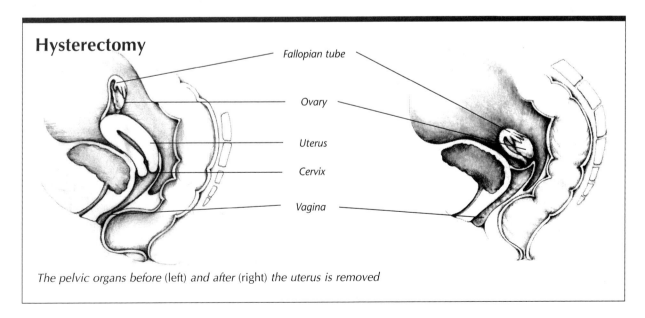

Hysterectomy

Fallopian tube

Ovary

Uterus

Cervix

Vagina

The pelvic organs before (left) *and after* (right) *the uterus is removed*

inside the abdomen and do part of the surgery. This procedure is called laparoscopically assisted vaginal hysterectomy (LAVH).

Tests are needed before the surgery. Your blood and urine will be tested. You may be given one or more enemas. Your abdominal and pelvic areas may be shaved. Antibiotics usually are given to prevent infection. A needle may be placed in your arm or wrist. It is attached to a tube that will supply your body with fluids, medication, or blood. This is called an intravenous (IV) line. Monitors will be attached to your body before anesthesia is given. You may be given a general anesthesia, which makes you unconscious, or a regional one, which blocks out feeling in the lower part of your body.

Risks

As with any surgery, problems may occur. These could include thrombophlebitis (blood clots in the veins or lungs), severe infection, bleeding after surgery, bowel blockage, injury to the urinary tract, problems related to anesthesia, or even death. Even though the risks of hysterectomy are among the lowest of any major surgery, you and your doctor must weigh the benefits and risks.

After Surgery

The length of stay in the hospital after surgery varies by type of surgery. You can expect to have some pain for the first few days. Normal activities, including sex, usually can be resumed in about 6 weeks. Meanwhile, don't douche or put anything in the vagina.

As you recover, activities such as driving, sports, and light physical work may be increased gradually. You and your doctor can plan your return to normal activities, including your return to work, at a rate best suited to your own recovery. If you can do an activity without pain and fatigue, it should be okay. If activity causes pain, discuss it with your doctor.

The surgery can have other effects that are both physical and emotional. Some last briefly, and others are long-term. You should be aware of these effects before having a hysterectomy.

Physical

After a hysterectomy, a woman's periods will stop. She can no longer get pregnant. If the ovaries are left in place, though, they still produce hormones. A woman who still has her ovaries will not have the symptoms that often occur with menopause, such as hot flushes. The ovaries still produce eggs, too, but because the eggs are not fertilized, they dissolve in the abdomen.

Uterine fibroids account for about 30% of all hysterectomies performed in the United States. Endometriosis, which accounts for 18%, is the second most common condition leading to hysterectomy.

If the ovaries also are removed with the uterus before menopause, there are hormone-related effects. It is as though the body goes through menopause all at once, rather than over a few years as is normal. Symptoms can usually be treated with the hormone estrogen.

Emotional

Many women have a brief emotional reaction to the loss of the uterus. This response depends on a number of factors: how well they were prepared for the surgery, its timing, the reason for having it, and whether the problem is cured. Women who are affected by the early loss of their ability to have children may feel depressed. If problems persist, discuss them with your doctor.

Hysterectomy and Sex

Some women may notice a change in their sexual response after a hysterectomy. Because the uterus has been removed, uterine contractions that may have been felt during orgasm will no longer occur. Some women have a heightened response, however. In part, this is because they no longer have to worry about getting pregnant and may be relieved of discomfort.

If the ovaries have not been removed, the outer genitals and the vagina are not affected. In this case, a woman's sexual activity is usually not impaired. If the ovaries are removed with the uterus, vaginal dryness may be a problem during sex. Use of estrogen can help relieve dryness.

If the procedure required making the vagina shorter, deep thrusting during sex may be painful. Being on top during sex or bringing your legs closer together may help.

In the past, it was thought that a hysterectomy may impair sexual function. Recent studies have shown that many women actually report an improvement in sexual functioning, including increased desire and frequency of sex and a decrease in painful sex.

▶ HYSTEROSALPINGOGRAPHY

Hysterosalpingography (HSG) is a procedure used to diagnose certain problems of the uterus and fallopian tubes. HSG most often is used to see if a woman's tubes are partly or fully blocked. This is a common cause of infertility. HSG also is used to help find the cause of repeated miscarriage.

Why Is HSG Done?

With HSG, the doctor can check for blockage or growths inside the uterus and tubes. This may help your doctor find the cause of infertility or repeated pregnancy loss (repeated miscarriage).

Partial or complete blockage of a tube can prevent a fertilized egg from moving into the uterus. Tubal blockage may result from scarring from a past infection, endometriosis, or surgery. Blockage of one or both fallopian tubes causes about 35% of cases of infertility in women.

HSG also is done to detect growths or scarring inside the uterus or problems in its size or shape. This can be the cause of repeated pregnancy loss.

What to Expect

HSG will be done in a special X-ray area in the hospital, clinic, or doctor's office. It is best to have HSG during the first half (days 1–14) of a woman's menstrual cycle. This timing reduces the chance that a woman may be pregnant during the procedure.

HSG is not done in a woman who:

▶ Is pregnant

▶ Has a pelvic infection

▶ Has an allergy to the dye used in the procedure

▶ Is having heavy uterine bleeding

To reduce pain during the procedure, you may want to take pain medication in advance. Discuss this with your doctor. He or she also may want you to take an antibiotic before HSG.

You will not be able to drive right after an HSG. Arrange to have someone take you home.

The Procedure

For HSG, a special fluid is placed into the uterus and tubes. The fluid shows up in contrast to these structures on an X-ray screen. This highlights their inner size and shape.

For the procedure, you will be asked to lie on your back with your feet placed as for a pelvic exam. A device called a speculum is inserted into the vagina to hold the walls of the vagina apart and allow a view of the cervix. The cervix is cleaned and the end of the cervix may be injected with local anesthesia. You may feel a pinch or tug as this is done.

A device is inserted to hold the cervix steady. A thin tube then is passed through the cervical opening to the lower part of the uterus.

An X-ray machine is placed over the abdomen. This allows the doctor to see the fluid inside your organs on a screen.

The fluid slowly is placed through the thin tube into the uterus and fallopian tubes. The fluid causes the uterus to stretch. This may cause uterine cramping. Also, if the tubes are blocked, the fluid will cause the tubes to stretch. This may cause pain.

X-ray images are made as the fluid fills the uterus and tubes. You may be asked to change positions a number of times for X-rays. If there is no blockage, the fluid will spill slowly out the far ends of the tubes. After it spills out of the tube, the fluid is absorbed by the cells lining the abdomen.

After the Procedure

Many women have minor side effects after having HSG. These are not serious and go away after a day or two in most cases. Side effects may include:

▶ Sticky vaginal discharge as some of the fluid drains out of the uterus

▶ Cramps

▶ Feeling dizzy, faint, or sick to your stomach

▶ Slight vaginal bleeding

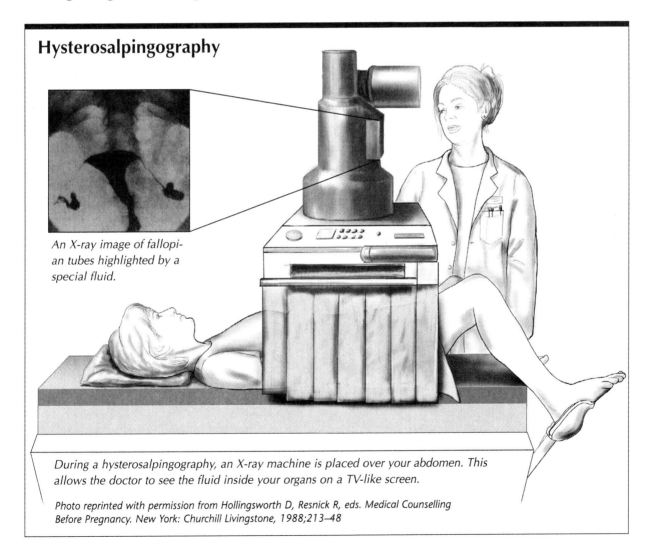

Hysterosalpingography

An X-ray image of fallopian tubes highlighted by a special fluid.

During a hysterosalpingography, an X-ray machine is placed over your abdomen. This allows the doctor to see the fluid inside your organs on a TV-like screen.

Photo reprinted with permission from Hollingsworth D, Resnick R, eds. Medical Counselling Before Pregnancy. New York: Churchill Livingstone, 1988;213–48

Talk to your doctor about what kind of medications you can take to relieve these symptoms. A pad can be used for the vaginal discharge. Do not use a tampon. If the discharge gets on your underwear or clothing, it may stain.

Your doctor may prescribe antibiotics for a few days after the procedure. Make sure you take all of the antibiotics, even if you feel fine.

Risks and Complications

Severe problems are rare. They may include an allergic reaction to the fluid, uterine injury, or pelvic infection. Call your doctor if you have any of the following symptoms:

▶ Vomiting

▶ Fainting

▶ Severe abdominal pain or cramping

▶ Heavy vaginal bleeding

▶ Fever or chills

Some women may have an allergic reaction to the fluid used in HSG. Symptoms include hives, itching, and low blood pressure. Call your doctor if you have any of these symptoms.

Test Results

Your doctor will discuss the results of your test with you. Based on the results, further tests may be needed. If a problem is found, your doctor will talk with you about a treatment plan.

▶ See also *Adhesions, Infertility, Miscarriage, Uterine Bleeding*

▶ HYSTEROSCOPY

Hysteroscopy is a way to look inside the uterus. A hysteroscope is a thin, telescope-like device that is inserted into the uterus through the vagina and cervix. It may help a doctor diagnose or treat a uterine problem.

Uses of Hysteroscopy

Hysteroscopy is minor surgery that may be done in a doctor's office or operating room with local, regional, or general anesthesia. In some cases, little or no anesthesia is needed. The procedure poses little risk for most women. Hysteroscopy may be used for diagnosis, treatment, or both.

Diagnostic Hysteroscopy

Hysteroscopy can be used to diagnose some problems in the uterus. It also can be used to confirm the results of other tests, such as hysterosalpingography (HSG).

The hysteroscope is sometimes used with other instruments or techniques. For instance, it may be done before dilation and curettage (D&C) or at the same time as laparoscopy. In a D&C, the cervix is widened (dilation) and part of the lining of the uterus is removed (curettage). In laparoscopy, a slender, telescope-like device is inserted into the abdomen through a tiny incision (cut) made through or just below the navel. Hysteroscopy also may be used for other conditions, such as infertility, repeated miscarriages, adhesions, abnormal growths, and displaced IUDs.

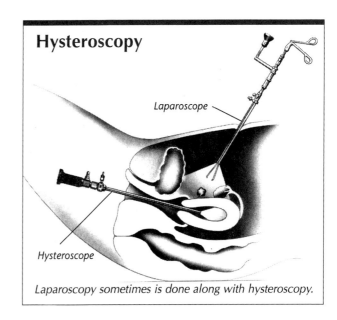

Hysteroscopy

Laparoscope

Hysteroscope

Laparoscopy sometimes is done along with hysteroscopy.

Operative Hysteroscopy

When hysteroscopy is used to diagnose certain conditions, it may be used to correct them as well. For instance, uterine adhesions or fibroids often can be removed through the hysteroscope. Sometimes hysteroscopy can be used instead of open abdominal surgery. Often it will be done in an operating room with general anesthesia.

The hysteroscope is used with endometrial ablation—a procedure in which the lining of the uterus is destroyed to treat some causes of heavy bleeding. After this is done, a woman can no longer have children. For this procedure, the hysteroscope is sometimes used with other instruments, such as a laser or a resectoscope. The resectoscope is a specially designed telescope with a wire loop or a rollerball at the end. Using electric current, any of these tips can be used to destroy the uterine lining. Endometrial ablation is done in an outpatient setting in most cases.

What to Expect

Hysteroscopy is a safe procedure. Problems such as injury to the cervix or the uterus, infection, heavy bleeding, or side effects of the anesthesia occur in less than 1% of cases.

Before Surgery

Hysteroscopy is best done during the first week or so after a menstrual period. This allows a better view of the inside of the uterus.

If you are having a hysteroscopy in a hospital, you may be asked not to eat or drink for a certain time before the procedure. Some routine lab tests may be done. You will be asked to empty your bladder. Then your vaginal area will be cleansed with an antiseptic.

Anesthesia

Hysteroscopy may be performed with local, regional, or general anesthesia. The type used depends on a number of factors. This includes whether other procedures are being done at the same time. Where you have your surgery—in your doctor's office or in the hospital—also may affect the kind of pain relief used. You will want to discuss your options with your doctor.

The Procedure

Before a hysteroscopy, the opening of your cervix may need to be dilated (made wider) with a special device. The hysteroscope then is inserted through the vagina and cervix and into the uterus.

A liquid or gas may be released through the hysteroscope to expand the uterus so that the inside can be seen better. A light shone through the device allows the doctor to view the inside of the uterus and the openings of the fallopian tubes into the uterine cavity. If surgery is to be done, small instruments will be inserted through the hysteroscope.

For more complicated procedures, a laparoscope may be used at the same time to view the outside of the uterus. In this case, a gas is flowed into the abdomen. The gas expands the abdomen. This creates a space inside by raising the wall of the abdomen and moving it away from the internal organs. This makes the organs easier to see. Most of this gas is removed at the end of the procedure. This procedure is not done in the office.

Recovery

If local anesthesia was used, you will be able to go home in a short time. If regional or general anesthesia was used, you may need to be watched for some time before you go home.

You may feel a pain in your shoulders if laparoscopy was done with hysteroscopy, or if gas was used during hysteroscopy to inflate the uterus. In most cases, the pain passes quickly as the gas is absorbed. You may feel faint or sick or you may have slight vaginal bleeding and cramps for a day or two. Check with your doctor before using tampons, douching, or having sex.

Warning Signs

Get in touch with your doctor if you have:

- A fever
- Severe abdominal pain
- Heavy vaginal bleeding or discharge

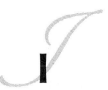

❱ INCOMPETENT CERVIX

During pregnancy, as the baby grows and gets heavier, it presses on the cervix. The cervix may start to open (dilate) too soon, before the baby is ready to be born. This condition is called incompetent cervix and it can lead to miscarriage. It doesn't cause the pain or contractions of normal labor.

There's no foolproof way for doctors to diagnose an incompetent cervix. Symptoms include:

❱ Spotting or bleeding

❱ A bloody, thick, or mucus-like vaginal discharge

❱ A feeling of pressure or weight in the lower abdomen.

An incompetent cervix occurs in only 1–2% of pregnancies. Almost 25% of babies lost (miscarriage) in the second trimester are because of an incompetent cervix. Some possible causes of this condition include:

❱ Previous surgery on the cervix

❱ Damage during a difficult birth

❱ Malformed cervix or uterus from a birth defect

If you have an incompetent cervix, your doctor will monitor you closely. He or she may decide to put stitches around the opening in your cervix to keep it closed. Also, you may be told to cut down on activity or to stay in bed until the baby is born.

❱ INFERTILITY

❱ See also *Assisted Reproductive Technologies Polycystic Ovary Syndrome, Preconceptional Care*

Many couples who want to have a child have not been able to do so. About 15% of couples in the United States are infertile. Couples may be infertile if they have not been able to conceive after 12 months of having sex without the use of birth control.

If you and your partner are trying to have a child and can't, you should think about having an infertility evaluation. Tests are done to find the cause of the problem. Based on the results of these tests, treatment may be needed.

Conception

For healthy, young couples, the odds are about 25% that a woman will conceive during any one menstrual cycle. This figure starts to decline in a woman's late 20s and early 30s and drops even more after age 35. A man's fertility also declines with age, but not as early.

A woman's menstrual cycle is about 28 days. Ovulation is the release of an egg from one of the ovaries. It occurs about 14 days after the first day of your last period in a 28-day cycle. Once an egg is released, it is able to be fertilized for about 12–24 hours. Conception can occur if you have sex during or near the time of ovulation.

When the man ejaculates during sex, his semen is released into the vagina. Semen is the fluid that carries the sperm. Sperm travel up through the cervix and out into the tubes. Sperm can live in the woman's fallopian tubes for 1–2 days. If the sperm and egg join, fertilization occurs.

The fertilized egg then moves through the tube into the uterus. It becomes attached there and begins to grow. All of these events must take place for pregnancy to occur. If there is a problem in this chain of events, infertility may result.

Testing

Infertility may be caused by more than one factor. You and your partner will receive care as a couple. Some causes are easily found and treated, while others are not. In some cases, no cause can be found in either partner.

The decision to begin testing depends on a number of factors, such as age of the couple and how long the couple has been trying to get pregnant. The basic workup can be finished within a few menstrual cycles in most cases. Ask your doctor about the costs involved. Find out whether they are covered by your insurance. The workup includes the following:

▶ Physical exam

▶ Medical history

▶ Semen analysis

▶ Check for ovulation

According to the American Society of Reproductive Medicine, infertility affects men and women equally. Problems with ovulation and sperm are the most common causes of infertility problems—they account for two thirds of cases.

❱ Tests to check uterus and for open tubes

❱ Discuss how often and when you have sex

Basic Workup for the Man

A semen analysis is a key part of the basic workup. It may need to be done more than once. The sample is obtained by masturbation. Sometimes it can be obtained at home. Sometimes it is obtained in a lab. Your doctor will give you specific instructions.

A man's sperm count does not decrease unless intercourse is more frequent than every 24 hours.

The semen sample is studied in the lab to count the number of sperm present. The doctor will study:

❱ Number

❱ Shape

❱ Movement

❱ Signs of infection

A man may be referred to a urologist (a doctor with special skill in treating problems of the urinary tract). The urologist will perform an exam, and tests may be done.

Basic Workup for the Woman

The workup begins with a physical exam and health history. The health history will focus on key points:

❱ Menstrual function, such as irregular bleeding and pain

❱ Pregnancy history

❱ Sexually transmitted disease (STD) history

❱ Birth control

Other tests, such as a Pap test and blood tests, may be done.

Tests

There are many ways to see if ovulation occurs. Some tests are done by the woman, and others are done by the doctor.

Urine Test. A way to predict ovulation is by using a urine test kit at home. This test measures luteinizing hormone (LH), a hormone that causes ovulation to occur. If the test result is positive, it means ovulation is about to occur. Sometimes these kits are used with basal body temperature charts.

Basal Body Temperature. After a woman ovulates, there is a small increase in body temperature. A woman takes her temperature by mouth every morning before she gets out of bed and records it on a chart. This record should be kept for 2–3 menstrual cycles to see if ovulation occurs.

Blood Test. After a woman ovulates, the ovaries produce the hormone progesterone. A blood test taken in the second half of the menstrual cycle can measure progesterone to show if ovulation has occurred.

Endometrial Biopsy. The lining of the uterus (endometrium) changes at ovulation. Sometimes a biopsy (getting a sample of the tissue) is done in this area to find out whether and when ovulation has occurred. A small plastic tube is inserted into the vagina and through the cervix. A sample of the lining is taken to check for ovulation and tissue response. This sample is later studied in a lab.

Postcoital Test. The postcoital (after sex) test examines the ability of sperm to enter and move into the cervical mucus just before the time of ovulation. The couple has intercourse close to the time of ovulation, and the cervical mucus is examined a few hours later. A postcoital test can also show if there is a reaction between the sperm and cervical mucus that could be causing infertility.

Procedures

The following tests may be done to look at a woman's reproductive organs:

- Hysterosalpingography (HSG)
- Transvaginal ultrasound
- Hysteroscopy
- Laparoscopy

These tests check if the uterus is normal and tubes are open. The tests you have depend on your factors and symptoms.

Treatments

Medical treatment may be needed to help you become pregnant. If so, you should be aware of what is involved. Some treatments require a great deal of expense and effort from both partners.

If the cause of infertility is with one partner, then that partner can be treated. Medication may be given, surgery may be needed, or assisted reproductive technologies may be used. In some cases, treatments are combined to improve results. For instance, medication and insemination may be used at the same time.

Before you have treatment, you should know the expected success rates and how success is defined. Some clinics define success based on the number of live births. Others define success based on the number of pregnancies achieved. Discuss with your doctor the success rates of your options.

Ovulation Induction

If the woman does not ovulate, she may be given certain medications to cause ovulation to occur (induce). She also can be given medication to increase (stimulate) the number of eggs released.

The medication used most often is clomiphene citrate. It is a pill given by mouth to cause ovulation to occur in women who have problems with ovulation. A number of treatment cycles may be needed, and dosage and medication may need to be altered.

If pregnancy does not occur after several treatment cycles of clomiphene citrate, medication may be given by injection. This medication is called human menopausal gonadotropin (hMG). It stimulates the ovaries to mature and produce eggs. Taking this medication may result in more than one egg being released each month. Blood tests and ultrasound often are used to monitor hMG treatment.

Most women who take ovulation-induction drugs respond to the treatment and begin to ovulate regularly. If no other problems need treatment, more than half become pregnant within 6 cycles. If a woman still hasn't started ovulating, she may have special tests done to find out why.

Multiple pregnancy may occur with the use of these drugs. The risk is higher with some drugs than with others. Rarely, a condition called ovarian hyperstimulation syndrome may occur.

Surgery

Surgery may be done to open tubes or repair other problems of the reproductive organs. It may be done to remove growths such as polyps or fibroids. Surgery also may be done to remove scarring that occurred as a result of a previous surgery, infection, or endometriosis. If endometriosis is found, surgery may be done to treat it. Success rates depend on the nature and extent of the problem.

Assisted Reproductive Technologies

Assisted reproductive technology (ART) includes treatments that involve a lab treating and using human eggs and sperm or embryos to help an infertile couple conceive a child.

Other Choices

You and your partner should give careful thought to all your options. You may want to think about other choices, adoption, or child-free living. Discuss your feelings with your partner. Sometimes counseling can help to sort out these feelings. Support groups with other infertile couples also may help.

About one third of infertility cases are because of factors that affect women, and about one third because of factors that affect men. For the remaining infertile couples, a combination of problems in both partners causes the infertility. Infertility cannot be explained in almost 20% of infertile couples.

▶ INTRAUTERINE DEVICES

The intrauterine device (IUD) is a type of birth control. It is a small, plastic device that is inserted and left inside the uterus to prevent pregnancy.

How the IUD Works

The IUD causes a reaction inside the uterus and fallopian tubes. This can interfere with the egg being fertilized or attaching to the wall of the uterus.

Although there have been several types of IUDs, currently only two are available in the United States—the hormonal and the copper. Both IUDs are T-shaped and made of plastic, but they work in different ways. The hormonal IUD releases a small amount of the hormone progesterone into the uterus. The copper IUD has a thin copper wire on it that releases a small amount of copper into the uterus.

The hormonal IUD must be replaced every year. The copper IUD can remain in your body for up to 10 years. Your health, medical problems, and preference will help you and your doctor decide which IUD will work best for you.

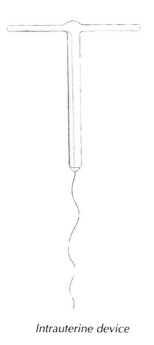

Intrauterine device

Benefits

The IUD has many benefits over other birth control methods:

▶ Easy to use—you don't have to remember to insert it before sex or to take a pill every day.

▶ Does not interfere with sexual intercourse, daily activities, or menstruation. You can use a tampon with the IUD. Vigorous physical activity, such as jogging or dancing, will not dislodge it.

▶ Once it's in place, you cannot feel it and neither can your partner.

Is the IUD Effective?

The IUD is a highly effective method of contraception. It is one of the safest methods of reversible birth control for women—it can be removed if you decide to become pregnant.

The IUD will protect against pregnancy over 98% of the time. This means only 1 or 2 women out of 100 may become pregnant each year with an IUD properly in place. The IUD is more effective than some other forms of birth control, such as the condom or diaphragm. In fact, it is only slightly less effective than the birth control pill.

Choosing the IUD

The IUD is best suited for women who have given birth to at least one child. If you've had children, the IUD is easier to insert and is more likely to stay in place.

For some women, certain conditions can increase the chance of having problems with the IUD. The IUD may not be a good method of birth control for women who have:

- Had a pelvic infection

- Had an ectopic pregnancy

- Severe pain during menstrual periods

- Abnormal vaginal bleeding

- Multiple sexual partners or a high risk for sexually transmitted diseases (STDs)

Talk to your doctor openly about your medical history and your current sexual practices. He or she can help you make a decision whether the IUD is right for you.

Insertion

Your doctor will perform a routine exam to make sure you're able to use an IUD. It should include:

- Reviewing your medical history to determine any possible risks

- A pregnancy test

- Taking some fluid or tissue from your vagina and cervix to check for infection

You may be asked to read and sign a consent form. Make sure you understand everything about the IUD to be inserted. If you have questions, ask your doctor to explain more to help you understand. The IUD is often inserted during or right after your menstrual period.

The doctor puts the IUD in a long, slender, plastic tube. He or she places it into the vagina and guides it through the cervix into the uterus. The IUD is then pushed out of the plastic tube into the uterus. The IUD springs open into place, and the tube is withdrawn.

Insertion of the IUD does not require anesthesia, although you may have some discomfort. Taking over-the-counter pain relief medication before the procedure may help.

Once the IUD is inserted, the doctor or nurse will show you how to check that it stays in place. Each IUD comes with a string or "tail" made of a thin plastic thread. After insertion, the tail is trimmed so that 1–2 inches hang out of the cervix inside

There is little or no increased risk of infertility among IUD users who are having a sexual relationship with only one person. When use of the IUD is stopped, the chance of pregnancy is no different than in women who stop using other methods of birth control.

If a woman using an IUD becomes pregnant, there is a 2–3% chance that the pregnancy will be ectopic.

your vagina. You will be able to tell the placement of the IUD by the location of this string. The string will not bother you, but your partner may feel it with his penis. This will not interfere with his sexual feeling.

It is important to check the string regularly. To do this, you must insert a finger into your vagina and feel around for the string. You can do this at any time, but doing it right after your menstrual period is easy to remember. If you feel the string is shorter or longer than it used to be—or if you don't feel the string at all—call your doctor. The IUD may have slipped out of place. Use another form of birth control until your IUD is checked.

A doctor must remove the IUD. Do not try to remove it yourself.

Years ago, IUDs did not require the approval of the U.S. Food and Drug Administration (FDA). One such IUD was the Dalkon Shield. Insertion of the Dalkon Shield was painful, and there was a high rate of infection among users. This was because of the braided tail, which was a haven for bacteria. Because of all of the side effects and problems, the device was banned in 1975. Since the Dalkon Shield incident, IUDs must now pass FDA approval before they are put on the market.

Concerns and Risks

Some women have some cramping and spotting during the first few weeks after the IUD is inserted. These symptoms are common and should disappear within a month.

There are warning signs that there may be a problem with your IUD. Be aware of these symptoms and call your doctor if you notice any one of them.

Serious complications from the use of an IUD are rare. However, some women do have problems. These problems usually happen during, or soon after, insertion:

▶ *Expulsion:* The IUD can be expelled (or pushed) out of the uterus into the vagina. If this happens, it is no longer effective.

▶ *Perforation:* The IUD can perforate (or pierce) the wall of the uterus during insertion. This is very rare and occurs in only about 2 out of every 1,000 insertions.

▶ *Pregnancy:* Rarely, pregnancy may occur while a woman is using an IUD. If the IUD is still in place, there can be risks to the mother and fetus. These include miscarriage, infection, and ectopic pregnancy.

▶ *Infections:* Infections in the uterus or fallopian tubes can occur after insertion. This may cause scarring in the reproductive organs, making it harder to become pregnant at a later date.

▶ *Painful periods:* Menstrual cramps may increase.

Although the IUD is an effective protection against pregnancy, it does not pro-

Warning Signs

These signs may signal there is a problem with your IUD. Call your doctor if you have any of the following symptoms:

▶ Severe abdominal pain

▶ Pain during intercourse

▶ Bleeding or spotting that occurs between periods, after intercourse, or that lasts more than a few months

▶ A missed period or other signs of pregnancy

▶ Unusual vaginal discharge

▶ A change in length or position of the string

tect against STDs. If you and your partner have other sexual partners, use a latex condom every time you have sex.

▶ IRRITABLE BOWEL SYNDROME

Irritable bowel syndrome (IBS) is a disorder of the intestines. It may cause pain, cramping, gas, bloating, and changes in bowel habits. IBS is quite common and affects more women than men.

Some people with IBS may be constipated. Some have diarrhea (loose stools). Some have both at different times. They may find it difficult or painful to move their bowels.

No one knows exactly what causes IBS, but it often seems related to stress. When the colon (large intestine) is examined, it shows no signs of disease. The symptoms of IBS are sometimes mistaken for problems of the reproductive system.

To diagnose IBS your doctor will rule out other causes of the symptoms. A sample of your stool will be checked. X-rays may be taken. Your doctor may want to view your colon through a flexible tube that is inserted into the anus. This is called sigmoidoscopy.

To treat IBS, your doctor may prescribe drugs to help stop diarrhea or relax the colon. Ways to manage stress and changes in your diet also may be advised.

Taking a fiber supplement or eating foods that are high in fiber may help manage IBS.

▶ KEGEL EXERCISES

Pelvic muscle exercises are better known as Kegel exercises. They are used to strengthen the muscles that surround the openings of the urethra, vagina, and rectum. Just like doing sit-ups to flatten your abdomen, these exercises only work when the right muscles are used, the "squeeze" is held long enough, and enough repetitions are done.

Your doctor or nurse can help you learn the correct way to do Kegel exercises. First, he or she will ask you to squeeze your vaginal muscles around his or her finger during the pelvic exam to check whether you are using the proper muscles. At home, when you begin the exercise program, you will want to place a

320

hand on your abdomen to make sure you don't squeeze the muscles of your abdominal wall. It's also important not to squeeze your thighs or buttocks. Squeeze your pelvic muscles for 10 seconds, 10–20 times in a row, 2–3 times a day. To improve your ability to hold urine, perform Kegel exercises regularly for at least 6 weeks.

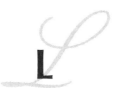

L

▶ See also *Preterm Labor*

▶ LABOR

Most women give birth between 38 and 42 weeks of pregnancy. However, there is no way to know exactly when you will go into labor. Birth often occurs within 2 weeks before or after your expected due date.

Making Plans

As you plan for the birth of your baby, you can take steps to help your labor go more smoothly. It is best to discuss your questions about labor with your health care team before the time comes:

▶ When should I call my doctor?

▶ How can I reach the doctor or nurse after office hours?

▶ Should I go directly to the hospital or call the office first?

▶ Are there any special steps I should follow when I think I'm in labor?

What women tend to think of as "labor" is really just the first stage of labor. The baby's birth happens in the second stage. The placenta is delivered during the third stage.

Before it's time to go to the hospital, there are many things to think about. You may not have time to think about them once labor begins, so it is best to consider them ahead of time:

▶ *Distance*—how far do you live from the hospital?

▶ *Transportation*—is there someone who can take you at any time, or do you have to call and find someone?

▶ *Time of day*—depending on where you live, will it take longer during rush hours than at other times of the day or night?

▶ *Home arrangements*—do you have other children to take to a babysitter's home, or do you have to make any other special arrangements?

▶ *Work arrangements*—do you have a plan for how your workload will be covered and for letting your co-workers know when you have had the baby?

It may be a good idea to rehearse going to the hospital to get a sense of how long it could take. Plan a different route you can follow to the hospital if there are delays on the regular route.

How Labor Begins

No one knows exactly what causes labor to start, although changes in hormones may play a role. Most women can tell when they are in labor. But sometimes it is hard to tell when labor begins.

As labor begins, the cervix opens (dilates). The uterus, which is a muscle, contracts at regular intervals. When it contracts, the abdomen becomes hard. Between the contractions, the uterus relaxes and becomes soft. Even up to the start of labor and during early labor, the baby will continue to move.

Certain changes also may signal that labor is beginning (Table 17). You may or may not notice some of these signs before labor begins.

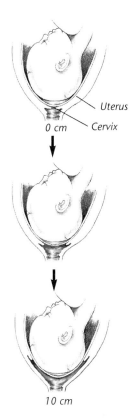

Dilation is the amount that the cervix has opened. It is measured in centimeters, from 0 centimeters (no dilation) to 10 centimeters (full dilation).

Table 17. Signs that You Are Approaching Labor

Sign	What It Is	When It Happens
Feeling as if the baby has dropped lower in your belly	*Lightening.* This is known as "baby dropping." The baby's head has settled deep into your pelvis.	From a few weeks to a few hours before labor begins
Increase in vaginal discharge (clear, pink, or slightly bloody)	*Show.* A thick mucus plug has accumulated at the cervix during pregnancy. When the cervix begins to dilate, the plug is pushed into the vagina.	A few days before labor begins or at the onset of labor
Discharge of watery fluid from your vagina in a trickle or a gush	*Rupture of membranes.* The fluid-filled amniotic sac that surrounds the baby during pregnancy breaks (your "water breaks").	From several hours before labor begins to any time during labor
A regular pattern of cramps that may feel like a bad backache or menstrual cramps	*Contractions.* Your uterus is tightening and relaxing. These contractions increase as labor begins and may cause pain as the cervix opens and the baby moves through the birth canal.	At the onset of labor

True Versus False Labor

You may have periods of "false" labor, or irregular contractions of your uterus, before "true" labor begins. These are called Braxton Hicks contractions. They are normal but can be painful at times. You might notice them more at the end of the day.

It can be hard to tell false labor from true labor. Table 18 lists some differences between true labor and false labor. Usually, false contractions are less regular and not as strong as true labor. Sometimes the only way to tell the difference is by having a vaginal exam to find changes in your cervix that signal the onset of labor.

One good way to tell the difference is to time the contractions. Note how long it is from the start of one contraction to the start of the next one. Keep a record for an hour. It may be hard to time labor pains accurately if the contractions are slight. If you think you're in labor, call your doctor's office or the hospital.

The following are other signs that should prompt you to call your doctor or go to the hospital:

▶ Your membranes rupture (your "water breaks"), even if you are not having any contractions

▶ You are bleeding from the vagina like a period (other than bloody mucus)

▶ You have constant, severe pain with no relief between contractions

▶ You notice the baby is moving less often

Table 18. Differences Between False Labor and True Labor

Type of Change	False Labor	True Labor
Timing of contractions	Often are irregular and do not get closer together (called Braxton Hicks contractions)	Come at regular intervals and, as time goes on, get closer together. Lasts about 30–70 seconds
Change with movement	Contractions may stop when you walk or rest, or may even stop with a change of position	Contractions continue, despite movement
Strength of contractions	Usually weak and do not get much stronger (may be strong and then weak)	Increase in strength steadily
Pain of contractions	Usually felt only in the front	Usually starts in the back and moves to the front

▶ LABOR INDUCTION

▶ See also *Fetal Monitoring, Postterm Pregnancy*

Sometimes the baby needs a little urging to help labor along. Using medications or other methods to bring on labor is called labor induction. If keeping a pregnancy going is more risky than delivering the baby, then labor may be induced. Some of the methods used to induce labor also can speed up a labor that's not going well. Labor may be induced if:

▶ Your amniotic sac has ruptured

▶ Your pregnancy is prolonged, or postterm (more than 42 weeks)

▶ You have high blood pressure caused by your pregnancy

▶ You have health problems such as diabetes or lung disease that could harm your baby

▶ You have chorioamnionitis (an infection in the uterus)

Labor induction carries some risks. It should be done only to protect the health of the mother or the baby. Your baby may be monitored with electronic fetal monitoring if labor is induced. There are four methods for starting labor:

According to the National Center for Health Statistics, the rate of induction of labor in the United States has increased from 90 per 1,000 live births in 1989 to 184 per 1,000 live births in 1997.

1. *Stripping the membranes.* Your doctor inserts a gloved finger through your cervix. Next, he or she sweeps the finger over the thin membranes that connect the amniotic sac to the wall of your uterus. You may feel some intense cramping and spotting when this is done. Stripping the membranes causes your body to release prostaglandins. These are hormones that ripen the cervix and may cause contractions.

2. *Ripening or dilating the cervix.* If your cervix is not ready for labor, steps can be taken to make it soft and able to stretch for labor. Certain medications or devices may be used to soften and dilate your cervix.

3. *Rupturing the amniotic sac.* If it hasn't broken already, breaking your water can get contractions started or make them stronger. Your doctor may make a small hole in the amniotic sac. You may feel discomfort as this is done. Most women go into labor within hours of their water breaking. Another method may be used if labor does not occur. That's because you and your baby are at risk for infection once the amniotic sac has broken.

4. *Oxytocin.* This is a hormone that causes contractions. When oxytocin is used to induce labor or make contractions stronger, it flows into your bloodstream through an intravenous (IV) tube in your arm. A pump hooked up to the IV controls the amount you are given.

▶ See also *Ectopic Pregnancy, Endometriosis, Hysterectomy, Infertility, Ovarian Cysts, Uterine Fibroids*

▶ LAPAROSCOPY

To diagnose certain problems, a doctor needs to look directly into the abdomen and at the reproductive organs. This can be done with laparoscopy.

The word laparoscopy comes from the Greek words that mean "look into the abdomen." A laparoscope is a small telescope that is inserted into the abdomen through a small incision (cut). It brings light into the abdomen so the doctor can see inside. Laparoscopy usually is done on an outpatient basis—you don't have to stay in the hospital overnight.

Laparoscopy often is used to diagnose the cause of abdominal pain. If the doctor finds that he or she can treat the condition during the procedure, diagnostic laparoscopy can turn in to operative laparoscopy. This procedure is used to treat many health problems. Before undergoing laparoscopy, you and your doctor will discuss the procedure and any other treatment.

In the past, most surgery involving reproductive organs was done by laparotomy. Laparotomy involves opening the abdomen to operate on reproductive organs. Now, many of these same procedures are done through the laparoscope. There are many benefits to laparoscopy—a shorter hospital stay, smaller incisions, and a shorter recovery.

The Procedure

You will be given medication to block the pain before the doctor begins the laparoscopy. The anesthesia used depends on the type of procedure, your doctor's advice, and your personal choice. General anesthesia usually is used so that you will not be awake. If local or regional anesthesia is used, you will be awake.

After the anesthesia is given, a small cut is made below or inside the navel. A gas, such as carbon dioxide or nitrous oxide, is usually put into the abdomen. The gas swells the abdomen so the pelvic reproductive organs can be seen more clearly.

Your body will be tilted slightly with your feet raised higher than your head. This shifts some of the abdominal organs toward the chest and out of the way.

The laparoscope is placed through the cut. Another cut often is made above the pubic region. Through this cut, an instrument is used to move the organs into view. One to

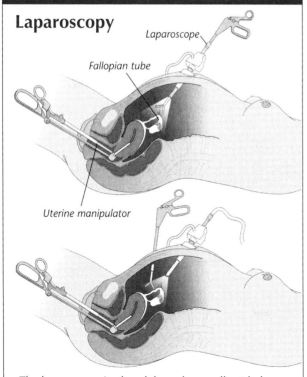

Laparoscopy

Laparoscope

Fallopian tube

Uterine manipulator

The laparoscope is placed through a small cut below or inside the navel (top). A second instrument may be inserted through another cut to move the organs into view (bottom).

four small cuts may be made, ¼ to ½-inch wide. An instrument may be placed in the uterus through the vagina as well in order to move the uterus during the procedure.

Usually, the laparoscope projects images of the surgery onto a television screen. This makes the image larger and easier for the doctor to see. These images can be photographed for later viewing.

Other surgical instruments can be inserted through the scope or through another small cut. Various types of instruments can be used:

▶ Mechanical surgical instruments, such as scissors, forceps, and clamps

▶ Electrosurgical instruments that use electric current through the laparoscope to perform surgery

▶ Lasers that use a high-energy light beam to perform the same procedures as electrosurgery

After the procedure, the instruments are removed and the gas released. The cuts are then closed, usually with stitches that dissolve. In a few hours you can go home. Plan to have someone take you home and stay with you, at least for a while.

There are many reasons why your doctor may use laparoscopy. For instance, it can be used to diagnose and treat endometriosis, ovarian cysts, ectopic pregnancy, and fibroids.

Possible Problems

Although problems seldom occur with laparoscopy, there can be some complications. You may have some bleeding, reactions to the anesthesia, or injury to other organs. The most common organs injured during the procedure are the blood vessels that surround the lower abdomen, the bowel, and the urinary tract. A follow-up laparotomy may be needed, which will require that you be admitted to the hospital. There is also a risk of infection after the procedure.

More common problems include:

▶ Nausea

▶ Pain around the cuts made in your abdomen

▶ Scratchy throat if a breathing tube was used during general anesthesia

▶ Abdominal cramps

▶ Discharge (like your period) that lasts a few days

▶ Swollen abdomen

▶ Tender navel

▶ Shoulder pain

Call your doctor right away if you are bleeding from the incision, if you have a fever, or if you are unable to urinate.

Recovery

The recovery time from laparoscopy is much shorter than that from regular surgery. It is safe to resume normal activities as soon as you feel up to it, usually within a few days. If you are sexually active, talk with your doctor about when you can have sex again.

See also *Hysterectomy, Laparoscopy*

LAPAROSCOPICALLY ASSISTED VAGINAL HYSTERECTOMY

To treat certain problems of the uterus, your doctor may suggest a procedure called laparoscopically assisted vaginal hysterectomy (LAVH). LAVH combines laparoscopy and hysterectomy. Laparoscopy is used to look directly into the abdomen at the reproductive organs. Hysterectomy is surgery to remove the uterus. Your doctor may suggest using laparoscopy to see inside the abdomen and help with the surgery.

What is LAVH?

LAVH is a special form of hysterectomy—removal of the uterus. The uterus is a reproductive organ in the lower abdomen. It holds the fetus during pregnancy. When a woman is not pregnant, the uterus sheds its lining each month during her menstrual period.

The uterus can be removed in two ways. When it is removed through a cut (incision) in the abdomen, the procedure is called an abdominal hysterectomy. When it is removed through the vagina, it is called a vaginal hysterectomy. After a vaginal hysterectomy, women often have less pain, a shorter hospital stay, and a quicker recovery than after an abdominal hysterectomy. Sometimes, a laparoscope allows a vaginal hysterectomy to be done when it could not be done safely otherwise.

LAVH involves the use of a small, telescopelike device called a laparoscope. The laparoscope is inserted into the abdomen through a small cut. It brings light into the abdomen so that your doctor can see inside. He or she views the pelvic organs on a special TV-like screen.

During laparoscopy, other small cuts are made in the abdomen. These cuts allow your doctor to insert other devices to help move organs into view, perform parts of the surgery, and remove the uterus through the vagina.

The laparoscope also can be used before hysterectomy to look at the pelvic organs to help your doctor see what condi-

In the United States, almost 600,000 hysterectomies are performed each year. This makes it the second most often performed major surgical procedure among reproductive-aged women; cesarean delivery is the first.

tions are present. He or she can then decide whether the uterus can be removed through the vagina.

Reasons for LAVH

Hysterectomy may be offered as a treatment option for problems with the uterus. Following are reasons to perform LAVH:

- *Adhesions.* Adhesions are bands of scar tissue that can cause the pelvic organs to stick together. They may occur in the abdomen because of past surgeries or pelvic infection. Your doctor can cut adhesions with the use of a laparoscope to free the uterus. This allows the uterus to be removed through the vagina.

- *Endometriosis.* In this condition, patches of tissue that normally line the uterus grow outside the uterus and become attached to other pelvic organs. This may lead to cysts and severe adhesions. Your doctor may want to use a laparoscope to treat the endometriosis and to do your hysterectomy.

- *Fibroids.* Fibroids are benign (not cancer) growths on the uterus. If they are large, they can make it hard for your doctor to remove the uterus through the vagina. Using the laparoscope may help.

- *Salpingo-oophorectomy.* If the ovaries and fallopian tubes also are removed during hysterectomy it is called salpingo-oophorectomy. Removing the tubes and ovaries through the vagina may be difficult, but a laparoscope can help.

You and your doctor will discuss whether LAVH is the best approach for you. If you have any questions about LAVH, ask your doctor.

The Procedure

Before LAVH, certain steps will be taken to prepare you for the procedure. Your pelvic area and abdomen may be shaved. You will be given an intravenous (IV) line and anesthesia (pain relief). You will not be awake during the surgery.

During LAVH, you will lie on your back as for a pelvic exam. The procedure most often follows these basic steps:

1. Your doctor will make a small cut near the navel. The laparoscope is inserted through this cut into the abdomen. A harmless gas also is put into your abdomen through this incision. The gas expands the space around your pelvic organs so that your doctor has enough room to look at and move them. The doctor can see your pelvic organs on a special TV-like screen.

Seventy four percent of hysterectomies are done on women between the ages of 30 and 54 years.

2. Your doctor may make one or more other small cuts (¼ to ½-inch wide) in the abdomen. These cuts are used to insert devices to move the pelvic organs and help remove the uterus. Devices that may be used include scissors, forceps (grasping device), clamps, or a special stapling device. Some use an electric tool to cut tissue or stop bleeding.

3. A cut is made where the uterus joins the vagina. The bladder and rectum are gently pushed off the uterus. Then, the uterus is removed through the cut.

4. The cuts in the abdomen and the vagina are closed with stitches.

After LAVH, you will have some small scars on your abdomen. In some cases, an abdominal hysterectomy may be required if an LAVH could not be done.

Benefits

The main reason for LAVH is to allow the uterus to be removed safely through the vagina if a standard vaginal hysterectomy cannot be done. With LAVH, there may be less discomfort than if you had an abdominal hysterectomy. You likely will get better quickly and be able to go back to your normal activities sooner after LAVH than after abdominal hysterectomy.

Risks

There are some risks that may occur with any surgery. These may include:

Almost 25% of women is the United States will undergo a hysterectomy by the time they are 60 years of age.

▶ Bleeding

▶ Infection

▶ Problems from the anesthesia

▶ Blood clots in the veins or lungs

▶ Death (very rare)

LAVH can take longer than other types of hysterectomy. This means that you may need more anesthesia than you would with other forms of hysterectomy. Laparoscopy also increases the risk of damage to other organs, such as blood vessels, intestines, or the urinary tract.

After Surgery

Hysterectomy is a major surgery, no matter how it is done. You will have some pain. You may need to stay in the hospital for a few days. After you leave the hospital, you will need to rest and take care of yourself. Plan to take some time off from your job or your work at home.

Because of the stitches in your vagina, you will have some vaginal bleeding or discharge. You should not have sex for a few weeks after the surgery. Do not douche or put anything, such as a tampon, into your vagina during this time. Your doctor will tell you when healing is complete. Make sure you know the warning signs of a problem.

> **Warning Signs**
>
> Call your doctor if you have:
>
> ▶ Fever or chills
>
> ▶ Heavy bleeding or vaginal discharge
>
> ▶ Severe pain
>
> ▶ Redness or discharge from the abdominal cuts
>
> ▶ Difficulty with urination or bowel movements
>
> ▶ Shortness of breath or chest pain

▶ LOOP ELECTROSURGICAL EXCISION PROCEDURE

▶ See also *Cervical Disorders*

Cells on the cervix grow and shed all the time. Sometimes these cells change and become abnormal. This may be an early warning that cancer may occur. When tests show that you have abnormal cells on your cervix, your doctor may suggest the loop electrosurgical excision procedure (LEEP). LEEP is used to remove the abnormal cells from your cervix.

The Cervix

The cervix is covered by a thin layer of tissue like your skin. The cells that make up this tissue grow all the time. During this growth, the cells at the bottom layer slowly move to the surface of the cervix. When these cells reach the surface, they are shed as a normal process.

When this normal process is changed in some way, cells become abnormal. This condition is known as dysplasia. In mild forms, this condition may go away on its own. If it is severe or does not go away, it may lead to cancer of the cervix. Other factors such as smoking and being exposed to sexually transmitted diseases (STDs) also increase the risk of cancer of the cervix.

A Pap test detects changes in the cervix. Other tests, such as colposcopy and biopsy, also are used.

Treating Dysplasia

Abnormal cells can be removed with LEEP. This allows new healthy cells to grow. LEEP is just one way to treat dysplasia. Dysplasia also can be treated with other procedures such as cryosurgery, electrocautery, laser, or cone biopsy. The decision of which method to use depends on how much cervical tissue needs to be removed and where on the cervix the abnormal cells are located.

The LEEP Procedure

LEEP uses a thin wire loop that acts like a scalpel (surgical knife). An electric current is passed through the loop, which cuts away a thin layer of the surface cells.

The procedure should be done when you're not having your menstrual period. This allows a better view of the cervix. In most cases, LEEP is done in a doctor's office or in a clinic on an outpatient basis. It should take only a few minutes.

You may be given pain relief before the doctor begins. During the procedure you will lie on your back and place your legs in stirrups. The doctor then will insert a speculum into your vagina in the same way as for a pelvic exam.

Loop Electrosurgical Excision Procedure

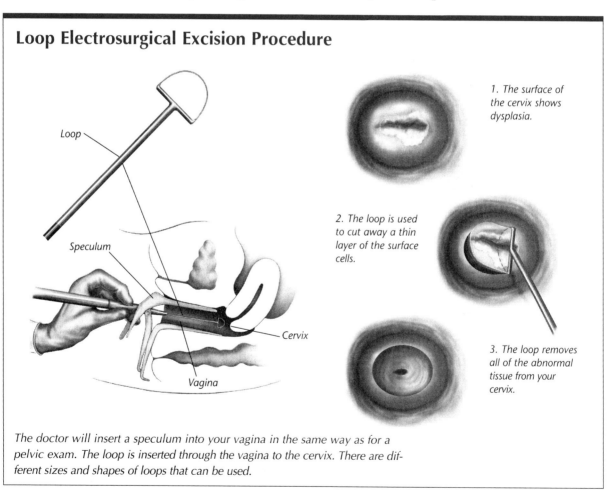

Loop

Speculum

Cervix

Vagina

1. The surface of the cervix shows dysplasia.

2. The loop is used to cut away a thin layer of the surface cells.

3. The loop removes all of the abnormal tissue from your cervix.

The doctor will insert a speculum into your vagina in the same way as for a pelvic exam. The loop is inserted through the vagina to the cervix. There are different sizes and shapes of loops that can be used.

A solution is applied to your cervix to show the abnormal cells. Colposcopy will be used to magnify the cervix during the surgery.

Your cervix will be numbed with local anesthesia. It is given through a needle attached to a syringe. You will remain awake during the procedure. You may feel a dull ache or cramp.

The loop is inserted through the vagina to the cervix. There are different sizes and shapes of loops that can be used. After the procedure, a special paste may be applied to your cervix to stop any bleeding. The tissue that is removed will be studied in a lab to confirm the diagnosis.

Warning Signs

You should contact your doctor if you have any of the following:

- Heavy bleeding (more than your normal period)
- Bleeding with clots
- Severe abdominal pain
- Fever (higher than 100.4°F)
- Foul-smelling discharge

Risks

Although problems seldom occur with LEEP, there can be some complications. You may feel faint during the procedure or have some bleeding. Electrocautery may be used to control bleeding. There is also a risk of infection after the procedure. These complications are rare and can be treated easily.

Your Recovery

It may take a few weeks for your cervix to heal. While your cervix heals, you may have:

- Vaginal bleeding (less than a normal menstrual flow)
- Mild cramping
- A brownish-black discharge (from the paste used)

For a few weeks after the procedure, you should not have sex or use tampons or douches. If you have any discomfort, your doctor may prescribe pain relief.

Staying Healthy

After the procedure, you will need to see your doctor for follow-up visits during the year. At these visits your doctor will check the health of your cervix. After 1 year of normal results, you may return to having exams once a year. If you have another abnormal Pap test, you may need more treatment.

By making a few lifestyle changes after the procedure, you can help protect the health of your cervix:

▶ Have regular pelvic exams and Pap tests.

▶ Stop smoking—smoking increases your risk of cancer of the cervix.

▶ If you have more than one sexual partner, limit your number of partners and use condoms to reduce your risk of STDs.

▶ See also *Cancer, Smoking* in *"Women's Wellness"*

▶ LUNG CANCER

Lung cancer is the number one cancer killer of women. Since 1987, more women have died each year of lung cancer than of breast cancer, which had been the major cause of cancer death in women for the past 40 years. In 1999 alone, more than 65,000 women died of lung cancer. Most lung cancer is caused by cigarette smoking. Women who smoke are 12 times more likely to get lung cancer than women who have never smoked. Second-hand smoke also increases your risk of lung cancer. Lung cancer has many warning signs:

▶ A cough that won't go away

▶ Sputum (phlegm) streaked with blood

▶ Chest pain

▶ Hoarseness

Lung cancer deaths among women increased 150% between 1974 and 1994. Deaths for men increased 20%.

▶ Loss of appetite

▶ Shortness of breath

▶ Fever

▶ Repeat attacks of pneumonia or bronchitis

If you have any of these symptoms, see your doctor. They also may be signs of other lung conditions.

If you smoke, the best way to reduce your chance of getting lung cancer is to stop smoking. Once you stop, your risks begin to decrease right away. In a few years, your risk of getting lung cancer is reduced to nearly that of a nonsmoker.

Lung cancer is hard to detect. There are no tests to detect it when symptoms are not present. Once symptoms occur, chest X-rays and exams of the bronchial passages (airways) help your doctor diagnose lung cancer. Survival rates for lung cancer are low. It is important to find and treat it early.

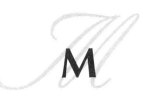

MAGNETIC RESONANCE IMAGING

In magnetic resonance imaging (MRI), a strong magnetic field is used to view internal organs and structures of your body. Magnetic resonance imaging is useful for diagnosing brain growths and damage, such as stroke. This technique also is used to diagnose problems in other parts of the body, such as uterine fibroids and pelvic pain. In patients with breast cancer, doctors may use MRI to gauge the extent of the tumor.

During an MRI, you will lie on a table that slides into a tube containing a large magnet. The magnet reflects signals off of your body. A computer then processes these signals to show "slices" of your body.

You will not feel pain during an MRI, but must lie very still for 30 minutes or more to be sure the images are clear. Inside the tube, you will hear a loud knocking sound as the scanner does its job. Magnetic resonance imaging is a very safe procedure. People who feel anxious in small spaces may be given a sedative to help them relax.

> See also *Pelvic Pain, Stroke, Uterine Fibroids*

Although a MRI is not known to harm the fetus when used during pregnancy, it is not recommended for use in the first 3 months.

MASTURBATION

Masturbation is stimulating your own genitals for sexual pleasure. It is a healthy way to explore your body's reactions and to release sexual tension. By masturbating, many people learn what feels good to them.

To masturbate, some women may stroke their clitoris or rub, squeeze, and fondle other parts of their body. Some women like to use a device to stimulate themselves. Masturbation often leads to orgasm, but not always.

It is common to start masturbating in childhood or the teen years. Masturbation can help satisfy your sex drive when you do not have a partner, or when you choose not to have sex with a person. Even people who have regular sex with a partner sometimes masturbate alone. Masturbation can be part of lovemaking between a couple, as well.

Masturbation is not harmful. Myths linger about masturbation causing acne or other problems, but they are untrue. It is a safe way to meet your sexual needs.

▶ See also *Birth Defects, Genetic Disorders*

▶ MATERNAL SERUM SCREENING

A maternal serum screening test is a blood test that gives information about a pregnant woman's risk of having a baby with certain birth defects, such as Down syndrome or spina bifida. It tests for products from the pregnancy that are also in the woman's blood (serum).

A screening test is a test that is performed when there are no symptoms or known risk factors present. It is not a diagnostic test. A screening test can only assess your risk of having a baby with a certain birth defect. A diagnostic test usually can show whether your baby has the birth defect or not. If your screening test shows a higher-than-average risk for having a baby with a certain defect, further tests may be used for diagnosis. Most women with abnormal screening tests have normal babies.

Your doctor may offer you a maternal serum screening test. The decision to have one of these tests is a personal one.

Who Should Be Tested

Maternal serum screening tests can find a higher-than-average risk of open neural tube defects and Down syndrome. Diagnostic tests usually can find the problem itself and will be offered to women who have abnormal screening test results. If a woman is already at an increased risk of having a baby with one of these problems, she may be offered the diagnostic test first rather than having the screening test. These risk factors may include:

Neural tube defects are the second most common serious fetal defect in the United States, with congenital heart defects being the most common.

▶ Being 35 years old or older when the baby is due

▶ Family or personal history of birth defects

▶ Previous child with a birth defect

▶ Use of certain medicines around the time of conception

▶ Insulin-dependent diabetes prior to pregnancy

Maternal Serum Screening Tests

Alpha-Fetoprotein Test

Alpha-fetoprotein (AFP) is a protein produced by a growing fetus. It is present in amniotic fluid, fetal blood, and, in smaller amounts, in the woman's blood.

The AFP test usually is performed at 15–18 weeks of pregnancy. This is when the test is most accurate. For the test, a small amount of blood is taken from a vein in the woman's arm. Results usually are available in about a week.

At 15–18 weeks, AFP levels are higher than normal in the maternal serum of many women (80%) carrying fetuses with open fetal defects. Other causes of high AFP levels include:

▶ Fetus is older than was thought

▶ Twins

AFP levels are lower than normal in most Down syndrome fetuses. Table 19 shows the test results that mean a higher-than-average risk of open fetal defects and Down syndrome.

Multiple Marker Screening Tests

Adding certain tests to the AFP test can give more information about your risk of having a baby with Down syndrome than the AFP test alone. These are called multiple marker screening (MMS) tests. The best combination of tests is not yet known. Most doctors who use multiple tests use two or three tests together.

Besides measuring AFP, MMS tests measure other substances in the woman's blood that come from the pregnancy. Two that might be measured are human chorionic gonadotropin (hCG) and estriol. Human chorionic gonadotropin is a hormone produced by the placenta. Levels of hCG are *higher* than normal in most pregnancies with a fetus with Down syndrome. Estriol is produced mostly in the placenta and in the liver of the fetus. Estriol levels are *lower* than normal in most pregnancies with a fetus with Down syndrome.

MMS tests also are performed at 15–18 weeks of pregnancy. Like the AFP test, a small amount of blood is taken

Table 19. Maternal Serum Screening Test Results Showing Risk of Open Fetal Defects and Down Syndrome

Condition	Type of Test*		
	AFP	*hCG*	*Estriol*
Open fetal defects	⇑	normal	normal
Down syndrome	⇓	⇑	⇓

*hCG and estriol are tested with AFP in the multiple marker screening test. They are not used alone to assess risk of birth defects.

⇑ = levels higher than normal.

⇓ = levels lower than normal.

from a vein in the woman's arm. Usually the same blood sample is used for all the tests. Results usually are available within a week.

What Do the Test Results Mean?

If AFP levels are normal or if your MMS results are normal, your risk of having a baby with either an open fetal defect or Down syndrome is low. There is still a chance, however, that the risk of a defect in your baby was not detected by the screening test.

Risk of Open Fetal Defects

Your baby may be at higher-than-average risk for open fetal defects if your AFP levels are high. Your doctor may offer you diagnostic tests to find the reason for a high level of AFP.

The first test you may be offered is an ultrasound exam. Ultrasound can confirm that the fetus has a heartbeat. A high AFP level could mean that the fetus has died, although this is rare. Ultrasound also can help show whether the estimated gestational age (the age of the fetus) is correct. If the pregnancy is further along than was thought, this may change the interpretation of the results of your test. Ultrasound may reveal that you have twins. It often can determine whether the fetus has an open fetal defect. In about half the cases, ultrasound explains why AFP levels are high.

If no reason for high AFP levels is found with ultrasound, you may be offered amniocentesis to measure AFP in the amniotic fluid. Amniocentesis is a good test for diagnosing an open fetal defect but does not diagnose closed defects. Only a small number of patients whose maternal serum screening test shows high AFP levels will have a baby with an open fetal defect. Your doctor can be more precise about your risk based on your results.

Risk of Down Syndrome

You are at increased risk for having a baby with Down syndrome if your AFP levels are lower than normal. If you had MMS tests and your AFP and estriol levels are lower than normal and your hCG levels are higher than normal, you also may be at higher risk.

The results will compare your risk of having a fetus with Down syndrome with the risk of an average 35-year-old woman. If your risk is the same or greater than that of a 35-year-old woman, amniocentesis will be offered.

An ultrasound exam can help show whether the estimated gestational age is correct. Ultrasound cannot tell if the fetus does not have Down syndrome.

Down syndrome occurs in 1 out of every 800 births. Unlike neural tube defects, the risk of Down syndrome increases with the mother's age.

If after ultrasound your results still show an increased risk of Down syndrome, you will be offered amniocentesis. This test can find most cases of Down syndrome. Only about 1–2% of patients whose MMS tests show an increased risk for Down syndrome will have a baby with Down syndrome.

MMS tests are better at predicting the risk of Down syndrome than the AFP test alone. If your MMS tests show very low levels of all three tests, your fetus may have a rare chromosomal problem called trisomy 18. If your test gives this result, you also may be offered amniocentesis.

False Results

No test is perfect. Not every abnormal result of a screening test will mean that your baby has a birth defect. An abnormal result may mean that the fetus was older or younger than thought or that there is more than one fetus. Sometimes there is no explanation for an abnormal screening test, and amniocentesis will show that your baby does not have the birth defect. If amniocentesis shows that your baby will have a birth defect, though, you will receive counseling about what this will mean for your family.

Not every normal result of a screening test will mean that your baby does not have a birth defect. Not all cases of open fetal defects or Down syndrome can be predicted. These tests do not give information about all the possible problems the baby might have. Some problems cannot be predicted by testing.

▶ MENSTRUAL HYGIENE PRODUCTS

▶ See also *Menstruation, Toxic Shock Syndrome*

During an average menstrual cycle, a woman loses anywhere from 2 tablespoons to more than 1/2 cup of blood.

Having a menstrual period is a normal and regular event in a woman's life. The average woman will have menstrual periods from about ages 12 to 51 years. There are many products you can use while having your period.

Sanitary Pads

Types of Pads

Pads are worn inside your underwear to collect menstrual flow. They come in different sizes, thicknesses, and styles. The choice is based on your comfort and the amount of your flow.

Regular maxi. Regular maxi pads are the traditional rectangular-shaped sanitary pads. They are about a half-inch thick. You should choose a maxi pad for medium-flow to heavy-flow days.

Thin maxi. Thin maxi pads are not as thick as regular maxi pads. Thin maxi pads are for lighter-flow days. Ultra thin maxi pads also are available. They may absorb more slowly than regular or thin maxi pads. Some ultra thin pads contain a gel that is very absorbent. Ultra thin pads are becoming more popular because they absorb well and are less bulky—making them more comfortable to wear for some women.

Long. Long—or "super"—pads are 1–4 inches longer than regular maxi pads. Long pads often are used for extra protection during the night or for heavy-flow days.

Options

Some pads have tabs called "wings" that wrap around and attach to the underside of your underwear with an adhesive. Winged pads usually are the same size as regular pads. The wings help hold the pad more firmly in place and help protect your underwear.

Deodorant pads also are available. These pads contain perfume. Some women notice that the perfume irritates the skin. If you are concerned about the smell of menstrual blood, you can control any smell by changing the pad often. Scented powder also can be irritating and should not be used on the pad. If you notice a bad or unusual odor during your period, see your doctor—it may be a sign of a vaginal infection.

Things to Consider

Absorbency and a comfortable fit are the main features women look for when buying menstrual products. Because the amount of menstrual flow is not the same every day, to find the best absorbency you may want to use several different types of pads during your period. To prevent leakage and odor, pads should be changed long before they become soaked.

Trying a variety of pads will help you find the most comfortable fit. If your pad does not stay in place, you may want to try one with wings. If your thighs become sore from rubbing on the pad, try a pad without wings or one that is narrower. If leakage is a problem, try a pad that is longer or more absorbent. If the pad does not feel soft enough, try a product with a clothlike feel.

Pads may slip out of place. They cannot be worn while swimming and may be bothersome while doing physical activities such as exercising. If this is a concern, you may wish to use a tampon.

Panty Liners

Panty liners—or panty shields—are shorter and thinner than maxi pads. They are made to use on light-flow days or along with tampons. Women sometimes wear panty liners to collect everyday (nonmenstrual) vaginal secretions. This shouldn't be necessary. Some vaginal discharge is normal. Cotton underwear will help absorb these normal secretions. If you find you need to wear a pad or panty liner every day, contact your doctor. You may have an infection.

Tampons

Types of Tampons

Unlike pads, tampons include a rating on the package for their absorbency. The absorbency of the tampon you use should vary based on the amount of your flow. For heavy-flow days, you may need "super" or "super plus." As your menstrual flow gets lighter, you may want to use "regular" or "junior" tampons. For absorbency, 1 gram is equal to about ¼ teaspoon of fluid:

▶ *Junior*—absorbs up to 6 grams

▶ *Regular*—absorbs 6–9 grams

▶ *Super*—absorbs 9–12 grams

▶ *Super plus*—absorbs 12–15 grams

The claim that tampon makers add the toxin asbestos to tampons is not true. According to the U.S. Food and Drug Administration, asbestos is not found in tampons and there are no reports that tampon use causes excessive bleeding.

You can tell how absorbent a tampon is by how often you need to change it. You should need to change a tampon after 4–6 hours of use. If your tampon does not need to be changed in 4–6 hours, it may be too absorbent. Switch to a less absorbent one. Your tampon also is too absorbent if it is hard to pull out, if your vagina feels dry, or if the tampon shreds when it is removed. A tampon should not be left in place longer than 24 hours.

Tampons come with a variety of applicators. The basic choices are plastic with a covered tip, cardboard with an exposed tip, and cardboard with a covered tip. There are also smaller tampons with applicators that need to be put together before being used. These smaller, pocket-sized tampons are easier to carry. Some brands of tampons do not have an applicator and are inserted into the vagina with your fingers.

Things to Consider

A tampon is comfortable to wear—once inserted, you should not feel it. If you can feel the tampon in place, it may be too

How to Use a Tampon

1. Wash your hands and find a comfortable position—either squat with knees bent and far apart or stand with one foot on the toilet seat.

2. To insert a tampon, use your thumb and middle finger to hold the applicator at the bottom of the outer tube. The removal string should be hanging down from the end of the tube.

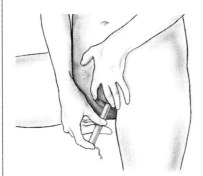

3. Put the rounded end of the tampon into the vaginal opening. The tip should point toward your lower back. Relax your vaginal muscles. Gently slide the applicator into the vagina toward the lower back.

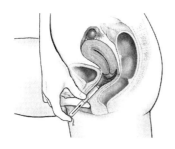

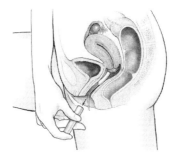

4. Hold the outer tube of the applicator firmly. With your index finger, push the inner tube all the way into the outer tube.

5. Remove both tubes and throw them away. The tampon should be comfortable inside your vagina, with the removal string hanging outside the vagina.

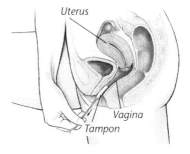

Uterus

Vagina

Tampon

6. When the tampon is inserted properly, you should not feel it. If it feels uncomfortable, it may not be placed far enough inside. If this happens, just remove the tampon by pulling the string and try again.

long or be placed improperly. Try to replace it by inserting the applicator deeper. If this doesn't work, try another size.

Tampons are a good choice for active women. They can be worn while swimming and don't interfere with exercise.

Tampons should be inserted carefully to avoid irritation. There should not be an odor when a tampon is in place. An unusual odor may be a sign of infection. It also might be a sign that you forgot to remove your tampon. If you notice an odor, see your doctor.

Tampons may be more difficult to remove on light-flow days because they absorb vaginal secretions along with menstrual fluid. If this is a problem for you, switch to a less absorbent tampon or a panty liner.

A rare, but serious, condition called toxic shock syndrome (TSS) can be related to tampon use. The risk of TSS increases with higher-absorbency tampons. To lower your risk of TSS, choose a tampon with the lowest absorbency to meet your needs.

The symptoms of TSS are a high fever, chills, vomiting, diarrhea, dizziness, fainting, and a rash that looks like a sunburn. If you have symptoms of TSS while using a tampon, remove it and see a doctor right away.

Other Options

Three new methods of menstrual protection are now available to use with or instead of the more traditional products:

1. *Disposable cup*—looks like a diaphragm and is worn the same way, inserted high in the vagina. The disposable cup collects, but doesn't absorb, your menstrual flow. It can be worn for about twice as long as a tampon on heavy-flow to medium-flow days.

2. *Reusable rubber cup*—inserted into the lower vagina to collect menstrual flow instead of absorbing it. The cup can hold 1 ounce (equal to about 6 teaspoons) of menstrual fluid. It should be emptied several times a day. The cup can be washed and reused for up to 10 years.

3. *Small pad*—a 2½-inch absorbent roll designed to be worn between the vaginal lips (labia). The tiny pad is made only for light-flow days, for temporary vaginal discharge, or for slight urine loss.

▶ MENSTRUAL CRAMPS

▶ See also *Dysmenorrhea*

Menstrual cramps are caused by the muscle of the uterus contracting. These contractions and the pain that results are caused by prostaglandins—natural substances produced by the inner lining of the uterus. Drugs such as ibuprofen relieve menstrual cramps by affecting the amount of prostaglandins. Some of these drugs can be obtained without a doctor's prescription.

Less commonly, menstrual pain may result from a tumor, an infection, or a condition called endometriosis. In these cases, the cause of the pain must be found and treated.

Most often, severe menstrual cramps can and should be treated. If your symptoms are severe enough to interfere with your work or ability to sleep, your doctor may be able to help.

Every body is different. Some women have just a few cramps, some have a lot, and some have none. The intensity of cramps varies and they may not occur before or during every period.

▶ See also *Dilation and Curettage*

▶ MISCARRIAGE

Often, the loss of a pregnancy is a miscarriage (often called spontaneous abortion by doctors). For many women, miscarriage involves more than the loss of a fetus. It also results in feelings of loss and grief.

Factors

Miscarriages occur in about 15–20% of all pregnancies. Most occur in the first 13 weeks, or first trimester. Some miscarriages take place before a woman misses a menstrual period or is even aware that she is pregnant.

The process of fertilization—in which the male sperm and the female egg join—is complex. Miscarriage can be caused by any one of a number of things before, during, or after this process. Often this is nature's way of ending a pregnancy in which the fetus was not growing as it should and would not have been able to survive.

The cause of miscarriage often is not known. Most factors that cause a miscarriage are genetic. Sometimes a miscarriage is caused by the mother's health problems.

Studies have shown that 80–90% of women who have had a miscarriage will go on to have a successful next pregnancy.

Genetic Factors

More than half of miscarriages that occur in the first 13 weeks of pregnancy are caused by problems with the chromosomes of the fetus. Chromosomes are tiny structures inside the center of the body's cells. Each chromosome carries many genes. Genes decide all of a person's physical traits, such as sex, hair and eye color, and blood type.

Miscarriages can result from an abnormal number or structure of chromosomes. The genes they carry may be abnormal, also. Most chromosomal abnormalities are not inherited (passed on from the parents). They happen by chance and are not likely to occur again in a later pregnancy. In most cases, there is nothing wrong with the mother's or father's health. Some genetic problems, though, are passed on from the mother or the father. These problems may relate to the age of the parents.

Factors of the Mother's Health

Problems with a woman's uterus or cervix (opening of the uterus) can lead to miscarriage. These problems most often occur in the second trimester (14–26 weeks) of pregnancy. Problems include an abnormally shaped uterus or an incompetent cervix. An incompetent cervix begins to widen and open too early, in the middle part of pregnancy, without any pain or other signs of labor.

If the mother has a chronic disease, such as diabetes that is not controlled, she may have a higher risk for miscarriage. Infections of the genital tract often cause no symptoms but may affect the uterus and fetus and, as a result, end the pregnancy. Problems with the mother's hormones also can cause very early miscarriage.

Lifestyle Factors

Pregnant women who smoke are more likely to have vaginal bleeding during pregnancy. Their risk of miscarriage is higher than that of women who don't smoke. Heavy alcohol use also increases the risk of miscarriage. This is especially true in early pregnancy, when the major organs of the fetus are being formed. Using illegal drugs, especially cocaine, also increases the risk.

What Doesn't Cause Miscarriage

Most aspects of daily life do not increase the risk of miscarriage. For instance, there is no proof that working, exercising, having sex, or having used birth control pills before getting pregnant increases a woman's risk. The upset stomach that is so common in early pregnancy also does not increase the risk. In fact, women who have severe stomach upset may have a lower risk of miscarriage.

Often women who have had a miscarriage believe that it was caused by a recent fall, blow, or even a fright. In fact, in most miscarriages the fetus died some weeks before the miscarriage occurred.

Symptoms of Miscarriage

Bleeding is the most common sign of miscarriage. Many women who have vaginal spotting or bleeding during the early months of pregnancy have healthy babies. Some of these women, though, will miscarry. This is why bleeding during early pregnancy is called threatened miscarriage. It does not mean that it is certain that the pregnancy will end in a miscarriage, but it might.

If you bleed while you are pregnant, you and your doctor will need to be watchful for a few days. In the very early stages, it is hard to tell if the pregnancy is going to miscarry.

Sometimes mild cramping of the lower stomach or a low backache may occur along with bleeding. Bleeding may persist, become heavy, or occur along

Warning Signs of Miscarriage

Call your doctor if you have:

- Spotting or bleeding without pain

- Heavy or persistent bleeding with abdominal pain or cramping

- A gush of fluid from your vagina but no pain or bleeding. You may need to be examined to see if your membranes have broken.

If you have heavy bleeding and think you have passed fetal tissue, place it in a clean container and take it to the doctor for inspection. Your doctor will want to examine you to see whether your cervix has dilated. If it has, miscarriage is certain.

with a pain like menstrual cramps or breaking of the amniotic sac (fluid-filled sac that surrounds the fetus in the mother's uterus). When the cervix has dilated (opened) and fetal tissue is lost, a miscarriage is certain.

If your doctor does not think that a miscarriage has occurred, you may be asked to rest and to avoid having sex. Although these measures have not been proven to prevent miscarriage, they may help reduce bleeding and discomfort.

After a Miscarriage

Often when miscarriage occurs early in pregnancy, tissue is left in the uterus. If there is concern about heavy bleeding or infection, this tissue will be removed. The tissue can be part of the fetus, part of the placenta (tissue that connects the mother and fetus), or both.

The tissue that remains may be removed by dilation and curettage (D&C) or suction curettage. With these methods, the cervix may be widened if needed. The tissue then is gently removed from the lining of the uterus. These procedures are done in the office, emergency room, or surgical center. They often do not require a hospital stay.

Your doctor may want to see you in a few weeks to check on your progress. You can expect spotting and some discomfort for a few days. You should call your doctor right away if you have any of the following:

▶ Heavy bleeding

▶ Fever

▶ Chills

▶ Severe pain

Your recovery will take some time. If you are beyond 13 weeks of pregnancy, you may still look pregnant, and your breasts may leak milk. Light exercise is good, but increase your activity slowly. Consult with your doctor about which exercises are best and how often you should do them. It is safe to have sex after the bleeding stops.

You can ovulate and become pregnant as soon as 2 weeks after an early miscarriage. If you do not wish to become pregnant again right away, be sure to use birth control.

If your blood is Rh negative, you should ask your doctor whether you need a blood product called Rh immune globulin (RhIG). This prevents you from developing antibodies that could affect a future Rh-positive baby. If you have had a number

Pregnant women who don't want to give up their morning cup of coffee or tea may be in luck. A recent study found that moderate caffeine intake (less than 5 cups of coffee per day) does not increase the risk of miscarriage.

of miscarriages in a row, your doctor may order a few tests to look for a cause.

Feeling the Loss

The death of a baby—whether before or after birth—is a profound tragedy. If you have lost a baby at any stage of pregnancy or during or after delivery, you are going through an emotionally painful time. Not only is this kind of loss usually sudden, but to many parents, it also seems so unfair that the baby they've been hoping and waiting for should be taken from them.

Grief can cause you to blame yourself although you did nothing wrong. You might find yourself thinking about the early days of your pregnancy, searching for a clue that would explain the loss. You also may find yourself angry at your partner or other loved ones for no good reason. Other signs of emotional stress might include headaches, loss of appetite, sleeplessness, fatigue, and trouble concentrating.

Grief is a normal and necessary response to the loss of your baby. Through grieving, you gradually learn to let go of the ties you have formed with your fetus or newborn and go on with your life.

For a mother, this bond can be very strong. It often begins well before birth, sometimes even before conception, and grows throughout pregnancy. Your baby becomes a person in your mind. You imagine whom the baby looks like and what the baby will be like. This bond is often greatly strengthened around 16–20 weeks of pregnancy, when you first feel your baby move. Techniques such as ultrasound (in which sound waves are used to create a picture of the fetus) may have enhanced this bond by letting you actually see the fetus.

A father also can feel a strong tie to his unborn child. His feelings may be different from a mother's, because he does not experience the pregnancy in the same way, but a father also feels the death of a baby as a profound loss.

Both of you may have intense feelings of grief, even if you lose a pregnancy in the first few months. Everyone grieves in a different way and at a different pace. It may take anywhere from several months to a few years to learn how to cope with a loss. Counseling can greatly help you and your family come to terms with this sad and painful event and go on with your lives.

The hurt will never vanish completely, but it will not always dominate your life and your thoughts. Eventually you'll be able to talk and think about the baby more easily and with less pain. And one day you'll find yourself doing more of the things you used to do—enjoying favorite activities, renewing friendships, and looking forward to the future.

Other Signs of Grieving

As you grieve, you may have other feelings or physical symptoms that also are natural and normal:

- *Aches and pains in the breasts and arms*
- *A tight feeling in the chest or throat*
- *Headaches*
- *Trouble sleeping*
- *Loss of appetite*
- *Tiredness*

If you have concerns about what you are feeling, either emotionally or physically, talk with your doctor.

Repeated Miscarriage

Three or more miscarriages in a row may be called repeated miscarriage (or habitual abortion). Women who have had repeated miscarriages need special tests to try to find the reason for them.

After several miscarriages, you may wonder whether you will ever be able to have a healthy baby. Be hopeful. The chances of having a successful pregnancy are good even after more than one miscarriage.

Because repeated miscarriage has many possible causes, your doctor will need a great deal of information to diagnose the problem. You will be asked about your medical history and past pregnancies, as well as your lifestyle and work setting. A complete physical exam, including a pelvic exam, also is important.

Your doctor also may suggest some or all of these tests:

▸ Blood tests for possible problems with hormones or the immune system

▸ Chromosomal testing of both you and your partner

▸ Genital tract cultures for the presence of infection

▸ Chromosomal testing of tissue from the miscarriage, if available

Procedures that might also be done include:

▸ Endometrial biopsy

▸ Hysterosalpingography

▸ Hysteroscopy

▸ Laparoscopy

▸ Ultrasound

About 10–15% of women who have had repeated miscarriages have problems with their uterus.

Special Care for Future Pregnancies

Sometimes the problem that caused the miscarriages can be treated. Surgery may be effective for some problems of the uterus and cervix. Treatment with antibiotics can cure infections. Hormone treatment may help in some cases.

If chromosomal problems are found in the parents, your doctor may advise genetic counseling. A genetic counselor can help you and your partner understand what risks a genetic problem might pose for future pregnancies. The fetus can be tested for some problems in future pregnancies by amniocentesis or chorionic villus sampling.

What You Can Do

If you have had repeated miscarriage, future pregnancies should be planned, diagnosed early, and watched carefully. You can improve your chances of having a successful pregnancy in the future by doing the following things:

▶ Have a complete medical workup before you try to get pregnant again. It may be that the cause of the miscarriages can be found and treated by your doctor.

▶ If you think that you might be pregnant, see your doctor right away. The sooner you seek prenatal care, the sooner you can receive any special care that you may need.

▶ Follow your doctor's instructions. He or she will tell you what you need to do to keep yourself and your fetus as healthy as possible.

▶ MOLAR PREGNANCY

Molar pregnancy (a "mole"), also called gestational trophoblastic disease (GTD), is rare. It results in the growth of abnormal tissue, not an embryo. In the United States, molar pregnancy occurs in 1 of every 1,000–1,200 pregnancies.

Both normal pregnancies and molar pregnancies develop from a fertilized egg. In a mole, though, the fertilized egg does not grow as it should. A genetic error causes abnormal cells to grow and form a mass of tissue.

Women who are older than 40 years or who have had two or more miscarriages are at increased risk of molar pregnancy.

Types of Molar Pregnancy

There are two kinds of molar pregnancy—complete and partial. The mass in a complete mole is made up of all abnormal cells that would have become the placenta in a normal pregnancy. There is no fetus. In a partial mole, the mass may contain both these cells and, often, an abnormal fetus that has severe defects.

Symptoms and Diagnosis

Most molar pregnancies cause symptoms that signal a problem. The most common symptom of a mole is vaginal bleeding during the first trimester. Other signs of moles, such as a uterus that is too large for the stage of the pregnancy or enlarged ovaries, can be found only by your doctor. If your doctor suspects a mole, he or she may order a blood test that measures the level of a hormone called human chorionic gonadotropin (hCG). This hormone is produced by the body during pregnancy or molar pregnancy.

Your doctor can find out whether you have a molar pregnancy by using ultrasound. If a molar pregnancy is found, a series of tests will be done to check for other medical problems that sometimes occur along with a mole. These problems might include preeclampsia (a condition of pregnancy in which there is high blood pressure and swelling) and hyperthyroidism (overactive thyroid gland). These problems are treated by removing the mole.

Treatment

The cervix is dilated, either under general or local anesthesia, and the mole is removed. About 80% of women whose moles are removed require no more treatment. They do need careful follow-up, though. For about 6 months to 1 year after the mole is removed, you should receive routine tests for hCG. These tests can tell your doctor whether the treatment was a success.

After a mole has been removed, abnormal cells may remain. This is called persistent GTD and it is rare. It also can occur after a normal pregnancy. One sign of persistent GTD is an hCG level that remains high after the mole has been removed. Sometimes chemotherapy may be needed to remove the molar pregnancy if it persists. In some cases, hysterectomy may be done. Cure rates are close to 100% for persistent GTD.

If you have had a molar pregnancy, your doctor most likely will advise you to wait 6 months to 1 year before trying to become pregnant again. It is safe to use birth control pills during this time. The chances of having another molar pregnancy are low (about 1%).

Very rarely a molar pregnancy may turn into a choriocarcinoma, a rare pregnancy-related form of cancer that can spread to other organs. There is a high success rate for treating this type of cancer if it is found early.

▶ MORNING SICKNESS

Nausea and vomiting are common during pregnancy, especially during the first part of pregnancy. This often is called "morning sickness," although it can occur at any time of the day.

Most cases of nausea and vomiting are not harmful. When nausea and vomiting are severe and persist, though, they can affect your health.

What Causes Nausea?

While you are pregnant, nausea and vomiting can occur as your body goes through many changes. Although no one is certain what causes the nausea and vomiting, increasing levels of hormones during pregnancy may play a role.

In most women, symptoms of nausea and vomiting are mild and go away after the middle of pregnancy. But some cases of nausea and vomiting are severe. This condition is called hyperemesis gravidarum. It can lead to loss of weight and body fluids.

Effects on Pregnancy

Most mild cases of nausea and vomiting do not harm you or your baby's health. Morning sickness does not mean your baby is sick.

Morning sickness can become more of a problem if you can't keep any foods or fluids down and begin to lose weight. If your nausea and vomiting are severe, call your doctor.

What You Can Do

Until the nausea and vomiting go away, there are some things you can do that might help you feel better:

- Get up slowly in the morning and sit on the side of the bed for a few minutes.

- Eat dry toast or crackers before you get out of bed in the morning.

- Get plenty of fresh air. Take a short walk or try sleeping with a window open.

- Drink fluids often during the day. Herbal teas and cold drinks that are bubbly or sweet may help.

- Eat five or six small meals each day. Try not to let your stomach get empty, and sit upright after meals.

- Avoid smells that bother you.

- Eat foods that are low fat and easy to digest. The BRATT diet (bananas, rice, applesauce, toast, and tea) may help. This diet will provide vital nutrients that will replace what you have lost.

Prenatal vitamins and iron may cause nausea. Ginger, acupuncture, motion sickness bands, or hypnosis may help relieve symptoms. Talk with your doctor before taking any medication or trying any treatment.

Medical Treatment

If your nausea and vomiting are severe, you may need medical treatment. If your doctor suspects that you have hyperemesis gravidarum, you may need to stay in the hospital for a while.

See also *High Blood Pressure During Pregnancy, Preterm Labor*

Call Your Doctor If You:

▶ Have a small amount of dark colored urine

▶ Can't keep down liquids

▶ Are dizzy or faint on standing up

▶ Have a racing or pounding heart

▶ Vomit blood

Your doctor may give you fluids through an intravenous (IV) line. You also may be treated with antinausea medications. In most cases, you will not be allowed to eat any food until the vomiting stops. Your doctor may suggest that you rest in a dimly lit room where it is quiet and private. This type of treatment in the hospital often relieves symptoms.

▶ MULTIPLE PREGNANCY

Being pregnant with more than one baby is called a multiple pregnancy. A multiple pregnancy can be twins (two babies), triplets (three babies), or more. Today, twins are born once in about every 41 births.

Having twins can bring great joy and rewards to a family. Sometimes, however, it can also pose a risk to the mother and her babies. Complications can occur that require special care.

Facts About Twins

Twins can be either identical or fraternal. Most are fraternal twins—each develops from a separate egg and sperm. Fraternal twins each have their own placenta and amniotic sac. Because each twin develops from the union of a different egg and a different sperm, these twins may not look alike. The twins can be boys, girls, or one of each.

Identical twins are more rare. They occur when one fertilized egg splits early in pregnancy and develops into two fetuses. Identical twins may share a placenta, but each baby usually has its own amniotic sac. Identical twins are the same sex and have the same blood type, hair color, and eye color, and they look very much alike.

Some families are more likely than others to have twins. Women who take fertility drugs also have a higher chance of having twins. Because these drugs can cause more than one egg to be released from the ovaries at once, multiple fertilizations become more likely.

Diagnosis

Most twins are diagnosed before delivery. Your doctor may tell you that you are carrying twins if:

◗ Your uterus grows more quickly or is larger than expected.

◗ More than one fetal heartbeat can be heard.

◗ You feel more fetal movement than you did in any pregnancies you had before.

◗ An ultrasound exam done for other reasons detects twins.

How Twins Are Formed

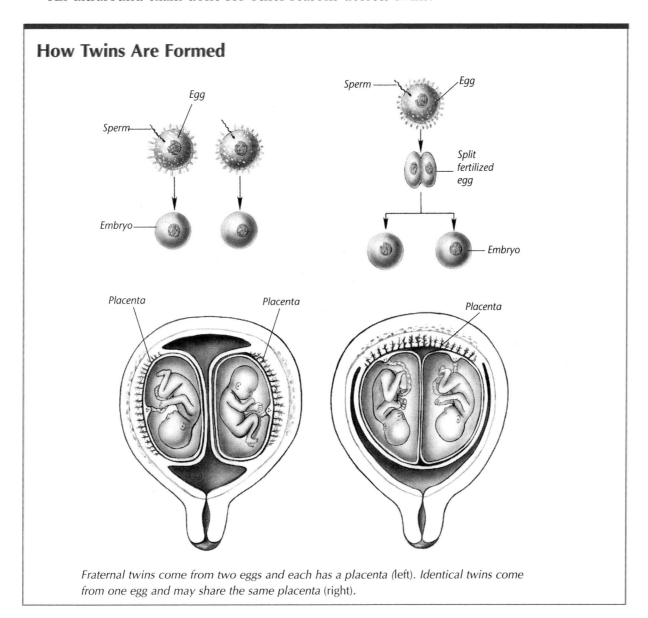

Fraternal twins come from two eggs and each has a placenta (left). Identical twins come from one egg and may share the same placenta (right).

The rate of multiple pregnancies is increasing with the use of assisted reproductive technologies. They now make up about 3% of all pregnancies.

Some twins are found when other prenatal tests are done. If a twin pregnancy is suspected, an ultrasound may be done to confirm it. The test also may be able to tell if the twins are identical or fraternal.

Prenatal Care

You will need special prenatal care with twins. You will need to see your doctor more often and you may have more medical tests. Plan to take childbirth classes during your fourth to sixth months of pregnancy. Ask about special classes for parents expecting twins. If there isn't one convenient for you, talk to your doctor about getting one started.

Nutrition

When pregnant with twins, you will need to eat more than if you were carrying one baby. Eating well and gaining weight are important for your health and the health of your twins. Your body must nourish the babies and meet your energy needs as well. You will need to eat about 2,700 calories every day.

Your doctor will prescribe extra vitamins and minerals to help your babies grow. Anemia (iron-poor blood) is more common in women pregnant with twins, so it's especially important to take your prenatal vitamins and iron as prescribed. Folic acid also is important for twins. It is hard to get all the folic acid you need just from your diet, so you should take folic acid along with the prenatal vitamin.

You should gain more weight when carrying twins than if you were having only one baby. Plan to gain 35–45 pounds. In the first half of pregnancy, you should gain about 1 pound a week. In the second half, aim for a little over 1 pound each week. If you are underweight, you may need to gain more.

Rest

Twins can make you more uncomfortable than usual during pregnancy because the uterus becomes much larger. Resting during the day will help give you energy. Avoid standing for long periods and lifting heavy objects. Talk with your doctor about your job or your work at home. Some women will be told to restrict their activity because of pregnancy complications. You may even need to stay in bed for several weeks. Talk to your doctor about what kind of activity is right for you.

Complications

The risk of certain complications is higher in a twin pregnancy. The mother is more likely to develop high blood pressure or anemia, and the babies are more likely to be born small. The mother also is more likely to go into preterm labor. Sometimes these problems can be prevented with early detection and care. The more babies you are carrying, the more complications you are likely to encounter.

Preterm Labor

Preterm labor is labor that starts before the end of 37 weeks of pregnancy. This can result in preterm birth, the most common problem of multiple pregnancy. About half of all twins are born preterm. When babies are preterm, they often have problems breathing and eating. They will have to stay in the hospital nursery longer than usual. Extremely preterm babies can die, even with the best of care. In others, problems can occur as they grow and develop.

If preterm labor is found early enough, delivery can sometimes be postponed. This will give your babies extra time to grow and mature. Even a few more days can make a big difference.

Bed rest at home or in the hospital has not been proved to prevent preterm delivery of a multiple pregnancy. Hospitalization may be needed to manage problems that occur more often in multiple pregnancies.

Premature Rupture of Membranes

The membranes that hold the amniotic fluid rupture (break) at the start of labor. Sometimes the membranes rupture or leak before labor. This is called premature rupture of membranes. When one or both of the sacs rupture early, the mother is at high risk of preterm labor and infection.

If you have premature rupture of membranes or preterm labor, you may be given injections of a steroid medication. This can help the babies' lungs work better.

Hypertension

High blood pressure that occurs for the first time in pregnancy is called pregnancy-induced hypertension. A sign of hypertension is swelling. Many women have some swelling, especially in their feet and legs, at the end of the day. Too much or sudden swelling may be more serious. If it is not treated, hypertension can cause seizures and threaten your life.

Growth Problems

Twins are more likely to have growth problems. Intrauterine growth restriction (IUGR) is the term for slow growth of babies during pregnancy. Ultrasound often is used to check the growth of each baby. Sometimes, all the babies will be smaller than normal.

Twins are called discordant if one is much smaller than the other. This may be due to one twin getting more blood and having more amniotic fluid than the other, poor functioning of the placenta, or birth defects. The smaller baby is more likely to have problems during pregnancy and after birth. Ultrasound will be used to check each baby's growth and the amount of amniotic fluid. Early delivery may be needed if either baby shows signs of having problems before term.

A condition that can cause one twin to be smaller than the other is twin–twin transfusion syndrome (TTS). TTS can develop when twins share a placenta. The blood passes from one twin to the other through their shared placenta. This can be dangerous for both twins. The twin that gives the blood will be very small and have too little amniotic fluid. The other twin can have too much blood and amniotic fluid and becomes too large. Your doctor will use ultrasound to check the amount of amniotic fluid. Some of the extra fluid may need to be removed. If TTS is severe, the twins may have to be delivered early.

Fetal Loss

In some twin pregnancies, one of the babies dies. In early pregnancy, this is called the vanishing twin. If this happens, you may have some spotting or bleeding from your vagina. This does not harm you or the other baby.

Death of one of the babies is more serious in later pregnancy. Losing a baby when you are still pregnant with another can be very hard for you and your family. It can help to talk with your doctor, nurse, or a counselor about your feelings.

Monitoring Twin Pregnancy

Many techniques are used to check the well-being of your babies. They may be done to confirm other test results or to provide further information. When problems arise, these tests can help to find them early.

Your doctor may use various ways to check your pregnancy:

- Repeat ultrasound to check the babies' growth

- Examine your cervix for changes that may show early signs of preterm labor

- Count your babies' movements, called kick counts

- Examine the babies' heart rate, body movement, muscle tone, and the amount of amniotic fluid by ultrasound

- Measure the babies' heart rate in response to their own movements (called a nonstress test)

Sometimes, amniocentesis is needed. Amniotic fluid contains a substance that shows the maturity of the babies' lungs. In the late months of pregnancy, amniocentesis may be used to decide if the babies' lungs are developed enough for them to be born safely.

The vanishing twin occurs most often in twin pregnancy, but also has occurred in pregnancies with more than two fetuses. It is not clear how often vanishing twin occurs, but one study reported a vanishing twin rate of 21.2%. If this occurs, it does not harm the mother and the outlook for the surviving twin is excellent.

Delivery

In some cases, twins can be delivered by vaginal birth. In others, a cesarean birth may be needed, in which the baby is delivered through a cut made in your abdomen and uterus. How your babies are born depends on certain factors:

 ▶ Position of each baby

 ▶ Weight of each baby

 ▶ Your health

 ▶ Health of the babies

Labor may take longer with twins, especially the pushing stage. Babies usually are born several minutes apart in a vaginal delivery, but it can take longer.

Twins usually can be born vaginally if they are both are in the head-down position. A vaginal birth also may be possible when the lower twin is in the head-down position but the higher twin is not. Once the first twin is born, the other twin can sometimes be turned or delivered with feet or buttocks' first. When this can't be done, the second twin is delivered by cesarean birth. When the lower twin is not in the head-down position, both twins often are delivered by cesarean birth. Cesarean delivery also may be needed when either of the babies is having problems.

Both fetuses will be monitored nonstop during labor. After delivery of the first twin, ultrasonography may be used to track the heart rate and position of the second twin before he or she is delivered.

Caring for Your Newborn Twins

Most twins do well at birth and can be cared for like any other healthy baby. However, if the babies are born early, they may need special medical care to breathe, eat, and keep warm. Preterm and small twins may be cared for in a special nursery called a neonatal intensive care unit at the hospital.

Many women wonder if they can breastfeed more than one baby. The answer is yes. Mother's milk is the best food for any infant. It has the right amount of all the nutrients the baby needs. When you breastfeed, your milk supply will increase to meet the amount needed by your babies. You will need to eat healthy foods and drink plenty of liquids. Women who breastfeed need at least 500 extra calories a day. If your babies are premature, you can pump and store your milk until they are strong enough to nurse from the breast. You may find it helpful to talk with a lactation specialist who is trained to teach women about breastfeeding.

Caring for twins can be stressful at times. Get as much rest as you can. Let others take care of the daily chores while you care for yourself and your new babies. Enjoy the special time you have with each one.

▶ **See also** *Birth Control, Reproductive Process* in *"Women's Bodies"*

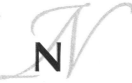

▶ NATURAL FAMILY PLANNING

Natural family planning is another name for the method of birth control that used to be called "rhythm method" or "safe period." More recently it also has been called "fertility awareness." It isn't a single method but a variety of methods. Each is designed to help a couple find out which days during a woman's menstrual cycle she is likely to be fertile or able to become pregnant. Using this method requires the couple to abstain from sexual intercourse during the fertile period in order to avoid a pregnancy. If pregnancy is desired, they need to know the best days for conception.

Natural family planning by periodic abstinence requires neither drugs nor devices. It is thus especially attractive to couples who, for whatever reason, don't want to interfere with reproduction in an artificial way.

Using periodic abstinence as a method of contraception (to prevent pregnancy) means a couple must refrain from sex at certain times during each month. This may lessen the spontaneity of sex. Also, it often is not as effective in practice as other methods of contraception—barrier methods, intrauterine devices, or oral contraceptives. Periodic abstinence can, however, be used by couples along with barrier methods of contraception.

These are things you should consider if you are planning to use periodic abstinence as a method of family planning. If you are thinking about using one of the methods of periodic abstinence, you will need details—ask your doctor about further information and instructions.

How Does It Work?

Methods of periodic abstinence help the couple determine when ovulation, or the release of an egg from the woman's ovary, is likely to occur. It is based on the assumption that the egg is released almost 2 weeks before the woman's next expected menstrual period. The egg remains able to be fertilized for about 24 hours after it is released. Sperm retain their capacity to fertilize an egg for about 48 hours. If the couple wishes to avoid a pregnancy, they avoid having intercourse during the "fertile period," or the time around expected ovulation. The "safe period"

The failure rate is as high as 25–26% in women using periodic abstinence or spermicide alone to prevent pregnancy. Of women using condoms, 15% had failure during the first 12 months of use. Of those using no method, there was an 85% failure rate.

includes those days in the menstrual cycle when intercourse is less likely to lead to pregnancy.

Based on the menstrual cycle of the "average" woman, the 10 or 11 days before the menstrual period, the days during the period, and about 2 days afterward are the "safe period." From the third day after menstruation for about 12 consecutive days is the "fertile period." Intercourse is avoided during this time because ovulation can occur. Ten days before the next expected menstrual period, the safe period starts again. But it is important to keep in mind that no woman is truly average—menstrual cycles normally vary quite a bit.

What Are the Methods?

There are three principal methods of family planning by periodic abstinence:

1. Basal body temperature method

2. Ovulation method

3. Symptothermal method

Basal Body Temperature Method

The temperature method of periodic abstinence is based on the fact that most women experience a slight but detectable increase in their normal body temperature just after ovulation. A woman using this method takes her temperature every morning before getting out of bed. She then records it on a graph. In this way she is able to detect the increase in body temperature that signals ovulation has occurred. A couple using this method abstains from sexual intercourse from the end of the menstrual period until 3 days after the increase in temperature is recorded.

The temperature method can be quite effective in preventing an unwanted pregnancy if it is used carefully and consistently. But there also are disadvantages:

▶ The time during which sexual activity is allowed is limited.

▶ You must take your temperature every day.

▶ Temperature readings may be affected by fever, restless sleep, or exertion.

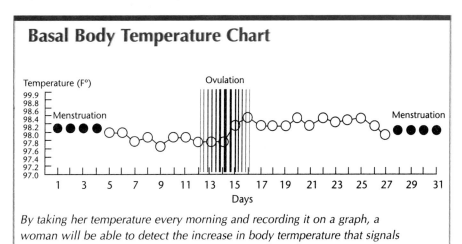

Basal Body Temperature Chart

By taking her temperature every morning and recording it on a graph, a woman will be able to detect the increase in body termperature that signals ovulation has occurred.

Ovulation Chart

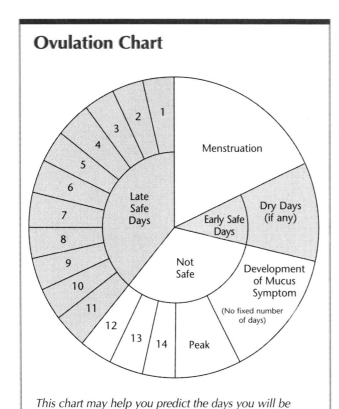

This chart may help you predict the days you will be ovulating. You produce more cervical mucus just before ovulation—about halfway through your menstrual cycle.

Ovulation Method

The ovulation method involves changes in how much mucus is produced by the cervix (mouth of the uterus) and in how it feels. Women who use this method learn to recognize the changes that occur around the time of ovulation. To do this, a woman checks regularly for mucus at the opening of the vagina and assesses it for such changes.

For example, for most women the vagina is dry for a time just after menstruation. Then a rather sticky mucus appears. Just before ovulation the mucus becomes increasingly wet and slippery and looks a little like raw egg white. The day of greatest wetness, called the "peak" day, often coincides with ovulation. Just after the "peak" day, the mucus becomes thick again or may even disappear, and the feeling of dryness reoccurs.

The "safe" days, those days on which intercourse is allowed for couples avoiding pregnancy, are the 10 or 11 days at the end of the cycle and the dry days, if any, that occur just after menstruation. The "fertile" period, during which abstinence should be practiced, starts with the development of the first signs of mucus and continues until 4 days after the "peak" day.

Although the days of bleeding are considered relatively infertile, pregnancy can occur during menstruation. It is possible for mucus production to overlap the menstrual period, thus creating a favorable environment for sperm. An experienced user of the method is able to detect these changes.

The ovulation method has advantage over the temperature method in that it does not require the use of a thermometer and can be used by women whose menstrual cycles are slightly irregular. However, false readings may be produced by certain factors:

▶ Vaginal infection

▶ Sexual excitement

▶ The use of lubricants for sexual intercourse

Thus, care must be taken in interpreting the changes. When first learning this method, instruction by a trained teacher is strongly advised.

Symptothermal Method

The symptothermal method combines the temperature and ovulation methods. In addition to taking the temperature and checking for mucus changes, other signs of impending ovulation are observed:

▶ Breast tenderness

▶ Abdominal cramps

▶ Vaginal spotting

▶ A change in the position and firmness of the cervix

This method requires that you abstain from sexual intercourse from the day you first notice feelings of vaginal wetness until the third day after the increase in temperature—or the fourth day after the "peak" day of mucus production.

The symptothermal method can be more effective than either of the other two methods because it uses a variety of signs instead of relying on just one. It is subject to some of the same limitations as the temperature and ovulation methods.

▶ NUTRITION DURING PREGNANCY

▶ **See also** *Breastfeeding*

A balanced diet is a basic part of good health at all times in your life. During pregnancy, diet is even more important. The foods you eat are the main source of the nutrients for your baby. As your baby grows, you will need more of most nutrients.

Before You Become Pregnant

Before you are pregnant is the best time to begin eating a healthy diet. Eating right before you become pregnant can help make sure that you and your baby start out with the nutrients you both need.

If you are planning to become pregnant, visit your doctor. Getting good health care before you are pregnant will help you throughout your pregnancy. As part of your visit, you will be asked about your lifestyle. This includes your diet. You and your doctor will discuss how to eat right before and during your pregnancy and how much weight you should gain.

Table 20. How Much Weight Can You Expect To Gain in Pregnancy?

Weight Status	Weight Gain (pounds)
Underweight	28–40
Normal weight	25–35
Overweight	15–25
Carrying twins	35–45

Weight Gain

Pregnant women are sometimes concerned about gaining too much weight. Keep in mind that your diet is the main source of energy for your baby. That means you have to eat more while pregnant. When you are pregnant, you need about 300 calories more a day than you usually eat.

How much weight you gain during pregnancy depends on your weight before pregnancy (Table 20). A healthy gain for most women is between 25 and 35 pounds. If you are overweight, you should gain less, but some weight gain is normal. If you are underweight, you should gain more. Discuss with your doctor or nurse the amount of weight you can expect to gain.

You are likely to gain about 3–5 pounds in the first 3 months. You may then gain 1–2 pounds each week in the rest of the pregnancy. Your weight gain is not all fat. It's mostly from retaining water in your body and from the weight of the growing baby. Gaining the right amount of weight is an important part of a healthy pregnancy.

Where Does the Weight Go?

In most women, 25–35 pounds is a good amount of weight to gain during pregnancy. Your body must store nutrients and increase the amount of blood and other fluids it makes. Here's how much weight an average woman gains in parts of her body during pregnancy:

Baby	7½ pounds
Your breasts	2 pounds
Maternal stores (your body's protein, fat, and other nutrients)	7 pounds
Placenta	1½ pounds
Uterus	2 pounds
Amniotic fluid (the water around the baby)	2 pounds
Your blood	4 pounds
Your body fluids	4 pounds

A Healthy Diet

The first step toward healthy eating is to look at the foods in your daily diet. Early in pregnancy, some women find that their appetite comes and goes. You still should try to eat a variety of foods each day.

Having healthy snacks that you can eat during the day is a good way to get the nutrients and extra calories you need. You may find that regular snacks and smaller meals are better than three big meals a day.

Eating healthy also means avoiding things that may be harmful. This includes drinking alcohol (beer, wine, or mixed drinks), which may cause birth defects. You also should stop smoking, especially if you smoke instead of eating to try to control your weight.

Try to plan your meals. Planning meals in advance can help ensure you and your family eat a balanced diet.

Meal Planning

For help in choosing what to eat, refer to the Food Guide Pyramid ("Women's Wellness"). It shows the number of servings a pregnant woman should have every day from each food group. Try to get all the servings you need during the day through meals and snacks. Table 21 gives tips on what kinds of foods you can eat to follow the Food Guide Pyramid.

Basic Nutrients

Every diet should include proteins, carbohydrates, vitamins, fats, and minerals. To be sure your diet gives you the right amount, you should know which foods are good sources of each.

The labels on food often have the letters RDA. This stands for Recommended Daily Allowance. RDAs are levels of nutrients you need every day. During pregnancy, the RDAs are higher for most nutrients. If you eat a mix of foods and eat enough servings of foods from the Food Guide Pyramid, you will be eating a very good diet. Table 22 shows the key nutrients you and your baby will need during your pregnancy.

Table 21. Daily Food Choices

Food Group	Number of Servings You Need Every Day	Example of Single Servings
Bread, Cereal, Rice, Pasta	9	1 slice of bread; 1 ounce of cold cereal; or ½ cup of cooked cereal, rice, or pasta
Vegetables	4	1 cup of salad greens, ½ cup of other cooked or raw vegetables, or ¾ cup of vegetable juice
Fruit	3	1 medium apple, banana, or orange; ¼ cup of raisins; or 4-ounce glass of orange juice
Poultry, Fish, Dry Beans, Meat, Eggs, and Nuts	3	2–3 ounces of cooked lean poultry, fish, or meat; 1 cup of cooked dry beans; or 1 egg
Milk, Yogurt, and Cheese	3	1 cup of milk or yogurt or 1 ounce of low-fat cheese

Extra Nutrients

You may need extra nutrients because you are pregnant. These may include iron, vitamins B_6 and B_{12}, and calcium. They can be given as single pills or as a combined pill. Sometimes a prenatal vitamin contains all you need. Ask your doctor or nurse how your needs can be best met.

Check with your doctor before taking any vitamins and herbs. They may be harmful during pregnancy.

Folic Acid

Folic acid is a type of vitamin that is key to the growth of your baby, especially during the first months of pregnancy. Not getting enough folic acid in your diet increases the risk of birth defects such as neural tube defects, which affect the spine and skull. Folic acid also is used to make the extra blood your body needs during pregnancy.

To help prevent neural tube defects, a woman should have 0.4 milligrams of folic acid daily before and during pregnancy. The best sources of folic acid in foods are listed in Table 22. Folic acid is added to breads and breakfast cereals along with other nutrients. It is hard to get all the folic acid you need just from your diet, so you should take a supplement with the right amount of this vitamin.

Table 22. Key Nutrients for You and Your Baby During Pregnancy

Nutrient	Why You and Your Baby Need It	Best Sources
Protein	Main "building block" for your baby's cells. Helps produce extra blood you need and provides extra stores of energy for labor and delivery. RDA = 60 grams	Meat, eggs, beans
Carbohydrates	Gives energy for you and your baby during pregnancy.	Bread, cereal, rice, potatoes, pasta
Calcium	Helps build strong bones and teeth. RDA = 1,200 milligrams (about four 8-ounce glasses of milk).	Milk, cheese, yogurt, sardines, spinach
Iron	Helps create the red blood cells that deliver oxygen to your baby and also prevents fatigue. RDA = 30 milligrams	Lean red meat, spinach, whole-grain breads and cereals
Vitamin A	Forms healthy skin and helps eyesight. Helps with bone growth.	Carrots; dark, leafy greens; sweet potatoes
Vitamin C	Promotes healthy gums, teeth, and bones. Helps your body absorb iron.	Citrus fruit, broccoli, tomatoes
Vitamin B_6	Helps form red blood cells. Helps body use protein, fat, and carbohydrates.	Beef liver, pork, ham; whole-grain cereals; bananas
Vitamin B_{12}	Maintains nervous system. Needed to form red blood cells.	Liver, meat, fish, poultry; milk (found only in animal foods—vegetarians should take a supplement)
Folic acid	Needed to produce blood and protein. Helps some enzymes function.	Green, leafy vegetables; dark yellow fruits and vegetables; liver; legumes and nuts
Fat	Provides long-term energy for growth. Should be 30% or less of your daily diet.	Meat, eggs, nuts, peanut butter, margarine

Women who have had a child with a spine or skull defect are more likely to have another child with this problem. These women need higher doses of folic acid—4 milligrams daily. It should be taken 1 month before pregnancy and during the first 3 months of pregnancy. Women who need 4 milligrams should take folic acid alone, not as a part of a multivitamin preparation. To get enough folic acid from multivitamins, a woman would be getting an overdose of the other vitamins.

Special Concerns

Vegetarian Diets

If you are a vegetarian, you can continue your diet during your pregnancy. You will need to plan your meals with care to ensure you get the nutrients you and your baby need. If your diet includes milk, cheese, and eggs, it will be easier to balance your daily nutrients.

If you are on a vegetarian diet, you may need to take supplements, such as vitamin B_{12} and vitamin D. These supplements will help you get all the nutrients you and your baby need.

Lactose Intolerance

Milk and other dairy products are the best sources of calcium in your diet. But some women have symptoms such as bloating, diarrhea, gas, and indigestion after drinking milk or eating dairy products. This is known as lactose intolerance.

If you are pregnant and lactose intolerant, make sure you are getting enough calcium. Talk with your doctor or dietitian. He or she may prescribe calcium supplements if you cannot get enough calcium from other foods that contain calcium. Calcium also can be found in sardines, salmon with bones, and spinach.

Pica

During pregnancy, some women feel strong urges to eat non-food items such as clay, ice, or laundry starch and cornstarch. This is called pica. Pica can be harmful to your pregnancy. It can affect your intake of nutrients and can lead to constipation and anemia (low blood count). Talk with your doctor if you have any of these urges. He or she may be able to suggest other things you can do when you feel the urge to eat non-food items.

O

▶ **See also** *Bone Mineral Density Testing, Hormone Replacement Therapy, Menopause* in "*Women's Bodies*," *Selective Estrogen Receptor Modulators*

▶ OSTEOPOROSIS

Bones go through a constant state of loss and regrowth. As a person ages, more loss than growth can occur. This can lead to a condition called osteoporosis. The bones then become thin and fragile and can break easily.

Osteoporosis can pose a special threat to women. Estrogen—a female hormone—protects against bone loss. As a woman nears menopause, her body produces less estrogen. This process begins long before menopause. By the time symptoms of osteoporosis show, a great deal of bone loss may have already occurred.

What Is Osteoporosis?

Bone is made up of calcium and protein. There are two types of bone—compact bone and spongy bone. Each bone in the body contains some of each type. Compact bone looks solid and hard and is found on the outer part of bones. Spongy bone is filled with holes, just like a sponge, and is found on the inside of bones. The first signs of osteoporosis are seen in bones that have a lot of spongy bone, such as the spine, hip, and wrist.

Once made, bone is always changing. Old bone is removed in a process called resorption, and new bone is formed in a process called formation. From childhood until age 30, bone is formed faster than it is broken down. The bones become large and more dense. After age 30, the process begins to reverse: bone is broken down faster than it is made. This process continues for the rest of your life. A small amount of bone loss after age 35 is normal in all women and men. It usually does not cause any problems. However, too much bone loss can result in osteoporosis.

In osteoporosis, bones become thin and brittle because more bone is lost than formed. The bones are still the same size, but the outside walls of compact bone become thinner, and the holes in spongy bone become larger. These changes greatly weaken the bone.

Signs of osteoporosis do not occur until a lot of bone is lost. Some of these symptoms are back pain or tenderness, a loss of height, and a slight curving of the upper back. As the spinal bones

More than 300,000 Americans older than 45 years are admitted to the hospital with hip fractures every year. Osteoporosis contributes to most of these injuries, especially in women. The rate of hip fractures is two to three times higher in women than men. A woman's risk of hip fracture is equal to her combined risk of breast, uterine, and ovarian cancer.

weaken, they slowly collapse under the weight of the upper body. This causes a curving of the spine—often called a "dowager's hump."

Osteoporosis affects at least 25 million Americans—most of whom are women. Each year, at least 1.2 million fractures related to osteoporosis occur in the United States. One third of women older than 65 will have a fracture of the spine. Fractures can be crippling and painful and cause lifelong disability. As many as 1 in 5 patients with a hip fracture dies within 6 months from problems caused by lack of activity, such as blood clots and pneumonia.

Risk Factors

Women are more at risk of osteoporosis because their bones are smaller and lighter than men's. The following factors can increase that risk:

▶ Menopause (bone loss increases after menopause because the ovaries stop making estrogen, which protects against bone loss)

▶ Removal of ovaries (if a woman has her ovaries removed before menopause, the sudden decrease in estrogen can result in rapid bone loss unless she takes estrogen)

▶ Diet low in calcium

▶ Race (white women and Asian women are at highest risk)

▶ Lack of exercise

▶ Slender build

▶ Eating disorders (anorexia nervosa or bulimia)

▶ Family history

▶ Some medications (for instance, diuretics ["water pills"], corticosteroids, anticonvulsants)

▶ Alcohol and tobacco use

▶ Hyperthyroidism

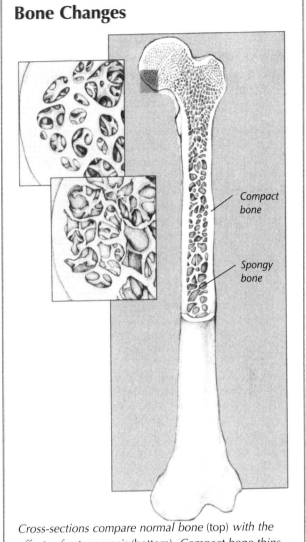

Bone Changes

Compact bone

Spongy bone

Cross-sections compare normal bone (top) with the effects of osteoporosis (bottom). Compact bone thins out and spaces around spongy bone become larger.

Effects of Osteoporosis

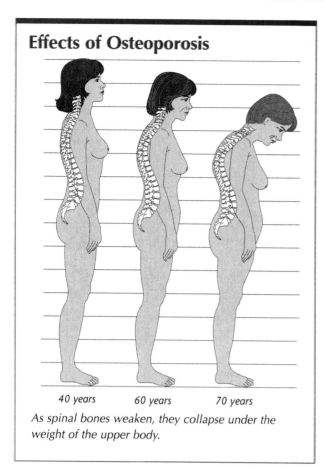

40 years   60 years   70 years

As spinal bones weaken, they collapse under the weight of the upper body.

Prevention

It is hard to grow new bone after it is lost, so prevention is important. To prevent osteoporosis, focus on building and keeping as much bone as you can. This can be done by exercising and eating enough calcium during your reproductive years. After menopause, your doctor may suggest hormone replacement therapy or some other drug to protect against bone loss.

Exercise

Exercise increases bone mass before menopause and slows bone loss after menopause. Just as muscles become stronger with regular exercise, so do bones. Bones are strengthened by having the muscles pull on them. Bone loss will occur any time the bones are not used. For example, it becomes worse in people who are bedridden for a long time. Active women have higher bone density than women who do not exercise.

Most aerobic exercise is good for the heart and bones. To help prevent bone loss, the exercise should be weight-bearing, such as low-impact or step aerobics, brisk walking, and tennis. Even walking several blocks each day will slow bone loss. It is never too late to start exercising, and even a little bit is better than none. If you have questions about the best exercise program for you, it may be wise to talk with your doctor or a professional who knows about health and exercise. Let him or her know if you have a physical problem that may limit your exercise.

Diet

Bone loss can increase if your diet is low in calcium. Calcium slows the rate of bone loss. If the amount of calcium in the bloodstream is too low, it will be taken from the bones to supply the rest of the body.

Good sources of calcium are dairy products, such as skim milk and yogurt. Other sources are leafy green vegetables, nuts, and seafood. A well-balanced diet is very healthy for bones.

Most women need more calcium on a daily basis. In fact, many women get only half the daily amount of calcium they need. It is hard to get enough calcium by diet alone without eating foods that are high in fat and calories. Thus, you may need to take calcium supplements. Not all calcium supplements prevent bone loss. Ask your pharmacist to suggest a supplement. Be aware, however, that your body can only absorb up to 750 milligrams of calcium at one time. If you take 800–1,500 milligrams per day, divide it into two doses.

Calcium cannot be absorbed without vitamin D. Milk that is fortified with vitamin D is one of the best sources. Another is sunlight. Being in the sun for just 15 minutes a day helps your skin produce vitamin D and activates vitamin D in your body. You also can use vitamin D supplements if you are not exposed to the sun. However, a woman should take in no more than the recommended daily amount of vitamin D, which is 400–800 International units (5–10 micrograms). Too much vitamin D can cause problems.

Birth Control Pills

Taking birth control pills (which contain estrogen) during your reproductive years can slow the rate of bone loss. One study found that women who had taken birth control pills had more bone than women who had never taken them. Birth control pills are safe for most women who do not smoke.

Hormone Replacement Therapy

Hormone replacement therapy restores estrogen and slows bone loss after menopause. Estrogen has been linked to a 50% decline in hip fractures and a 90% decline in spinal deformities. It also helps prevent heart disease and stroke. Estrogen can relieve other symptoms that occur around menopause, such as hot flushes (hot flashes).

To prevent osteoporosis, hormone replacement therapy should be started after a woman stops menstruating (or when the ovaries are removed). Starting estrogen at any time after menopause, though, can help prevent bone loss. Therapy must be thought of as long term. For a woman to continue to benefit, she must continue therapy. You and your doctor should decide whether this treatment is right for you.

Other Medications

If a woman does not take estrogen, there are other options for preventing osteoporosis. These include raloxifene and alendronate. Other options that may be used to slow bone breakdown are etidronate and calcitonin (given by injection or nasal spray). Slowing bone loss helps build strong bones.

Detection and Treatment

You should have a physical exam once a year. A yearly check of your height can help detect osteoporosis. You also can be given

About 10 million Americans have osteoporosis. Another 18 million Americans have bone mass low enough to put them at risk for the disorder.

a bone mineral density test. Once you know you have osteoporosis, these tests also can help your doctor check your rate of bone loss. They are helpful for some women, especially those at high risk or who do not take estrogen. Routine X-rays only show when much bone has already been lost.

Women with osteoporosis should try to reduce their risks of injuries from falls. They should:

▶ Use good posture

▶ Avoid twisting, bending, and lifting

▶ Make their home safe by using nonskid backing on throw rugs, making sure rooms are well lit, and using handrails by stairs and in the bathroom

▶ **See also** *Cancer*

▶ OVARIAN CANCER

Cancer of the ovary is a disease that affects one or both ovaries, the two organs on either side of the uterus. If cancer of the ovary is found and treated early, the cure rate is good. Patients whose cancer has not spread outside the ovary have an 80–95% chance of living 5 years or longer after treatment. Unfortunately, cancer of the ovary often has no symptoms in early stages. As a result, it often is found in advanced stages when it is harder to treat with success.

What Is Ovarian Cancer?

Normal, healthy cells that make up the body's tissues grow, divide, and replace themselves on a routine basis. Sometimes, though, cells develop abnormally and begin to grow out of control. When this happens, too much tissue is made and begins to form growths or tumors.

There are three types of ovarian cancer:

1. Epithelial

2. Germ cell tumors

3. Sex cord–stromal tumors

Epithelial cancers are the most common. About 90% of all ovarian cancers arise from epithelial cells. These are the cells that cover the surface of the ovaries. Most women who get epithelial ovarian cancers are older than 40 years.

About 10% of ovarian cancers are germ cell tumors. The rest are sex cord–stromal tumors. Both types tend to occur in women younger than 40 years. There is a good chance that they can be treated with success.

Recent studies have shown that genetic testing may be an effective way to screen high-risk women for ovarian cancer. A genetic link has been found in 5–10% of women who have close family members who have had ovarian, colon, or breast cancer. For instance, about 5–7% of all breast and ovarian cancer cases are linked to the presence of the BRCA 1 or BRCA 2 genes. Women who have a BRCA 1 gene mutation have a greater than 80% chance of developing breast cancer in their lifetime and about a 45% chance of developing ovarian cancer by age 70 years. BRCA 1 appears to have a higher risk of ovarian cancer than does BRCA 2.

Who Is at Risk?

Women of any age can have cancer of the ovary, but the risk increases with age. It occurs most often in women who are between 50 and 75 years old. It is less common in women younger than 40 years, and more common in white women.

Women who have had several children are less likely to get ovarian cancer. Those who have used birth control pills or are now using them also are less likely to get it.

Women may have a high risk of ovarian cancer if they:

▶ Did not have children

▶ Did not use birth control pills

▶ Have family members who have had ovarian cancer

A woman may have some or all of these risk factors and never have ovarian cancer. Even women with no risk factors should know the symptoms of ovarian cancer and have routine checkups.

Over the past 17 years, ovarian cancer deaths have increased in women 65 years and older and decreased in younger women. Factors such as improved treatment of early stage ovarian cancer (more common in younger women), and the use of birth control pills may have influenced the decrease among younger women.

Symptoms

Cancer of the ovary often does not have any symptoms in its early stage. There are few symptoms of the disease. As a result, the cancer may not be found until it's in an advanced stage. This makes it harder to treat.

When there are symptoms, they may be mild and hard to detect. The warning signs are:

▶ A sense of discomfort in the pelvic region

▶ Indigestion, gas, and bloating that can't be explained

▶ Abnormal bleeding

▶ Pain and swelling of the abdomen

▶ Loss of appetite

Most patients with these symptoms don't have a severe problem. They should be discussed with a doctor, though.

Screening

Currently, there is no effective way to screen for ovarian cancer. The best way to detect ovarian cancer at an early stage is by a pelvic and rectal exam. The doctor may be able to feel a tumor or cyst on one or both of the ovaries. Very few of these cysts will be cancerous. The cysts should be checked often for growth.

Finding a Better Screening Test

Two tests are being studied as methods for screening for cancer of the ovary before symptoms are present:

1. *Ultrasound exam.* This can be used to detect changes in the ovary. The exam shows if an ovary is enlarged. It also shows if a growth on an ovary is solid or filled with fluid. It does not give the doctor enough information to confirm a cancer, though.

2. *A blood test to detect an antibody called CA 125.* The antibody has been found in the blood of women with ovarian cancer and may be a sign of the disease. However, the CA 125 blood test may produce results that suggest that a woman has ovarian cancer when she really does not. This is because levels of CA 125 may be present in higher amounts in women with benign conditions such as fibroids, endometriosis, pelvic infections, or pregnancy. Also, some types of ovarian cancers do not increase CA 125 levels.

Neither of these tests can be relied on to screen for cancer of the ovary at this point. They need further study before they can be used to detect cancer.

The Pap test is a vital part of a routine checkup. It is not a good way to detect ovarian cancer, however.

Treatment

If a woman is thought to have ovarian cancer, surgery is needed. The surgeon will explore the extent of the disease, remove the cancer, and decide what other treatment is needed.

The disease will be staged as a result of this surgery. Treatment is based on the stage and how fast the cancer is spreading. The age, state of health, and wishes of the patient also are taken into account in planning treatment.

Surgery for most patients includes removing the uterus (hysterectomy) and the ovaries and fallopian tubes (salpingo-oophorectomy). Sometimes, some lymph nodes and parts of the bowel may have to be removed. Young women may have early tumors of certain types confined to only one ovary. The surgeon may remove only that ovary.

The surgery often is followed by chemotherapy or radiation. Chemotherapy often involves taking the drugs cisplatin or carboplatin along with other drugs.

▶ **See also** *Laparoscopy, Ovarian Cancer, Ultrasound Exam*

▶ OVARIAN CYSTS

The ovaries are two small organs, one on each side of a woman's uterus. It is normal for a small cyst (a fluid-filled sac or pouch) to develop on the ovaries. These cysts are harmless and in most cases go away on their own. Others may cause problems and need treatment.

Types of Ovarian Cysts

Ovarian cysts are quite common in women during their childbearing years. Most cysts result from the changes in hormone levels that occur during the menstrual cycle and the production and release of eggs from the ovaries. A woman can develop one cyst or many cysts. Ovarian cysts can vary in size—from as small as a pea to as big as a grapefruit.

There are different types of ovarian cysts, and each type causes a variety of symptoms. All cysts can bleed, rupture (burst), and twist and cause pain. Most cysts are benign (not cancerous). A few cysts, though, may turn out to be malignant (cancerous). For this reason, all cysts should be checked by your doctor.

Functional Cysts

The most common type of ovarian cyst is called a functional cyst. It develops from tissue that changes in the normal process of ovulation. There are two types of functional cysts—follicle and corpus luteum. Both of these cysts usually have no symptoms or minor ones when they occur. They disappear within a few months.

Dermoid Cysts

Dermoid cysts are made up of different kinds of tissue, such as skin, hair, fat, and teeth. They may be found on both ovaries. Dermoid cysts are often small and may not cause symptoms. They can, however, become large and cause symptoms.

Cystadenomas

Cystadenomas are cysts that develop from cells on the outer surface of the ovary. They are benign, but they can create problems. Cystadenomas can grow very large and interfere with abdominal organs and cause pain.

Endometriomas

Endometriomas are cysts that form when endometrial tissue grows in the ovaries. This tissue then responds to monthly changes in hormones. The tissue bleeds monthly, which may cause it to form a gradually growing cyst on the ovary. An endometrioma also is known as a "chocolate cyst" because it is filled with dark, reddish-brown blood.

An endometrioma often is linked to a condition known as endometriosis. It can be painful, especially during the menstrual period or during sexual intercourse.

Multiple Cysts

Women who do not ovulate regularly can develop multiple cysts. This is a disorder in which the ovaries are enlarged and contain many small cysts. It can be linked to a condition called polycystic ovary syndrome (PCOS). This condition may cause irregular menstrual periods, infertility, and increased body hair.

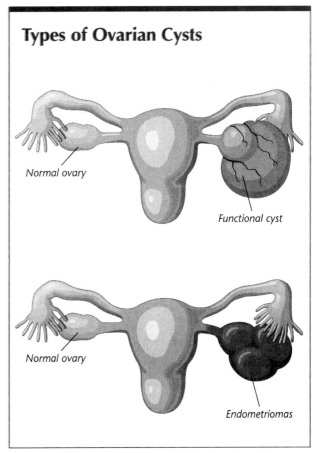

Types of Ovarian Cysts

Normal ovary

Functional cyst

Normal ovary

Endometriomas

Symptoms

Most ovarian cysts are small and do not cause symptoms. Some go away on their own. Some may cause symptoms because of twisting, bleeding, and rupture. They may cause a dull ache in the abdomen and pain during sexual intercourse.

Some cysts may be cancerous. The risk of ovarian cancer increases as you get older. Although ovarian cancer often has no symptoms in its early stages, you should be aware of its warning signs. If you have any of these symptoms, see your doctor. If ovarian cysts are found early, many of the problems caused by them can be treated.

Diagnosis

An ovarian cyst often is found during a routine pelvic exam. When your doctor detects an enlarged ovary, he or she may do other tests to confirm the diagnosis, such as:

▶ Ultrasound

▶ Laparoscopy

▶ Blood tests

Some of these tests provide further information about the cyst that is helpful in planning treatment. Some may be used only if there is a high risk of problems.

Treatment

If your cyst is not causing any symptoms, your doctor may simply monitor it for 1–2 months. Most functional cysts go away on their own over one or two menstrual cycles.

If your cyst is large or causing symptoms, your doctor may suggest treatment with hormones or surgery. The type of treatment depends on several factors:

▶ Size and type of cyst

▶ Your age

▶ Your symptoms

▶ Your desire to have children

Hormonal Therapy

Your doctor may prescribe oral contraceptives (birth control pills) to treat functional ovarian cysts. The hormones in birth control pills stop ovulation. This prevents follicles from developing and stops new cysts from forming. Birth control pills may not be right for every woman, especially for women who smoke

Many studies show a major decrease in the frequency of functional ovarian cysts that require surgery among women who take birth control pills with more than 35 micrograms of estrogen. Women who take the newer birth control pills with lower levels of hormones also have the same benefit.

cigarettes and are older than 35 years. Your doctor will help you decide if hormonal therapy is right for you.

Surgery

Your doctor may suggest surgery to remove the cyst. He or she will decide which type of treatment is best for you. The extent and type of surgery that is needed will depend on several factors. Sometimes, a cyst can be removed while leaving the ovary—called cystectomy. In other cases, one or both of the ovaries may have to be removed. Your doctor may not know which procedure is needed until the surgery begins.

▶ **See also:** *Female Reproductive System and Sexuality* in *"Women's Bodies"*

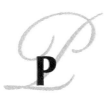

▶ PAIN DURING SEX

When a woman feels pain while having sexual intercourse, it is called dyspareunia. Painful sex is fairly common. Nearly 2 out of 3 women have it at some time during their lives. The pain can range from very mild to severe.

Why You May Feel Pain

Painful sex can have both physical and emotional causes. To understand why the pain occurs, you should know what happens to your body during sex. A woman's body follows a regular pattern when she has sex. There are four stages:

1. Desire

2. Arousal

3. Orgasm

4. Resolution

The arousal stage is important because this is when your vagina prepares itself for your partner to enter you. During this stage, the vagina and vulva become moist and the muscles of the opening of the vagina relax. If any part of this natural pattern does not happen, you may feel discomfort or pain with sex.

It is not always easy to discuss sexual problems with your doctor. Keep in mind that your health is a concern shared by both you and your doctor. If you can develop a physician–patient relationship based on mutual trust and respect, your doctor can help you feel comfortable and find the best method of treatment for you.

Types of Pain and What You Can Do

During sex a woman may feel pain in the vulva, at the opening of the vagina, within the vagina, or deep inside. Vulvar pain is pain felt on the surface (outside) of the vagina. Vaginal pain is felt within the vagina. Deep pain can occur in the lower back, pelvic region, uterus, and bladder.

Different types of pain have different causes. It's important to find the cause because you may have problems that need medication, surgery, or counseling.

Vulvar Pain

Pain can occur when some part of the vulva is touched. The vulva may be tender or irritated from using soaps or over-the-counter vaginal sprays or douches. Other causes include scars, cysts, or infections.

Vaginal Pain

Vaginal dryness. The most common cause of pain inside the vagina is lack of moisture. This can occur with certain medications, with certain medical conditions, or because you are not aroused. It can occur at certain times of your life such as during or just after pregnancy, while breastfeeding, or near or after menopause.

Around menopause, estrogen levels become lower. As a result, vaginal tissue may get thinner and drier. This may cause discomfort during sex. Some menopausal women take estrogen therapy to relieve the dryness. You also can buy water-soluble lubricants that help moisten the vagina.

Vaginal dryness can occur when you are not aroused enough during sex. You should discuss with your partner what makes you feel aroused. Often it is helpful for a couple to use a cream, jelly, or vaginal suppository to provide vaginal lubrication needed for sex. However, never use any kind of oil—such as petroleum jelly or baby or mineral oil—with latex condoms. These substances can dissolve the latex and cause the condom to break. Water-based cream or jelly is safe for use with condoms.

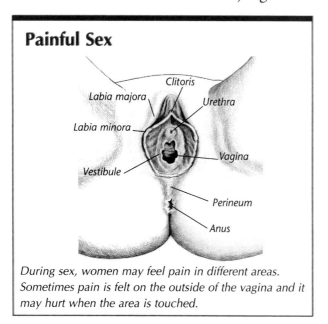

Painful Sex

Clitoris
Labia majora
Urethra
Labia minora
Vestibule
Vagina
Perineum
Anus

During sex, women may feel pain in different areas. Sometimes pain is felt on the outside of the vagina and it may hurt when the area is touched.

Vaginitis. Another cause of vaginal pain is vaginitis—an inflammation of the vagina. The most common symptoms of vaginitis are discharge, itching, and burning of the vagina and vulva. Vaginitis has many possible causes, such as yeast or bacterial infection. Vaginitis can be treated with medication that you take by mouth or place in the vagina.

Vaginismus. Vaginismus is a spasm of the muscles at the opening of the vagina. It causes pain when your partner tries to enter the vagina. In some cases, vaginismus is present the first time a woman has—or tries to have—sex. The pain also may occur during a pelvic exam.

Vaginismus can have many medical causes. These include:

▶ Scars in the vagina from injury, childbirth, or surgery

▶ Irritation from douches, spermicides, or the latex in condoms

▶ Infections of the vulva or vagina

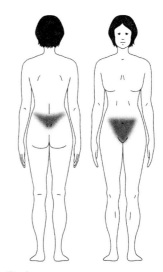

During sex, a woman may feel pain in different places (shaded areas).

Vaginismus also can be a response to a fear of some kind, such as being afraid of getting pregnant. It is sometimes caused by past pain or trauma, like from rape or sexual abuse. In most cases, this condition can be treated with success.

The doctor will examine you and may do some tests. During the exam, you may want to have a friend or family member in the room with you. This may help you feel more at ease. If you have any questions or concerns about the exam, talk to your doctor.

If your symptoms are caused by an infection, you will be given medication to help treat it. Surgery may be needed to treat other causes.

Deep Pain

Pain that starts deep inside may be a warning sign of an internal problem. Pain that happens when the penis touches the cervix can have many causes:

▶ Pelvic inflammatory disease

▶ Problems with the uterus

▶ Endometriosis

▶ A pelvic mass

▶ Bowel or bladder disease

▶ Scar tissue (adhesions)

▶ Ovarian cysts

A pelvic exam often gives clues about the causes of deep pain. Your doctor may suggest laparoscopy to look into your abdomen and at the reproductive organs. Laparoscopy also can be used to treat some of these problems.

How Emotions Play a Role

Pain during sex sometimes can be linked to a state of mind. Emotional factors, like memories or fears, can keep you from relaxing. Some women may feel guilty having sex. Or, some women may be afraid of getting pregnant or getting a sexually transmitted disease. Sometimes, a past bad sexual experience, such as rape or sexual abuse, may be the cause. All these factors may make it hard to relax during sex. This prevents arousal and lubrication.

Some women may feel pain during sex if they are having problems with their partner. It's a good idea to talk about your concerns with your partner and your doctor. Your doctor may suggest that you see a counselor to help you cope with your problems.

> See also *Chlamydia, Gonorrhea*

▶ PELVIC INFLAMMATORY DISEASE

Pelvic inflammatory disease (PID) is a broad term used to refer to infection of the uterus, fallopian tubes, or ovaries. It is a common but serious illness. About 1 million women are treated for PID in the United States each year. About 1 in 7 women are treated for PID at some point in their lives.

PID often can be treated with success, but the infection still may damage a woman's reproductive organs and cause long-term problems. Women who know how to protect themselves from this disease can lower their risk of getting it.

Causes of PID

PID most often affects sexually active women during their childbearing years. Most cases of PID are thought to stem from sexually transmitted diseases (STDs). The two most common STDs are gonorrhea and chlamydial infection. Without treatment, the same organisms that cause these diseases also can cause PID.

PID often forms in a two-stage process. First, the organisms infect the cervix (opening of the uterus). Then, in about 1 out of 10 women with an infection of the cervix, the organisms find their way to the uterus, tubes, or ovaries. It is not known just how these organisms travel from the cervix to these other sites.

Less often, PID occurs when infecting organisms enter the upper reproductive organs by one of three ways:

1. After an induced abortion (the planned termination of a pregnancy before the fetus can survive outside the uterus)

2. After giving birth

3. By insertion of an intrauterine device (IUD)

Dangers of PID

PID is a major cause of illness in young women. One quarter of the women who contract PID each year in the United States are hospitalized. Many of these women require surgery because of severe infection. And more than 150 women in the United States die from this infection each year.

PID is the most common preventable cause of infertility in the United States. The infection can cause scarring of the tissue inside the fallopian tubes. The scarring can damage or block the tubes. The more often a woman has PID, the greater are her chances of being infertile. The risk doubles with each bout of the disease.

PID also is a leading cause of ectopic pregnancy. Damage to a fallopian tube can cause a fertilized egg to attach to the inside of the tube and begin to grow there instead of inside the uterus. This can lead to bursting of the tube and bleeding into the abdomen, which requires emergency surgery and may result in death. About 70,000 women in the United States have an ectopic pregnancy each year. Half of these cases can be linked to prior PID.

PID also can lead to other long-term problems, such as:

▶ Forming of an abscess

▶ Frequent bouts of illness

▶ Chronic pain

▶ Physical disability

According to the Centers for Disease Control and Prevention, PID and its complications affect more than 750,000 women each year. The cost of treating PID and its complications is about $4 billion annually.

Who Is at Risk?

PID is most common in women younger than 25 years who have sex with more than one partner. Hospitalization for PID is more common among women who are single. Women who have had an STD or PID before have a higher risk of getting PID. Having an IUD inserted also may slightly increase the risk of PID. The risk is highest during the first few months after insertion. A woman whose partner has more than one sex partner also is at greater risk of getting PID.

Symptoms

PID may cause severe symptoms, minor symptoms, or no symptoms at all. Symptoms that may occur include:

- Vaginal discharge with a bad odor
- Painful urination
- Pain in the lower abdomen (often of a mild, aching nature)
- Abnormal uterine bleeding
- Fever and chills
- Nausea and vomiting

Any of these symptoms should prompt you to see your doctor, even more so if you have had PID before. The symptoms may signal a repeat infection.

Diagnosis

The diagnosis of PID is sometimes hard because the site of infection is not easy to examine. Also, the symptoms of PID may be like those of other conditions, such as appendicitis or ectopic pregnancy.

Your doctor will ask you questions about your medical history. Questions may include the sexual habits of both you and your partner, your use of birth control, and your symptoms. The doctor also may perform a pelvic exam to find out if your reproductive organs are tender or swollen. This will help find the site of the infection.

Your doctor may take samples of cells from your cervix to look for the organisms that cause gonorrhea and chlamydial infection. Blood tests may be done to look for signs of infection. Culdocentesis, a process in which a needle is inserted into the area behind the vagina, may help the doctor find out if there is pus in the abdominal cavity.

If the diagnosis is not certain, other methods may be used:

- *Laparoscopy*—A slender, telescopelike device is used to view the pelvic organs through a small incision (cut) made through or just below the navel.

- *Ultrasound*—An electronic device is moved over the stomach or placed in the vagina. The device creates echoes that are transformed into pictures that can be viewed on a TV-like screen. This can help find out if the tubes are swollen or an abscess is present.

Treatment

PID is first treated with antibiotics. In most cases, antibiotics alone can get rid of the infection. PID often is caused by more than one type of organism, and no one antibiotic kills all the organisms thought to cause PID. For this reason, two or more antibiotics often are taken to fight a wide range of organisms. Two antibiotics often used to treat PID are ampicillin and tetracycline.

Antibiotics can be given by mouth or intravenously (by vein). If you are given antibiotics by mouth to treat PID, finish all of the medication, even if your symptoms go away. In most cases, the drugs must be taken for 10–14 days to make sure that the infection is cleared up. This will help prevent it from coming back.

Often, your doctor will schedule a visit 2–3 days after starting treatment to check your progress. If your condition hasn't improved, you may need to be treated in a hospital.

Hospitalization also may be needed if the diagnosis is unknown and appendicitis or ectopic pregnancy cannot be ruled out. Patients with a very high fever or severe stomach problems may require hospitalization so antibiotics can be given by vein. If antibiotic treatment fails or if the doctor suspects a burst abscess, surgery may be needed.

As with any serious infection, getting rest is the best way to get better fast. Hot baths and heating pads applied to the lower back and stomach may help to relieve pain and discomfort. Pain medications also will help.

If you are treated for PID, your partner also should be examined and treated. You should not have sex until your treatment and your partner's treatment are complete and your follow-up test results show the infection has been cured. Unless your partner receives treatment, you may be infected again when you have sex.

Prevention

Because PID can affect a woman's health and fertility, prevention of this disease is key. Not having sex is the only sure way to prevent PID. However, women who are in sexual relationships with only one partner have very little risk of PID (if neither person was infected with an STD from a partner they had before). Using barrier methods of birth control also can help prevent STDs. Using spermicides with another barrier method like condoms helps even more.

Birth control pills may reduce a woman's risk of being hospitalized with PID by about 50%. A woman who is taking birth control pills also should use foam and condoms to further reduce her risk of PID if she has more than one sex partner.

Because most cases of PID are linked to STDs, treatment of a woman's sex partners is vital to prevent repeat infection. All recent sex partners should be checked and treated by a doctor as if they had both gonorrhea and chlamydial infection. A woman with PID should not have sex again until her sex partners have been treated.

▶ See also *Endometriosis, Menstrual Cramps, Pain During Sex*

▶ PELVIC PAIN

Many women have pain in their pelvic region at some point in their lives. Each woman responds to pain in her own way. Some women are bothered by pain more than others. You should discuss any pain with your doctor, but even more so if it disrupts your daily life, if it worsens over time, or if you've noticed a recent increase in pain.

Finding the cause of pelvic pain can be a long process. Often there is more than one reason for the pain, and its exact source can be hard to pin down.

Causes of Pelvic Pain

Pelvic pain is not always caused by problems with the reproductive organs. Gastrointestinal problems, such as irritable bowel syndrome (IBS), also can cause pelvic pain. In fact, IBS may be responsible for almost half of all cases of chronic pelvic pain.

The type and nature of pelvic pain—whether it comes and goes or is constant, whether it is short-term or long-term—will help your doctor detect the problem. Pelvic pain often is caused by a number of factors. Some of them are described here.

Acute Pain

Acute (sharp) pain starts over a short time (a few minutes to a few days). It often has one cause. Most often an exam and some tests can pinpoint the cause. Acute pain is a warning that something has gone wrong. The causes of acute pain need to be looked into and treated promptly.

Infection. Pelvic pain can be caused by an infection or inflammation. The infection does not have to be in the reproductive organs to cause pelvic pain. The source of the pain may be the bladder, bowel, or even the appendix.

Pelvic inflammatory disease (PID) is a broad term used to describe infection of the uterus, fallopian tubes, and ovaries. Most cases of PID are thought to come from sexually transmitted diseases (STDs). An STD is a disease spread through sexual contact. If an STD that affects the cervix is not treated, the infection can travel into the uterus and tubes and cause PID. Symptoms of PID include fever and pain in the lower stomach. The pain often is a mild ache, but it can be severe.

Vaginal infection (vaginitis) can sometimes be painful, mainly during and after sex. Many kinds of organisms can cause vaginal infections.

Infections of the urethra, bladder, or kidneys (urinary tract infections) may cause pain, too. Patients often feel pain during urination and a strong and frequent urge to urinate even when little urine is there. When pain also is felt in the back, the infection may have spread to the kidneys.

All of these causes of pain may require a visit to your doctor. A history will be taken, you will have a physical exam, and some tests may be done.

Ovarian Cysts. Sometimes a cyst may form on an ovary. A cyst is a sac filled with fluid. It is somewhat like a blister. Some cysts on the ovaries form as a result of the normal process of ovulation (release of an egg from the ovary). Often a cyst begins fairly quickly but goes away within a day or two. Some cysts can last a long time. These cysts often are felt as a dull ache or heaviness. Sometimes they cause pain during sex. Sharp pain can occur if a cyst leaks fluid or bleeds a little. This may happen around the middle of the menstrual cycle.

A pelvic exam often will detect a cyst. In some cases, pelvic ultrasound (a test in which sound waves are used to view the internal organs) is needed to be sure. Most small cysts will go away by themselves. Rarely, more severe, sharp, and constant pain happens when a large cyst twists. Large cysts and those that don't go away on their own within a few months may need to be removed by surgery.

Ectopic Pregnancy. A tubal or ectopic pregnancy is one that starts outside the uterus, often in one of the fallopian tubes. This happens most often in women who have some damage to their tubes. The pain often starts on one side of the abdomen after a missed period. Vaginal bleeding or spotting may occur with the pain. This problem needs urgent care and may require surgery. An ectopic pregnancy can lead to bursting of the tube and bleeding inside the abdomen. This can threaten your life.

Chronic Pain

Chronic pain can be either intermittent (it can come and go) or constant (it is there most of the time). Intermittent chronic pain often has a distinct cause. Constant chronic pain may be caused by more than one problem. An illness may start with intermittent pain that becomes constant.

Dysmenorrhea. Dysmenorrhea is a case of long-term, intermittent chronic pain. Although some mild pain is common during a woman's menstrual period, some women have severe pain with their periods. It may be caused by prostaglandin, a hormone made by the lining of the uterus (endometrium). It causes spasms or cramping of the uterus.

Endometriosis and Adenomyosis. Sometimes menstrual cramps can be a sign of disease. If cramps get worse over the years or stay strong beyond the first 1 or 2 days of flow, they may be due to a disease such as endometriosis or adenomyosis.

The cause of endometriosis and the reasons for pain during the menstrual cycle are not known for sure. Endometriosis often makes menstrual cramps worse. It can also cause pain at times other than during the menstrual cycle. Sometimes sex is painful. How severe the pain is, though, does not depend on the amount of endometriosis present. For instance, a small amount of endometriosis may cause a lot of pain, and a large amount may not.

Adenomyosis occurs when the endometrium buries itself in the muscle wall of the uterus. This can cause menstrual cramps. It also can cause pressure and bloating in the lower abdomen before periods and more bleeding during periods.

Ovulation Pain. Pain that is felt around the time of ovulation is sometimes called mittelschmerz (German for "middle pain"). Ovulation occurs in the middle part of the menstrual cycle. Pain can range from a mild pinch or twinge to something more severe. It can occur every month in some women. It is intense only now and then, though.

Constant Chronic Pain

Some women may feel pain almost every day. This may mean that a problem has gotten worse. Or it could mean that a person has become less able to cope with pain. The pain may then get worse even though the disease that started the problem hasn't changed.

Not being able to deal with pain is more likely when the pain disturbs work, physical activities, sexual relations, sleep, or family duties. Not knowing the cause of the pain can make it more stressful because you might fear severe illness.

When pain has been present for a long time, it affects your mental and physical health. In seeking the cause for pelvic pain, your doctor may ask you questions about the pain and its effect on your life and your emotions.

Other Causes of Pain

Adhesions or scar tissue can form as a result of the healing process. Scar tissue causes the surface of organs and structures inside the stomach to bind to each other. Endometriosis, surgery, or a severe infection such as PID can cause adhesions or scar tissue. Adhesions can involve the uterus, tubes, ovaries, and bowels. They can attach any of these structures to each other or to the sides of the pelvic area.

Fibroids may grow on the inside of the uterus, on its outer surface, or within the wall of the uterus. It is not known for certain what causes fibroids. Estrogen is thought to play a role in their growth, though.

Fibroids often cause no symptoms. When symptoms do occur, they may include heavier or more frequent menstrual periods and pain or pressure in the stomach or lower back.

Fibroids attached on a stem may become twisted and cause more acute symptoms.

Other causes of lower abdominal and pelvic pain include:

▶ Diverticulitis (inflammation of a pouch bulging from the wall of the colon)

▶ Irritable bowel syndrome (a condition that may cause alternating bouts of diarrhea and constipation and often seems to be related to stress)

▶ Kidney or bladder stones

▶ Appendicitis

▶ Muscle spasms or strain

Diagnosis

Because there are so many causes of pelvic pain, your doctor may use many tests to rule out likely causes of your pain. Although it may seem complex and time-consuming, this approach is the best way to find out what is causing the pain.

Your doctor may ask you to keep a journal in which you describe the exact nature of the pain. What you write down can help to rule out certain causes. Bring it with you when you see your doctor.

Your doctor may consult with or refer you to other specialists. It depends on what your doctor suspects may be the cause of the pain. The specialists may include doctors who deal with problems of the gastrointestinal, urinary, or neurologic systems.

Physical Factors

The evaluation begins with an exam. Cultures and blood tests are sometimes needed to look for infection.

Other studies are sometimes useful to find the cause of pain. They are often less helpful for evaluating chronic pain than for other gynecologic conditions, though. They include:

▶ *Ultrasound:* A test in which sound waves are reflected off the internal organs, producing an image that can be viewed on a screen

▶ *Computed tomography (CT):* A type of X-ray that shows internal organs and structures (sometimes called a "CAT scan")

▶ *Magnetic resonance imaging (MRI):* A method of viewing internal organs and structures by using a strong magnetic field

▶ *Intravenous pyelography (IVP):* A type of X-ray taken after fluid is injected into a vein and excreted by the kidneys

▶ *Barium enema:* A solution given through the rectum that helps problems in the colon show up on X-rays

Sometimes these tests are referred to as "imaging studies." This is because they are all used to make an image of the inside of the body, using sound waves, X-rays, or other techniques. These studies cannot always detect endometriosis or adhesions, which may be a cause of chronic pelvic pain.

Laparoscopy is the best way to assess endometriosis and some other problems. In this type of surgery, a slender device that transmits light is inserted through the navel while you are under anesthesia. This allows the doctor to see inside the body. Sometimes, treatment can be done at the same time. A doctor cannot be certain of a diagnosis of endometriosis unless surgery is done.

Psychologic Factors

Being in pain can put great strain on a woman and those close to her. Women who have depression in their family or who had a difficult childhood (especially when sexual abuse was involved) are more likely to have chronic pain.

For these reasons, your doctor may ask many questions about you and your family to see if there is a need for emotional help. Sometimes the doctor may suggest that you get counseling.

Mood and pain may be chemically linked in the brain. Chemical changes may make the brain less able to cope with pain or may block out pain signals. Treatment of chronic pain can sometimes be improved by using antidepressant medications. Antidepressants alter these signals.

Treatment

Acute pain or intermittent chronic pain often involves treatment of one specific condition. Treatment of constant chronic pain is not like that. Your doctor may talk to you about a few factors that may add to the pain, but may not know which one is the main cause. Treatment may involve a few medications at once, nondrug treatments, or surgery.

Medications

If you have had a problem such as a urinary tract infection or vaginitis before and

---

Pain Journal

A record of your pain will help your doctor find its cause. You may be asked to keep a pain journal so that more complete information can be obtained.

In your pain journal, note the following when you feel pain:

- What time of day is it?
- Is it at certain times of your monthly cycle? If so, when?
- Is it before, during, or after:
  —Eating?
  —Urination?
  —Bowel movement?
  —Sex?
  —Physical activity?
  —Sleep?

Describe the pain and note how long it lasts:

- Is it a sharp stab or a dull ache?
- Does it come in phases or is it steady?
- How long does it last?
- How intense is it?
- Does it always occur in the same place(s)?
- Is it mostly in one place or over a broad area?

it has come back, your doctor may prescribe medication over the phone. Most often, antibiotics or vaginal creams will reduce the pain of an infection within 1 or 2 days. Severe PID, though, may require days of treatment in the hospital. With some kinds of STDs, your sex partner must also be treated, even if there are no symptoms.

Drugs that reduce inflammation, such as ibuprofen, can be used to lessen the pain of dysmenorrhea. These drugs block the making of prostaglandins, which cause the uterus to contract. Ibuprofen can be bought over the counter. If it does not work, prescription drugs may help.

For other problems, treatment with hormones may help. Combination oral contraceptives (birth control pills) can be used to relieve pain from menstrual cramps. Other hormones can shrink some types of growths, such as endometriosis, fibroids, and certain types of benign tumors. Fibroids often return to their former size, though, when treatment is stopped.

Antidepressants have been used in some patients with pelvic pain when other treatments have not worked. They can help break the cycle in which the pain and the depression add to each other. The pain seems to be made more intense by depression.

Most people try to use as little pain medication as they can. When treating chronic pain, it is better to use a nonnarcotic pain medication as part of a routine. It is not a good idea to wait until the pain is severe before you take it. Pain medication may only take the edge off the pain. It may not get rid of it. It is best to avoid strong narcotic medication. It can lead to addiction or the need for higher doses.

Antibiotics only work against infections that are caused by bacteria. These drugs are not effective against viral infections. This is why your doctor will not always prescribe an antibiotic if you have an infection.

Surgery

Certain problems may be treated with surgery. The type of surgery depends on your exact problem. Some surgery, such as a laparoscopy, often can be done without a hospital stay. Some conditions outside the uterus can be treated by laparoscopy using laser or cautery. It often can be done at the same time that the diagnosis is made.

Some conditions inside the uterus can be treated with a hysteroscope (a thin telescope with a light). The hysteroscope is inserted through the cervix and into the uterus. Small growths may then be seen and removed.

Other times, major surgery, such as a hysterectomy (removal of the uterus), is needed. Sometimes, the fallopian tubes and the ovaries are removed also. Your doctor will discuss what options you have, based on your exact problem. Your doctor will also discuss with you the risks and benefits of these procedures and their chance of working.

Other Treatments

Heat therapy, muscle relaxants, nerve block, and relaxation exercises may all help to treat other causes of pelvic pain. If disorders of the bladder, bowel, or other organs are the cause of the pain, certain treatments will be used.

▶ See also *Kegel Exercises, Urinary Incontinence*

▶ PELVIC SUPPORT PROBLEMS

Many women have changes in their pelvic organs as they age. They may have a feeling of pelvic pressure or heaviness. It may feel like "something is falling out of the vagina." These symptoms may be caused by pelvic support problems. These problems may begin with childbirth. Women may notice them even more as they age.

The Pelvic Organs

The parts of the body affected by pelvic support problems include the urethra and bladder, the small intestine, the rectum, the uterus, and the vagina. The urethra and bladder lie in front of the vagina. The bladder receives and stores urine from the kidneys and expels it through the urethra (a short, narrow tube). The uterus is at the top of the vagina. Behind the uterus is a space within the pelvic cavity called the cul-de-sac. This space contains some of the small intestine. Along the back of this space is the rectum, which continues down the back of the vagina and ends at the anus. The perineum is the tissue between the opening of the vagina and the anus.

Almost 10% of women in the United States will have major surgery at some time in their lives to correct urinary incontinence or pelvic support problems.

The pelvic organs are held in place by three types of support:

1. Layers of connecting tissue called endopelvic fascia

2. Thickened parts of the fascia called ligaments

3. A paired group of muscles that lies on either side and around the openings of the urethra, vagina, and rectum

When the tissues that support the pelvic organs are stretched and damaged, the organ that they support may drop down and press against the wall of the vagina. This causes a bulge. Sometimes the organ will drop down so much that the bulge sticks out through the vaginal opening.

Causes

The main causes of pelvic support problems are childbirth and aging. As the baby passes through the vagina during childbirth, the fascia and ligaments may be damaged. They may become weak. In later years, when a woman goes through menopause, the loss of the female hormone estrogen may make these problems worse.

Sometimes pelvic support problems occur in women who have never had children. In these women, the cause may be:

▶ Weakening of the vaginal tissues after menopause

▶ Increases in abdominal pressure because of a chronic cough (often linked to smoking or lung disorders), heavy lifting, obesity, or constipation

▶ An inherited weakness of the tissues

Pelvic support problems are limited almost entirely to adult women. One of the main causes is vaginal childbirth.

Symptoms

The symptoms of pelvic support problems depend on which organs are involved. They can cause minor discomfort or major problems in the way the organs work. Symptoms include:

▶ Feeling of pelvic heaviness or fullness, or as though something is falling out of the vagina

▶ Pulling or aching feeling in the lower abdomen, groin, or lower back

▶ Leakage of urine or problems having a bowel movement

You may notice the symptoms after you have been standing for a long time or at the end of the day. They may be worsened by repeated coughing, lifting, or straining.

In severe cases, the pelvic organs may bulge into the vagina. This bulge may stick out of the vaginal opening, where it may be seen with a mirror or felt with the fingers. Sometimes a woman may need to push the organs back up into the vagina to empty the bladder or have a bowel movement.

The uterus may stick out through the vaginal opening. If the uterus or a part of the vaginal wall stays outside of the vaginal opening, it may become irritated. It may develop small sores or ulcers that bleed or become infected.

Types of Pelvic Support Problems

The main types of pelvic support problems include:

▶ *Cystocele*—bladder

▶ *Enterocele*—small intestine

▶ *Rectocele*—rectum

▶ *Uterine prolapse*—uterus

▶ *Vaginal prolapse*—vagina

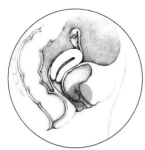

Cystocele

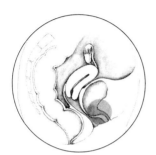

Cystourethrocele

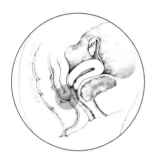

Enterocele

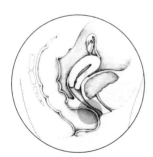

Rectocele

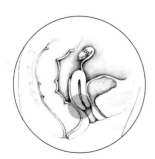

Uterine prolapse

Although each problem occurs in different pelvic organs, they often occur at the same time.

Cystocele

A cystocele occurs when the bladder drops from its normal place into the vagina. Some cystoceles cause urine to leak when you cough, sneeze, lift objects, or walk. Large cystoceles may partially close the urethra and cause problems with the passing of urine. If this occurs, you may have to strain or push the bladder up by reaching into the vagina to pass urine. If there is a very large cystocele and if the bladder loses some of its ability to contract, it may not completely empty.

Small cystoceles are common. In most cases, they do not cause problems with urination and do not need surgery. If a cystocele is causing symptoms, your doctor can suggest ways to relieve it.

The place where the bladder joins the urethra is called the bladder outlet or bladder neck. When the tissues that support the bladder neck are damaged, the bladder may drop and push against the vaginal wall. A dropped bladder neck is called a cystourethrocele. It may cause urine to leak.

Urine is more likely to leak when there is a sudden increase in abdominal pressure caused by walking, jumping, coughing, sneezing, laughing, lifting, or making sudden movements. The amount of urine lost may be only a few drops. In other cases, it may be enough to require changing clothes or wearing pads.

You should tell your doctor if you cannot control the leakage of urine. Sometimes leakage is not caused by a cystourethrocele. It may be caused by a urinary tract infection, bladder problems, or other medical conditions.

Enterocele

An enterocele forms when the intestine bulges into the upper vagina. To diagnose an enterocele, a doctor may place a finger in your vagina and a finger in your rectum while you are standing.

Rectocele

When the rectum bulges into or out of the vagina, it is called a rectocele. It is caused by a weakness of the back wall of the vagina. A large rectocele may make it hard to have a bowel movement, especially if you have constipation. Some women must push the bulge back into the vagina to have a bowel movement.

Uterine Prolapse

When the uterus drops down into the vagina, it is called uterine prolapse. The distance the uterus drops may vary. Mild degrees of prolapse are common. It often does not cause symptoms and does not need surgery.

Women with more severe forms of this condition often will have a feeling of pelvic pressure or a pulling feeling in the groin or lower back. The cervix (the opening of the uterus) may stick out from the vagina. This may cause discomfort or problems with sex. Uterine prolapse most often occurs when other pelvic organs are also out of place.

Vaginal Prolapse

Sometimes after hysterectomy (removal of the uterus), the top of the vagina loses its support and drops. This is called vaginal prolapse. The degree of prolapse varies. The top of the vagina may drop part of the way into the vagina and remain there, or it may extend part or all of the way through the vaginal opening. Most women who have vaginal prolapse also have an enterocele. Women who have complete vaginal prolapse also may have problems with bladder and bowel function.

Changes in the lower urinary tract may make older women more likely to have urine leakage, but almost all women can be treated with success.

Diagnosis

Proper diagnosis is key to treating pelvic support problems. Diagnosis is not always simple, though. The symptoms of pelvic support problems often mimic those of other conditions. In most cases, a woman with these symptoms will know that she has a problem, but the cause may be unclear. The exact cause of the problem must be found before the best treatment can be given.

To make an exact diagnosis, your doctor will take your medical history and do a thorough pelvic exam. You may be examined while you are lying down and again while you are standing. Your bladder function also may be tested.

If you have a problem with either passing or controlling urine, other tests may be needed:

▶ *Cystoscopy and urethroscopy*—the inside of the bladder and urethra is viewed through a small, lighted telescope

▶ *Cystometry*—the amount the bladder can hold and control is measured

▶ *Uroflowmetry*—urine flow is measured

Treatment

Treatment of pelvic support problems may involve special exercises or insertion of a special device called a pessary. These treatments may improve support. Your doctor may suggest a high-fiber diet or medications to soften the stool and make bowel movements easier. Keeping your weight under control, eating right, not smoking, and not doing activities that stress pelvic support muscles also can help. Hormones may be given to improve the quality of the tissues.

If you have pelvic support problems, remember to brace the pelvic support muscles when coughing, sneezing, laughing, or lifting. This helps reduce the amount of stress on these muscles.

Hormone Treatment

Estrogen is a hormone often prescribed to preserve or improve the quality of the pelvic tissues. It can be taken in a pill, skin patch, or vaginal cream. Sometimes a combination of these methods is used.

Hormone replacement therapy (HRT) may be used after a woman has gone through menopause. It eases her symptoms of menopause and protects her from heart disease and bone problems. If a woman still has a uterus, the hormone progesterone is given as well. Hormone replacement therapy may improve the results of surgery or pelvic exercises. Women who are not taking HRT may be prescribed an estrogen cream to help relieve symptoms.

Many women with pelvic support problems do not need further treatment. Some bladder control problems respond best to changes in voiding habits, diet, and medications. Others may be treated by surgery.

No form of treatment, even surgery, is certain to solve the problem. The chances for getting some degree of relief, though, are quite good.

Special Exercises

Exercises called Kegel exercises, or pelvic muscle exercises, are used to strengthen the muscles that surround the openings of the urethra, vagina, and rectum. Do these exercises three or more times a day. In time, you may be better able to hold urine.

Diet

The doctor may suggest that you drink fruit juices to help reduce the risk of bladder infection. You also may need to cut down on caffeine, which acts as a diuretic. It is found in coffee, tea, and soft drinks. A high-fiber diet may be prescribed to help with bowel control and to prevent constipation.

Medicines

Sometimes a medication that softens stools is prescribed along with a special diet to help control intestinal symptoms. A medication that puts bulk in the stool also may be given with a high-fiber diet.

There are special medicines that help to control urination. These drugs suppress bladder contractions. Other drugs will help prevent leakage by increasing the pressure inside the urethra. If there is a urinary tract infection, antibiotics may be needed. Some of these drugs have some side effects.

Surgical Repair

Pelvic support problems may be corrected by surgery. The type of support problem you have will decide whether surgery is done through the vagina or abdomen.

It is best to put off surgery for pelvic support problems until you have completed your family. This is because if you have uterine prolapse, your doctor may suggest that your uterus be removed as a part of the procedure. If the uterus is left in place, a later vaginal delivery may increase the chances that a cystocele or rectocele will recur. If you have severe pelvic support problems and wish to keep your uterus so that you might still have children, discuss this with your doctor.

If you decide to have surgery, you should be aware of the risks:

▶ The operation may fail to correct your symptoms, and more surgery may be needed later.

▶ Chronic pain, discomfort, or pain during sex may persist if they were present before the surgery.

▶ Surgery may not correct your urinary or bowel problems.

Your vagina may be smaller after surgery. It may not be shorter, though. It is not likely to be so small that you will not be able to have sex.

Surgery may relieve some, but not all, of the symptoms caused by pelvic support problems. In a few cases, symptoms may return. The doctor has to use the already weakened fascias, ligaments, and muscles that are within your pelvis to improve your pelvic support. In some cases, synthetic materials that the body accepts well may be used to help correct the problems. If you have had prior surgery or radiation, there is a much lower success rate.

If you smoke, you should stop before and after your surgery. You will heal and recover faster, especially in the incision area, if you do not smoke.

The factors that caused you to have prolapse in the first place can cause it to occur again. After surgery, you should not smoke, control your weight, avoid constipation, and avoid activities, such as heavy lifting, that put pressure on these muscles.

Special Devices

Sometimes surgery is too risky because of a woman's general health. In such cases, a pessary may be inserted into the vagina to support the pelvic organs. When a pessary is used, it must be removed, cleaned, and reinserted on a regular basis. If it is not cleaned, it might cause a bad-smelling discharge and ulcers in the vagina. If used correctly, a pessary can last for years.

There are many types of pessaries. Your doctor can fit you with the right one for you. It may take a few trials to get a good fit.

▶ PLACENTAL DISORDERS

▶ See also *Molar Pregnancy*

Heavy vaginal bleeding early or late in pregnancy can mean there is a problem with the placenta. The placenta is the tissue that provides nourishment to and takes away waste from the fetus. The most common disorders of the placenta are placenta previa, placental abruption, and placenta accreta.

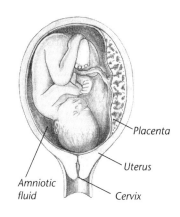

Normal pregnancy

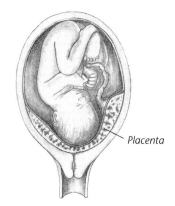

Placenta previa is when the placenta lies low in the uterus and blocks the cervix.

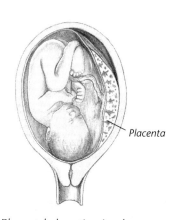

Placental abruption is when the placenta becomes detached from the uterine wall.

Placenta Previa

When the placenta lies low in the uterus, it may partly or completely cover the cervix. This is called placenta previa. It may cause vaginal bleeding. Placenta previa is serious and requires prompt care.

Placenta previa occurs in 1 woman in 200. It is more common in women who have had more than one child, who have had a cesarean birth or other surgery on the uterus, or who are carrying twins or triplets. Bleeding often occurs without pain. This is a frequent finding by ultrasound in early pregnancy. If it is still there after 24 weeks of pregnancy, there may be a problem.

Placental Abruption

The placenta may detach from the uterine wall before or during labor. This may cause vaginal bleeding. Only 1% of pregnant women have this problem. It usually occurs during the last 12 weeks of pregnancy. Stomach pain often occurs, even if there is no obvious bleeding.

When the placenta becomes detached, the fetus may get less oxygen. This can pose a danger to the fetus.

Placental abruption is more likely to occur in women who:

- Have already had children
- Are older than 35
- Have had abruption before
- Have sickle cell anemia
- Have high blood pressure
- Receive intense blows to the stomach
- Use cocaine
- Smoke

Placenta Accreta

In placenta accreta, cells from the placenta stick to or invade the wall of the uterus. Doctors can often detect placenta accreta during an ultrasound exam. Sometimes other tests are needed, as well.

Pregnant women with placenta accreta have a higher than normal risk of hemorrhage (serious bleeding) when they give birth. Women with placenta accreta have cesarean delivery rather than a vaginal birth to reduce the risk of losing too much blood. The woman's uterus may need to be removed at the same time. This is called a cesarean hysterectomy.

Other Disorders

Other types of placental disorders are placenta increta and placenta percreta. Placenta increta occurs when the placenta invades the uterine wall. Sometimes the placenta passes through the uterine wall. This is called placenta percreta.

▶ POLYCYSTIC OVARY SYNDROME

▶ See also *Amenorrhea, Hirsutism, Infertility*

Polycystic ovary syndrome (PCOS) is a disorder in which the ovaries are enlarged and contain many small cysts (fluid-filled sacs). Women with PCOS may have irregular or no menstrual periods. PCOS is a condition that can last many years and can have a major impact on a woman's health.

What Is PCOS?

Everyone has both male and female hormones. PCOS occurs as a result of an increase in the production of androgens (male hormones) by the ovaries and the adrenal glands. In PCOS, the ovaries often become enlarged and contain many small cysts. The increase in androgen causes irregular menstrual periods and may stop ovulation. Because of this, women continue to make estrogen, but they do not produce progesterone.

In some women, the presence of estrogen without progesterone increases the risk that the endometrium will grow too much. This is a condition known as endometrial hyperplasia. If untreated over a long time, endometrial hyperplasia may turn into cancer. PCOS is linked to other diseases that occur later in life, such as diabetes, atherosclerosis, and high blood pressure.

The symptoms of PCOS usually include:

▶ Irregular menstrual periods or no periods

▶ Excess hair on the face and body (known as hirsutism)

▶ Acne

▶ Obesity

▶ Infertility

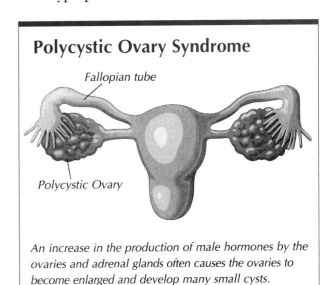

Polycystic Ovary Syndrome

Fallopian tube

Polycystic Ovary

An increase in the production of male hormones by the ovaries and adrenal glands often causes the ovaries to become enlarged and develop many small cysts.

Metformin

Another symptom of PCOS is resistance to insulin. The hormone insulin is produced by the pancreas and helps balance the amount of glucose in your blood. Glucose is a sugar that is the body's main source of fuel. If there is not enough insulin or the body resists its effect, conditions such as diabetes, obesity, or infertility can occur. Studies have shown metformin, a medication used to treat insulin resistance in people with type 2 diabetes mellitus, may help treat fertility problems and increase ovulation in obese women with PCOS.

Diagnosis and Treatment

To diagnose PCOS, your doctor will ask you questions about your health and your menstrual cycle. He or she also will perform a complete exam that may include blood tests and tests of blood pressure (often high with this condition). The type of treatment you receive depends on your symptoms and whether you want to become pregnant.

To treat irregular menstrual periods, your doctor may prescribe either the hormone progesterone or birth control pills. Women who wish to become pregnant may be given fertility drugs instead of birth control pills.

Your doctor also may prescribe birth control pills and other medications to help slow the growth of new excess body hair. It may take several months, however, for you to notice any results. To remove unwanted hair sooner, you may want to try electrolysis or other hair removal methods.

If you are overweight, losing weight can help relieve the symptoms of PCOS. Weight loss can also help lower the risk of other long-term conditions.

▶ See also *Dilation and Curettage, Hysteroscopy*

▶ POLYPS

Polyps are growths inside the body, attached to tissue by a stem. Most of the time they are small and benign (noncancerous). In women, polyps are mostly found in the vagina, cervix, or lining of the uterus.

Polyps in the vagina or on the cervix are often tear-shaped. They may be pink or red. The main symptom is vaginal bleeding. You are most likely to notice this blood during or after sexual intercourse. Polyps are not usually painful. Sometimes a woman doesn't know she has one until her doctor finds it during a routine exam. Polyps on the vagina or cervix often can be removed right in the doctor's office. You may be given a local anesthetic to numb the area.

Abnormal vaginal bleeding is a common sign of uterine polyps. Although many times there are no symptoms. Sometimes the polyps extend through the opening of the cervix, where your doctor can see them. If the polyps become twisted, they may get infected and cause a foul-smelling discharge. Often these polyps are treated with dilation and curettage, a procedure in which the doctor gently scrapes the uterine lining. When your doctor removes a polyp, the tissue may be checked for cancer cells, just to be safe. In rare cases, such as when a polyp shows signs of cancer, the whole uterus may be removed.

Polyps also can be diagnosed using other methods, such as an ultrasound exam or hysteroscopy. In an ultrasound exam, sound waves create pictures of the internal organs. In a hysteroscopy a thin device is inserted through the vagina and cervix so the doctor can see inside the uterus. This method also can be used to treat the polyps.

▶ POSTDATE PREGNANCY

▶ See also *Fetal Monitoring*

Waiting for the birth of a child is an exciting and anxious time. Most women give birth at term—between 38 and 42 weeks of pregnancy. About 10% of normal pregnancies go past 42 weeks. These are called postdate or postterm pregnancies. Postdate pregnancies seem to occur as often in women who have given birth before as in women with first pregnancies.

A Difficult Diagnosis

Pregnancy occurs around the time of ovulation. The average length of pregnancy is 280 days, or 40 weeks. When a pregnancy exceeds 294 days, or 42 weeks, it is postterm. The due date is counted from the first day of a woman's last menstrual period. It can be hard to predict the exact due date, though. Only 5% of babies are born on the exact due date.

The most important factor in diagnosing postterm pregnancy is knowing the age of the fetus. The timing of ovulation is the best method to set the age of the fetus, but it often isn't known. For this reason, doctors often use more than one method to check the age of the fetus. The methods used most often include:

▶ *Clinical exam*—The size of the uterus can be useful to assess the age of the fetus.

▶ *"Quickening"*—Pregnant women often first feel the fetus move, or "quicken," by 16–20 weeks of pregnancy.

▶ *Fetal heart tones*—The doctor often can hear fetal heart tones by 12 weeks of pregnancy using an electronic device.

▶ *Ultrasound*—This test can be used to estimate the age of a fetus within 1–2 weeks if it is done in the first half of pregnancy. Later in pregnancy, this method is not as precise.

Many women wonder why the doctor doesn't simply bring on labor at 42 weeks of pregnancy. First, there is a chance that the due date is off. Estimates can be wrong. Often, neither the mother nor her doctor can be sure that the fetus is fully mature and ready to be born. Second, in some women, the cervix is not ready for labor to start.

The due date should be set as early in pregnancy as possible. Later, it becomes harder to set the due date accurately. This is one reason why early prenatal care is important.

Risks

Beyond 42 weeks of pregnancy, risks to the health of the baby and mother increase. Problems occur in only a few postterm pregnancies, however. About 95% of babies born between 42 and 44 weeks of pregnancy are born without problems.

The postterm baby may be in danger for a number of reasons. Beyond 42 weeks of pregnancy, the placenta may not function as well. Also, as the baby grows, the amount of amniotic fluid may begin to decrease. Less amniotic fluid may cause the umbilical cord linking the baby to the placenta to become pinched as the baby moves or the mother's uterus contracts.

If pregnancy goes past 42 weeks, a baby has a higher risk of certain problems:

▶ *Dysmaturity syndrome*—The baby is malnourished and born with a long and lean body, an alert look on the face, lots of hair, long fingernails, and thin wrinkled skin.

▶ *Macrosomia*—The baby is larger than average, which may cause problems during and after delivery.

▶ *Meconium aspiration*—The baby inhales meconium. This blocks the airways, causing the baby to gasp for air. It requires treatment without delay.

Postterm pregnancy may increase the chance of cesarean birth. The risks to the mother are increased in cesarean birth. It is major surgery and requires anesthesia.

Even during a postterm pregnancy, you should continue to feel your baby move. Decreased fetal movement may be a sign that you need to call your doctor.

▶   See also *Depression*

▶ POSTPARTUM DEPRESSION

Having a baby is a joyous time for most women. After childbirth, though, many mothers feel sad, afraid, angry, or anxious. Most new mothers have these feelings in a mild form called postpartum blues. Sometimes these feelings are called "baby blues." Postpartum blues almost always go away in a few days.

About 10% of new mothers have a greater problem called postpartum depression. Postpartum depression lasts longer and is more intense. It often requires counseling and treatment. Postpartum depression can occur after any birth, not just the first.

Baby Blues

Many new mothers are surprised at how weak, alone, and upset they feel after giving birth. Their feelings don't seem to match the feelings they thought they would have. They wonder, "What have I got to be depressed about?" They fear that these feelings mean that they are bad mothers.

In fact, about 70–80% of women have baby blues after childbirth. About 2–3 days after birth, they begin to feel depressed, anxious, and upset. For no clear reason, they may feel angry with the new baby, their partners, or their other children. They:

 May cry for no clear reason

 May have trouble sleeping, eating, and making choices

 Almost always question whether they can handle caring for a baby

These feelings may come and go in the first few days after childbirth. This seems strange and scary at the time. The baby blues often go away in a few hours or a week or so without treatment.

Postpartum Depression

Women with postpartum depression have such strong feelings of sadness, anxiety, or despair that they have trouble coping with their daily tasks. Without treatment, postpartum depression may become worse or may last longer.

When To Suspect Postpartum Depression

A new mother may be developing—or already have—postpartum depression if she has any of the signs or symptoms below. Take steps right away to get help.

 The baby blues don't go away after 2 weeks.

 Strong feelings of depression and anger come 1–2 months after childbirth.

 Feelings of sadness, doubt, guilt, or helplessness seem to increase each week and get in the way of normal functions.

 She is not able to care for herself or her baby.

 She has trouble doing tasks at home or on the job.

 Her appetite changes.

 Things that used to bring her pleasure no longer do.

 Concern and worry about the baby are too intense, or interest in the baby is lacking.

 Anxiety or panic attacks occur. She may be afraid to be left alone in the house with the baby.

 She fears harming the baby. These feelings are almost never acted on by women with postpartum depression, but they can be scary. These feelings may lead to guilt, which makes the depression worse.

 She has thoughts of self-harm, maybe even suicide.

Postpartum depression is more likely to happen in women who lack the support of a partner or who have had:

▶ Postpartum depression before

▶ A psychiatric illness

▶ Recent stress, such as losing a loved one, family illness, or moving to a new city

Postpartum depression does not seem to relate to the mother's age or number of children she has had.

A few new mothers will develop a more severe mental illness. This happens in 1–3 cases for every 1,000 births. Women are more at risk if they have had manic depression (bipolar disorder) or schizophrenia or if family members have had these diseases.

Reasons for Postpartum Depression

Postpartum depression is likely to result from body, mind, and lifestyle factors combined. No two women have the same biologic makeup or life experiences. This may be why some women have postpartum depression and others don't. It also may help explain why a woman can cope with the demands of everyday life but find the stress of a new baby hard to handle.

Body Changes

The postpartum period is a time of great changes in the body. These changes can affect a woman's mood and behavior for days or weeks.

Levels of the hormones estrogen and progesterone decrease sharply in the hours after childbirth. This change may trigger depression in the same way that much smaller changes in hormone levels can trigger mood swings and tension before menstrual periods. Some women are more bothered by these changes than others. They may be more likely to have postpartum blues or depression.

Hormone levels produced by the thyroid also may decrease sharply after birth. If these levels are too low, the new mother may have depression-like symptoms, such as mood swings, nervousness, fatigue, trouble sleeping, and tension.

Many women feel very tired after giving birth. It can take weeks for a woman to regain her normal strength. Some women have their babies by cesarean birth. Because this is major surgery, it will take them longer to feel strong again.

Although postpartum depression is not the same for every woman, all of the symptoms can be equally upsetting. Many times a woman feels ashamed, guilty, and isolated. There are ways to treat this condition.

Also, new mothers seldom get the rest they need. In the hospital, sleep is disturbed by visitors, hospital routine, and the baby's feedings. At home, the baby's feedings and care must be done around the clock, along with household tasks. Fatigue and lack of sleep can go on for months. They can be a major reason for depression.

Emotional Aspects

Many emotional factors can affect a woman's self-esteem and the way she deals with stress. This can add to postpartum depression.

Feelings of doubt about the pregnancy are common. The pregnancy may not have been planned. Even when a pregnancy is planned, 9 months may not be enough time for a couple to adjust to the extra effort of caring for a baby.

The baby may be born early. This can cause stressful changes in home and work routines that the parents did not expect. If the baby is born with a birth defect, it may be even harder for the parents to adjust.

Mixed feelings sometimes arise from a woman's past. She may have lost her own mother early or had a poor relationship with her. This might cause her to be unsure about her feelings toward her new baby. She may fear that caring for the child will lead to pain, disappointment, or loss.

Feelings of loss are common after having a baby. This can add to depression. The loss can take many forms:

▶ *Loss of freedom.* This can include feelings of being trapped and tied down.

▶ *Loss of an old identity.* The mother may be used to someone else taking care of her or of being in control.

▶ *Loss of a slim figure and feelings of having sex appeal.*

Lifestyle Factors

A major factor in postpartum depression is lack of support from others. The steady support of a new mother's partner is a comfort during pregnancy and after the birth. It helps when partners are willing to assume household chores and share in childcare. If a woman lives alone or far away from her family, support may be lacking.

Breastfeeding problems can make a new mother feel depressed. New mothers need not feel guilty if they cannot breastfeed or if they decide to stop. The baby can be well nourished with formula. Your partner can help with some of the feedings. This can give you more time for yourself or for rest.

It's OK to feel overwhelmed. Childbirth brings many changes, and parenting may be a new role. When you're not feeling like yourself, these changes can seem like too much to cope with. Talk to your doctor for ways to feel better.

The Role of Myths

Women who have an idea of the "perfect mother" are more likely to feel let down and depressed when faced with the needs of day-to-day mothering. Three myths about being a mother are common:

Myth No. 1: Motherhood Is Instinctive. First-time mothers often believe that they should just know how to care for a newborn. In fact, new mothers need to learn mothering skills just as they learn any other life skill. It takes time and patience. It takes reading child care books, watching skilled child caregivers, and talking with other mothers. As a mother's skills grow, she will become more sure of herself.

Mothers also may believe that they must feel a certain way toward their newborns or they are not "maternal." In fact, some women feel very little for their infants at first. Mother love, like mothering skills, does not just happen. Bonding often takes days or even weeks. When the special feelings of motherhood begin to emerge, they should be nurtured.

Myth No. 2: The Perfect Baby. Most women dream about what their newborns will look like. When the baby arrives, it may not match the baby of their dreams.

Also, babies have distinct personalities right from birth. Some infants are easier to care for. Others are fussy, have upset stomachs, and are not easy to comfort. A new mother may find it hard to adjust to the baby.

Myth No. 3: The Perfect Mother. For some women, being perfect is a never-ending goal. A mother may think she is not living up to the ideal. She may feel that she is a failure.

Of course, no mother is perfect. It is not true that every woman can "have it all." Most women have trouble finding a balance between caring for a new baby and keeping up with household duties, other children, and a job. They often feel this way even with a lot support.

What You Can Do

If you are feeling depressed after the birth of your child, there are some things you can do to take care of yourself and your baby:

Find time to do something for yourself, even if it is only for 15–20 minutes a day. Try walking, taking a relaxing bath, reading, or meditating.

▶ Get plenty of rest. Don't try to do it all. Try to nap when the baby naps.

▶ Ask for help from family and friends, especially if you have other children. Have your partner help with feedings at night.

▶ Take special care of yourself. Shower and dress each day, and get out of the house. Get a babysitter or take the baby with you. Go for a walk, meet with a friend, and talk with other new mothers.

◗ Spend time with your partner. Tell him how you feel. Often just talking things out with someone you trust can provide relief.

Call your doctor if your feelings do not lessen after a few weeks and you have trouble coping. Blues that don't go away after a few weeks may be a sign of a more severe depression. Tell your doctor if you are afraid you might neglect or hurt your baby. Help is at hand. Your doctor can refer you to experts in treating depression. These experts will give emotional support, help you sort through your feelings, and help you make changes in your life.

There also are hotlines and support groups for women with postpartum depression. Talk to your doctor about finding help in your area.

You also may be given medication to treat depression. If you are breastfeeding your baby, be sure to talk with your doctor about any side effects of the medication.

Sometimes a mother may develop a more severe depression. She may need to stay in the hospital until she can take care of herself and her child again.

To get well, women with postpartum depression need realistic goals and support. Learn how to nurture yourself as well as your family. Small, daily things can make a big difference. It's important to take time for yourself, get out of the house, and reach out to family and friends. Do only what is needed, and let the rest go.

For more information on postpartum depression, contact:

*Postpartum Support
   International
927 N Kellogg,
Santa Barbara, CA 93111
Phone: (805) 967-7636
Fax: (805) 967-0608
Web Address: www.postpar
   tum.net*

◗ PRECONCEPTIONAL CARE

Becoming a parent is a major commitment filled with challenges, rewards, and choices. By making some plans and changes now, before you conceive, you are more likely to have a healthy pregnancy later. Some aspects of pregnancy are part of a natural process you cannot control. You can have a big impact on other aspects, however, especially lifestyle. A healthy lifestyle adds greatly to your health and that of your baby. Planning for pregnancy can help you prepare for the events ahead and promote a healthy lifestyle for your future.

Pregnancy is a major event. If you plan for it, you can make wise decisions that will benefit both your health and that of your baby. Good health before pregnancy can help you cope with the stress of pregnancy, labor, and delivery. It also can help ensure that neither you nor your baby is exposed to things that could be harmful during pregnancy. Getting good health care before you become pregnant—sometimes called preconceptional care—will help you throughout your pregnancy. It also provides a chance to find any risks and treat any medical problems you may have.

A Preconceptional Visit

If you are planning to become pregnant, you may wish to schedule a preconceptional visit with your health care provider. As part of your visit, you will be asked questions about your family and medical history, medications you take, your diet and lifestyle, and any past pregnancies. Your answers should be honest and open because they will help show whether you could need special care during pregnancy.

Your preconceptional visit is a time for you to ask questions. Don't hesitate to seek advice or discuss any concerns you might have. Your health care team is there to give information and guidance.

Family History

Some conditions occur more often in families. If a close member of your family has a history of a disorder, you may be at greater risk of having it, too. For example, you may be asked whether any member of your family has ever had diabetes, hypertension (high blood pressure), epilepsy (seizures), or mental retardation. You also may be asked if anyone in your family has a history of twin pregnancies.

Certain disorders can be inherited. These are called genetic disorders. Based on your age or family history, you may be advised to see a genetic counselor—someone with special training in inherited disorders. Genetic counseling can help couples be aware of their chances of having a child with an inherited disorder. It also can help pinpoint a pattern of inherited disorders, if one exists. Genetic counseling involves a detailed family history and sometimes a physical exam along with lab tests. Some genetic disorders can be detected by testing before you are pregnant.

Medical History

Some women have medical conditions, such as diabetes, high blood pressure, and epilepsy, that call for special care during pregnancy. The condition may be an illness you had before pregnancy. Because pregnancy puts new demands on your body, a health problem that is normally under control can change while you are pregnant. If you have certain medical conditions, they should be brought under control before you become pregnant. They may require you to see your doctor more often or get other special care. Changes in your lifestyle also may be necessary.

Even if you show no signs of having a genetic disorder, it's possible to be a "carrier" and pass it along to your baby.

Questions you may be asked about your medical history include:

▶ Do you have diabetes, high blood pressure, or epilepsy? If so, when did it begin?

▶ Are you or have you ever been anemic? If so, for how long?

▶ How old were you when you had your first period?

▶ Have you ever had surgery? If so, what type?

▶ What type of birth control do you use?

▶ Have you had any accidents? What type?

▶ Do you have any allergies?

Past Pregnancies

Another part of preconceptional care is a review of your obstetric history. You will be asked about any previous pregnancies and if you had any complications.

If you had a problem in a past pregnancy, that doesn't mean the problem will recur or that you shouldn't try to get pregnant again. Some problems recur, but most do not. Previous problems can be a sign that you may need special attention before and during your current pregnancy.

Some women worry that they will have trouble having a baby if they have had a miscarriage. One in five women who become pregnant are known to have a miscarriage at some point in that pregnancy, and many more that are not detected are thought to occur. Most of these women go on to have normal pregnancies the next time they conceive. A few women have recurrent miscarriages (three or more pregnancy losses in a row). Most likely, though, if you have one miscarriage you will not have others and will be able to have a normal, healthy baby.

Most doctors agree that having a previous pregnancy terminated (induced abortion) does not make it harder to get pregnant again, nor will it affect the outcome of a future pregnancy. However, not much is known about the risk for women who have had more than one abortion. It is possible that more than one abortion might increase the risk for a low-birth-weight or a preterm baby.

Let your doctor know if you had diabetes, high blood pressure, premature labor, preterm birth, or birth defects in a past pregnancy so he or she can keep a close eye on your health.

Medications

You will be asked about any medications you are taking, including those bought over the counter (such as aspirin, antihistamines, and diet pills). Some medications could affect your fetus and should not be taken while you're pregnant. For example, a prescription medication for acne called isotretinoin can cause

Many women use medications, remedies, and nutritional supplements to promote their health. Some drugs, herbs, and even vitamins can be harmful to your baby and shouldn't be taken while you are pregnant. Just because something is natural, doesn't mean it's safe.

birth defects, and medications for high blood pressure called ACE inhibitors can cause kidney problems in the fetus. If you're taking certain medications, you may need to switch to others before you try to get pregnant. You also will be asked if you're still taking birth control pills. It's a good idea to take any medications you are using with you to the preconceptional visit.

Questions you may be asked about other medications include:

▶ Do you take sedatives or tranquilizers?

▶ Do you use illegal drugs?

▶ Do you drink alcohol? This includes beer and wine.

▶ Do you smoke? How many packs a day?

Lifestyle

Diet

Eating right before you become pregnant can help make sure that you and your fetus start out with the nutrients you both need. A balanced diet is a basic part of good health at all times in your life. During pregnancy, diet is even more important. The foods you eat are the main source of the nutrients for your fetus. As the fetus develops and places new demands on your body, you will need more of most nutrients. If you already follow a healthy diet, you can easily make changes during pregnancy to get the extra calories you need.

Special Needs. There may be needs in your diet that should be met before you become pregnant. Certain factors can affect how your body uses nutrients. If any of the following factors apply to you, consult your doctor, because you may need to make some changes in your diet.

▶ Do you eat a strict vegetarian diet?

▶ Do you commonly run long distances or do strenuous exercises?

▶ Do you fast?

▶ Are you following a diet to lose weight?

▶ Do you have a history of anemia?

Folic acid may help prevent certain birth defects called neural tube defects. The U.S. Public Health Service has recommended that all reproductive-aged women take 0.4 mg of folic acid daily to reduce the risk of neural tube defects. It can be taken as a vitamin or can be found in certain foods such as leafy, dark-green vegetables; citrus fruits; beans; and bread.

Women who have had a previous pregnancy that involved a neural tube defect have a higher risk of it recurring in a future pregnancy and should take 10 times more folic acid than the amount recommended routinely. Such women should take 4 mg daily for 1 month before pregnancy and during the first 3 months of pregnancy. These women should take folic acid alone, not as a part of a multivitamin preparation. To get enough folic acid from multivitamins, a woman would be getting an overdose of the other vitamins.

Weight. Maintaining proper weight is important for your good health. The right eating habits and moderate exercise are crucial to keeping a healthy weight and fit body—both before and during pregnancy. Weighing too much is a health hazard. During pregnancy, being overweight is linked to high blood pressure or diabetes. Extreme obesity puts a strain on the heart that becomes an added burden during pregnancy. Women who weigh too little tend to have low-birth-weight babies. These babies have more problems than other babies during labor and after birth.

It's best not to try losing weight while you are pregnant or trying to become pregnant. A weight-loss diet could deny you and your baby the nutrients you both need. It is best to try to reach a healthy weight well before you become pregnant.

Exercise

Good health at any time in your life involves proper diet and getting enough exercise. What you can do in sports and exercise during pregnancy depends on your health and, in part, on how active you are before you become pregnant.

Ideally, you should be in shape and follow a regular exercise routine before you become pregnant. When starting an exercise program, decide whether you want to improve your heart and lung function, the tone of your body muscles, or both. Then, select exercises that will allow you to meet your goals. If you are not used to being active, you should start an exercise program gradually.

To get the best workout and strengthen your heart and lungs, you should exercise so your heart beats at a certain level called your target heart rate. Your target heart rate dictates how hard you should exercise.

Every time you exercise, you should begin with a 5- to 10-minute period of light activity, such as brisk walking, as a warm-up before each session. Once your body is warmed up, exercise for 20–30 minutes at your target heart rate. End with a cooldown period of at least 10 minutes by slowly reducing your activity to let your heart rate return to a normal level.

To tone your muscles or strengthen your heart you need to exercise at least three times a week. It does not have to be done

In 1998, the U.S. Food and Drug Administration required that all breads, flours, corn meals, pastas, rice, and other grain products be fortified with folic acid to help prevent neural tube defects. It is still a good idea to take a folic acid supplement if you are of child-bearing age. In order to get enough folic acid through diet, a woman would need to eat 10 slices of bread every day!

daily—some people's muscles cannot withstand hard exercise every day. Every other day is fine. But it is important that you keep up your routine throughout the year. If you stop for 6–8 weeks, you will need to start again at a lower level of exertion.

Substance Use

Tobacco, alcohol, and illegal drugs are addictive and can harm both you and your fetus. They can have bad effects on the fetus at a time when organs are forming, which can cause damage that can last a lifetime or even result in death. The misuse of prescription medications also can harm the fetus.

Used in combination, as these substances often are, they are even more dangerous. For the sake of your own health and that of your baby, now is a good time to quit or at least cut down your use of tobacco, alcohol, and illegal drugs.

It takes time and patience to quit a habit. This is especially true if you've had that habit for a long time. Don't be embarrassed. Ask your doctor to suggest ways to get through the withdrawal stage of quitting and to refer you to support groups. Your decision to quit may be one of the hardest things you've ever done, but it will be one of the most worthwhile.

If you live with someone who smokes, you are likely to breathe in harmful amounts of secondhand smoke. In turn, your developing baby will be exposed.

Environment

Some substances found in the environment or at the workplace can make it harder for a woman to become pregnant or can harm the fetus. If you are planning to become pregnant, it's a good idea to look closely at your workplace and surroundings. If you see that you could be exposed to a harmful substance, you can take steps to avoid it. The effects of most chemicals in the environment are not known, however.

Before you accept a job, find out from your employer whether you might be exposed to toxic substances, chemicals, or radiation. After you start a job, discuss your level of exposure to specific substances with your employee health division, personnel office, or union representative.

Radiation, a form of energy transmitted in waves that you cannot see, is used in some jobs. It also is used, in the form of X-rays, to diagnose and treat disease. Exposure to high levels of some kinds of radiation can make men and women less fertile and can affect the fetus of a pregnant woman. Women planning a pregnancy who are exposed to radiation in industrial and medical settings should ask for monthly readings that show how much radiation they have been exposed to. The amount of radiation in a chest X-ray will not hurt fertility or a fetus. Radiation to treat diseases such as cancer, however, is used in much larger amounts and can be harmful.

Exposure to lead or certain solvents, pesticides, or other chemicals can reduce your partner's fertility by killing or damaging his sperm. Unlike women, who are born with a complete supply of eggs for their whole lifetime, men make new sperm daily for most of their lives. Unless the damage to a man's reproductive system is very serious, he will probably be able to make healthy sperm again a short time after his exposure to the harmful material stops.

Infections

Infections can prove harmful to both the mother and the fetus. Some infections during pregnancy can cause serious birth defects or illness in the fetus. Some can be prevented by vaccination. Ask your doctor if there are immunizations (vaccinations) you should have (eg, measles, mumps, tetanus, polio, and rubella). Even if you were vaccinated as a child, you may not be immune now. If you're vaccinated before you become pregnant, you will be protected. The vaccine should be given at least 3 months before you try to conceive. During that time you should use birth control.

If you plan to travel to areas where you may come in contact with infectious diseases not found in this country, you may need to be vaccinated against them. If you are not using birth control, consult your doctor regarding possible effects during pregnancy.

Other infections that are harmful during pregnancy are those passed on by sexual contact—sexually transmitted diseases (STDs). STDs come in many types and forms and not only can affect your ability to conceive but also can infect and harm your baby. Some common STDs are chlamydia, gonorrhea, genital herpes, and human immunodeficiency virus (HIV).

The use of some birth control methods, such as condoms and spermicides, can lower the risk of getting an STD. When a woman is trying to get pregnant, she will be at a higher risk of getting an STD because she will not be using any birth control. This is especially true if she has sex with more than one partner.

If you think you may have an STD, see your doctor right away to be tested and treated. Your partner also should be treated, and you both should not have sex until you have completed treatment.

Are Your Immunizations Up-to-Date?

Although some vaccines are safe to receive during pregnancy, it's best to have all needed immunizations before you become pregnant. Women should have the following immunizations:

3 months before pregnancy

▶ Measles–mumps–rubella vaccine (once if not immune)

1 month before pregnancy

▶ Varicella vaccine*

Safe during pregnancy

▶ Tetanus–diphtheria booster (every 10 years)

▶ Hepatitis A vaccine*

▶ Hepatitis B vaccine*

▶ Influenza vaccine (if will be in the second or third trimester of pregnancy during flu season)

▶ Pneumococcal vaccine*

*These immunizations are given as needed based on risk factors. If you don't know whether you need one, check with your health care provider.

Later Childbearing

Most women in their mid-30s and older have healthy pregnancies and healthy babies. Even so, some questions arise for these women. They may have concerns about whether their age will affect their ability to become pregnant, their health, and the health of their babies. Although there is no absolute age that is unsafe for older women who want to become pregnant, there are some special concerns that these women should consider.

A woman's fertility gradually declines as she reaches her mid-30s and beyond. Therefore, women at this age may find it takes longer to get pregnant. As women get older, certain medical and obstetric problems also occur more often. Because pregnancy puts new demands on a woman's body, the risk of complications during pregnancy is higher for women with these problems. They are more likely to need to visit the doctor more often, to stay in the hospital before the birth of the baby, and to need special tests.

There's no set age that is unsafe for women to become pregnant. Most women older than age 35 can have a normal pregnancy and healthy baby.

▶ See also *Back Pain During Pregnancy, Morning Sickness*

▶ PREGNANCY CHANGES

Your body goes through many changes when you are pregnant. As your fetus grows, it is normal for you to have some discomforts. Some of these changes may occur only in the early weeks of pregnancy. Others may occur only at the end. Still others may appear early, then go away, only to return.

Backache

Backaches are common. They are usually caused by the strain put on your back by your growing uterus and by changes in your posture.

Try doing some of these things to help your back feel more comfortable:

▶ Change position.

▶ Wear low-heeled shoes.

▶ Avoid lifting heavy things or children.

▶ Do not bend over at the waist to pick things up. Squat down, bend your knees, and keep your back straight.

▶ Place one foot on a stool or box when you have to stand for a long time.

▶ Sleep on your side with one knee bent. Support your upper leg on a pillow.

▶ Apply heat, cold, or pressure to your back.

▶ Ask your doctor or nurse for special exercises you can do.

Severe back pain is not a normal part of pregnancy. It could be a sign of kidney infection or preterm labor. If you have pain in your back that doesn't go away or gets worse, call your doctor.

Breast Changes

Early in pregnancy, your breasts begin to grow and change to prepare for breastfeeding your baby. They will feel firm and tender. As your breasts grow, wear a bra that fits well and provides support.

Your nipples may stick out more and get darker. This will help your baby to breastfeed. Some women's nipples do not stick out but sink inward (retracted nipple). If you have retracted nipples and you plan to breastfeed, your doctor may suggest that you try massaging the nipples so they stick out.

Breathing Problems

As the fetus grows, the uterus takes up more room. Your lungs do not have as much room to expand, so you may be short of breath.

A few weeks before you give birth, the fetus's head will move down in the uterus, or "drop," and press against the cervix. This usually happens between 36–38 weeks of pregnancy in women who have not had a baby before, but may happen later. In women who have already had a baby, it may not happen until the start of labor. When the fetus drops, it will be easier to breathe.

If you are short of breath, here are some things to try:

❯ Sit up straight.

❯ Sleep propped up.

❯ Ask your doctor or childbirth educator about breathing exercises.

Constipation

At least half of all women are constipated at some point during pregnancy. Changes in hormones slow food's passage through your body. During the last part of pregnancy, your uterus may press on your rectum. This may add to the problem. Some things may help:

❯ Drink lots of liquids. Include fruit juices, such as prune juice.

❯ Eat foods high in fiber, such as raw fruits and vegetables and bran cereals.

❯ Exercise each day—just walking is fine.

To help relieve constipation, ask your doctor about taking a bulk-forming agent. These products absorb water and expand inside your body. That adds to the moisture in stool and makes it easier to pass. Don't take laxatives during pregnancy.

Hemorrhoids

Very often, pregnant women who are constipated also have hemorrhoids. Hemorrhoids are varicose (or swollen) veins in the rectum. They are often painful. Straining during bowel movements and having very hard stools may make hemorrhoids worse. Some products for treating pain from hemorrhoids and the tips about constipation should help.

Cramps

In the last part of pregnancy, you may have leg cramps. Stretching your legs before going to bed can help ease cramps. Avoid pointing your toes when stretching or exercising.

Frequent Urination

You will need to urinate often during the first 12–14 weeks of pregnancy. This feeling may go away in the middle of pregnancy. In the last few weeks, you may need to urinate more often again. If you also have pain, fever, or a change in the odor or color of your urine, you may have an infection. Contact your doctor right away.

Inability to Sleep

After the first few months, you may find it hard to sleep. This often happens in the last weeks of pregnancy. Your abdomen is large, and it is hard to get comfortable.

To get the rest you need:

- Take a warm bath at bedtime.

- Try the tips to relax that you learned in childbirth classes.

- Lie on your side with a pillow under your abdomen and another between your legs.

- Rest for short breaks during the day.

Indigestion

Indigestion also is called "heartburn," but it does not mean that anything is wrong with your heart. It is a burning feeling in the stomach that seems to rise up into the throat.

Changes that take place in your body during pregnancy may make indigestion worse. Changes in your hormone levels slow digestion and relax the muscle that keeps the digested food and acids in your stomach. Also, your growing uterus presses up on your stomach. For relief:

- Eat five or six small meals a day instead of three large ones.

- Avoid foods that you know cause gas.

- Sit up while eating.

- Wait an hour after eating before lying down. Do not eat before going to bed.

- Wait 2 hours after eating before exercising.
- Do not take any medicines, including antacids and baking soda, unless you first check with your doctor.

Lower Abdominal Pain

As the uterus grows, the muscles that support it are pulled and stretched. You may feel this as sharp pains or a dull ache in your abdomen. Resting and changing your position seem to help the most. The pains are most often felt between 18–24 weeks of pregnancy.

Nausea and Vomiting

Nausea and vomiting are common during the first 12–14 weeks of pregnancy, but sometimes happen throughout pregnancy. This is called "morning sickness," but it can occur any time during the day. It is common when the stomach is empty. Here are some tips to make you feel more comfortable:

- Eat dry toast or crackers before getting out of bed in the morning.
- Get up slowly and sit on the side of the bed for a few minutes.
- Eat five or six small meals each day. Try not to let your stomach get completely empty.
- Avoid unpleasant smells.
- Contact your doctor if nausea or vomiting is severe.
- Always check with your doctor before taking any medicines.

Morning sickness can become more of a problem if you can't keep any foods or fluids down and begin to lose weight. If your nausea and vomiting are severe, call your doctor.

Numbness and Tingling

As the uterus grows, it rests on some of your nerves. Some nerves also may get pressed if you are swollen from retaining water. This may cause numbness or tingling in the legs, toes, and sometimes the arms. It usually is not serious. It will go away after the baby is born.

Skin Changes

The hormones in your body often cause some normal changes on your skin. Some women have brownish, uneven marks around their eyes and over the nose and cheeks. This is called chloasma. These marks usually disappear or fade after delivery, when hormone levels go back to normal. Being in the sun tends to make the marks darker.

Many of the miracle creams or lotions sold to prevent stretch marks do not work. In fact, there is little you can do to keep them at bay. Keeping your weight gain within the limits your doctor suggests may help. Once your baby is born, these marks will slowly fade.

In many women, a line running from the top to the bottom of the abdomen becomes dark. This is called the linea nigra. In others, streaks or stretch marks may appear on the abdomen and breasts as they grow. This is caused by the skin tissue stretching to support the growing fetus. There is no way to prevent stretch marks. They may slowly fade after pregnancy.

Swelling

Some swelling (called edema) is normal in pregnancy. It happens most often in the legs and usually in the last few months. It may happen more often in the summer. Swollen hands and face may mean there is a problem. Let your doctor know if they swell. You can help reduce the swelling in your legs if you:

▶ Put your legs up when you can.

▶ Rest in bed on your side. Your left side is best.

▶ Limit salty foods.

▶ Wear support pantyhose or stockings.

Never take medicines (fluid pills) for the swelling unless your doctor has prescribed them.

Tiredness

You may often feel tired during pregnancy—especially in the beginning and at the end. If you get enough exercise and rest (including naps) and eat a healthy diet, you are likely to feel better.

Varicose Veins

You are more likely to have varicose veins if someone in your family had them. You can't prevent varicose veins, but there are ways to relieve the aches.

Varicose veins are swollen veins. They appear most often in the legs but can appear near the vulva and vagina. They are caused by pressure from your uterus on your veins. They often occur if you must stand or sit for a long time. They are usually not serious. They can be uncomfortable, though. You may have aching, sore legs.

For some relief:

▶ Put your legs up when you can.

▶ Lie down with your legs raised.

▶ Try not to stand for a long time.

▶ Do not wear anything that binds your legs, such as tight bands around stockings or socks.

- Try wearing support stockings, or your doctor can recommend special stockings.

- If you must sit a lot on the job, stand up and move around from time to time.

▶ PREGNANCY CHOICES

▶ See also *Abortion, Induced; Adoption*

Many women have mixed feelings when they find out that they are pregnant. They may wonder if they are ready and willing to accept all that comes with bringing up a child. When you find out you are pregnant, you have a number options. You can have the baby and raise it. You can have the baby and place it for adoption. Or, you can have an abortion (end the pregnancy).

Making a Decision

First, you need to be sure that you are pregnant. If the results of an over-the-counter pregnancy test are positive, you should go to a clinic or see a doctor to confirm that you are pregnant. The doctor will find out how far along you are and talk to you about your options.

You will need to think about many factors as you decide. Your health, values, beliefs, and circumstances will play a role. You should think about:

- Medical problems you may have—there may be a risk to the fetus or signs that something might go wrong with the pregnancy

- How far along you are in your pregnancy

- How much it costs to raise a child, pay for prenatal care and delivery, or have an abortion

- What your choice will mean for you

Talk with your doctor and with others that you trust, such as your partner, a friend, or a parent. If you need help finding someone to talk to about your options, a family planning clinic, a family services agency, or an adoption agency can guide you. Be sure that the counselor covers all of your options. Counseling at these places is free or costs very little in most cases.

Decide as early as you can. If you choose either to raise the baby or place it for adoption, it is best to begin prenatal care as soon as you can. If you choose to have an abortion, it is simpler and safer for you to have it as soon as possible. Explore your feelings to make sure that what you decide is right for you.

Raising a Child

There are many rewards that come with raising a child. It also demands much physical and emotional energy.

The better the support system you have, the easier it will be for you to raise a child. Think about:

▶ Will you need help with childcare?

▶ Is a partner or other family member there to help you?

▶ Will you have to change your living arrangements? If so, can you afford to do this?

If your income falls below a certain level, government programs, such as the Women, Infants and Children (WIC) program may be able to help. WIC provides food vouchers for nutritional foods for pregnant women and children up to a certain age.

Think about whether you are prepared for the long-term commitment. Raising a child can be stressful. You will have less time for yourself and may need to change your lifestyle. The demands of being a mother may make it harder to reach goals that you have set for yourself. For instance, you may need to change the amount of time you spend at your job or at school. You will have less time for other things. Keep in mind that the changes a baby brings to your life can bring you joy and comfort as well.

If you plan to have the baby, prenatal care—a program of care for a pregnant woman before the birth of her baby—is vital. Good prenatal care makes it more likely that you will have a healthy baby.

To find out more information about the WIC program in your area, visit the U.S. Department of Agriculture web site at www.fns.usda.gov/wic.

Adoption

In an adoption, a child legally gets new parents. A new birth certificate will be issued with the new parents' names on it. If you cannot raise or take care of a child, adoption may be a good option.

If you choose adoption, prenatal care is as vital as if you were going to raise the child yourself. Start care early and see your doctor regularly.

You may have a mixture of feelings when the baby is adopted—anger, grief, a sense of loss, or relief. These feelings may last for a long time. They could return to you on the child's birthday, even years after the baby has been adopted.

Counseling can help you come to terms with this decision. The agency that provides the adoption service or a local family services agency may offer counseling.

There are two kinds of adoption—open and closed. In open adoption, the birth mother and the adoptive parents know something about each other. They may meet and exchange names and addresses. In a closed adoption, the birth mother and adoptive parents do not meet or know each other's names.

Abortion

Abortion means removing a fetus from a woman's uterus before it can live outside the uterus. Almost all abortions are done in the first 12 weeks of pregnancy.

The decision to have an abortion needs to be made as early as possible. The type of procedure used and some of the risks depend on how long you have been pregnant. The doctor can explain the stage of development of the fetus to help you decide.

Your health may play a role in your decision. Some conditions might pose a risk to a woman during pregnancy.

Abortion is a personal decision. Because state laws about abortion change, ask your doctor or counselor what the law is in your state. If you are a minor, state law may require that your parent(s) or guardian be notified or give consent or that you seek permission from a court.

Changing Your Mind

If you were going to have and raise the child and then decide against it, you still can think about adoption. You can begin adoption procedures after birth. This is true even if the birth mother had not made this choice before the baby was born.

If a woman decides to place her child for adoption and then changes her mind after she signs the consent papers, she should check her state's laws. In some states, the consent cannot be changed. In other states, the birth mother can change her mind up to 30 days or even longer after she signs the consent forms.

A decision to have an abortion should be made as early in pregnancy as possible. If you decided to have the baby and later want to have an abortion, you need to discuss it with your doctor. After a certain point, you may not be able to have an abortion. The longer a woman waits to have an abortion, the more risk it carries for her.

◗ PREGNANCY REDUCTION

◗ See also *Multiple Pregnancy*

The risk of problems during pregnancy increases with the number of fetuses the mother is carrying. If the health of the mother or the fetuses is at risk, her doctor may talk to her about pregnancy reduction. Early in the pregnancy, the doctor can remove one or more of the embryos to increase the chances that the other(s) will be born healthy. Pregnancy reduction also may be offered in the case of twins if one of the fetuses is found to have major birth defects.

When a woman is carrying more than twins, it is called a "high-order multiple pregnancy." With the increased use of fertility drugs, multiple pregnancy has become more common. The drugs may cause several eggs to be released at once, instead of one.

Multiple pregnancies have a higher risk of problems. The babies may be very small and some may be impaired. There is a risk that some may die before birth. The mother may go into labor early, before the babies are fully developed. There are risks to the mother, too, such as very high blood pressure.

For the procedure, a needle is inserted through the woman's vagina or abdomen. The needle then is inserted into the embryo chosen for reduction. Medication is injected to stop the heartbeat of that fetus.

Women carrying many fetuses at once face some hard choices. In most cases, the choice to have a pregnancy reduction is done to try to improve the well-being of the most number of fetuses.

▶ PREGNANCY SIGNS AND SYMPTOMS

The first sign that you are pregnant usually is a missed menstrual period. A late period doesn't always mean that a baby's on the way, though. Not all women start their periods at the same time each month. Even if you usually have regular periods, stress, illness, or a change in your exercise or eating habits can delay menstruation. Thus, also be on the lookout for these other symptoms of early pregnancy:

▶ Spotting or a very light menstrual period

▶ Tender breasts

▶ Feeling very tired

▶ Upset stomach or nausea

▶ Feeling bloated

▶ Frequent urination

▶ Being moody

If you have missed your period and have one or more of these signs, you could be pregnant. This is true even if you have been using birth control. The next step: buy a home pregnancy test or visit your doctor's office or clinic.

Warning Signs in Early Pregnancy

Get medical help right away if you suspect you are pregnant or are in early pregnancy and have any of these symptoms:

▶ Cramps or severe abdominal pain

▶ Spotting that lasts more than 1 day

▶ Bleeding that's as heavy as a menstrual period or soaks a sanitary pad each hour

▶ Blood clots, bright red blood, or flesh-like tissue from your vagina

▶ Heavy, foul-smelling vaginal discharge

▶ Faintness or dizziness

▶ Painful urination

▶ Vomiting so severe that you can't keep any food or liquid down

PREGNANCY TESTS

Thanks to advances in testing, pregnancy can be confirmed as early as the first day of a missed period. Soon after conception, the developing placenta produces human chorionic gonadotropin (hCG). This hormone is released into the mother's urine and blood, where it is picked up by a pregnancy test.

These days, home pregnancy tests are simple to use and can be bought over the counter. Most tests involve urinating on a chemically treated stick or dipping it in a cup of your urine. If hCG is present, the chemicals in the stick will react to the hormone and produce a signal in the test's result window—a blue line, a pink dot, or a red "plus" sign, for instance.

The tests are accurate as long as you use them correctly. Still, they can give an incorrect (false-positive or false-negative) result if you are taking certain medications, if you don't follow the directions, or if you take the test too early. A false-positive result tells you that you are pregnant when you really aren't. A false-negative result tells you that you aren't pregnant when you really are.

If a home test result is negative but your period doesn't start in a couple of days or you develop other pregnancy symptoms, repeat the test or ask your doctor to give you a test. (See the doctor right away if you have vaginal bleeding or stomach pain, no matter what the test results show.) If a home test is positive, visit your doctor as soon as possible.

PREMENSTRUAL SYNDROME

See also *Reproductive Process* in *"Women's Bodies"*

Many women go through certain changes in the days or weeks before their menstrual periods start. When these changes cause problems, they are known as premenstrual syndrome (PMS). Up to 40% of women who menstruate report some symptoms of PMS. Although the cause of PMS is unknown, it can be treated to some degree in most women.

Symptoms of PMS

Women with PMS have symptoms in the second half of the cycle. Symptoms appear after ovulation (about day 14). Once their period starts, most women get rapid relief.

Discomforts range from breast tenderness to bloating to emotional changes and trouble coping with day-to-day stress. These changes occur before a woman's period. They usually go away when her period starts. The symptoms are cyclic in

Common Symptoms of PMS

Physical Symptoms

▶ Abdominal bloating

▶ Sore breasts

▶ Appetite changes and food cravings

▶ Swelling of hands and feet

▶ Headache

▶ Upset stomach

▶ Constipation

▶ Clumsiness

▶ Fatigue

▶ Hot flashes and dizziness (less common)

Emotional Symptoms

▶ Irritability

▶ Mood swings from sadness to anger

▶ Depression

▶ Being overly sensitive

▶ Crying spells

▶ Social withdrawal

▶ Forgetfulness

▶ Lack of concentration

▶ A change in sex drive

nature—that is, they appear and disappear at about the same time in a woman's menstrual cycle.

Most women with PMS have only some of these symptoms. Some women have more of the physical changes. Others have more of the emotional symptoms. The amount of discomfort varies from woman to woman.

How to Recognize PMS

PMS tends to follow a pattern of symptoms that occur at the same time in a woman's cycle. This general pattern occurs month after month. It may vary somewhat from month to month, though. For a woman to be diagnosed with PMS, her doctor needs to confirm a pattern of symptoms. He or she will ask if you have:

▶ Physical or emotional discomfort starting near the middle of the cycle with the most intense symptoms felt in the last 7 days before a woman's period starts?

▶ Relief of symptoms once the period starts?

▶ A symptom-free time between days 4 and 12 of the cycle?

Other Problems

Other problems that are not related to PMS can cause similar symptoms. These conditions do not have both the physical and emotional symptoms of PMS. These problems are sometimes found in women who think they might have PMS:

▶ *Depression and anxiety disorders.* These are the most common conditions confused with PMS. The symptoms of depression and anxiety are much like the emotional symptoms of PMS. Unlike PMS, depression does not have a symptom-free period. Many women with these conditions find that the symptoms worsen around the time of their menstrual flow, making them think that they may have PMS. Some women can have both PMS and depression. It is important to find out whether a woman has just PMS, just depression, or both because the treatments may differ.

▶ *Dysmenorrhea, or severe menstrual cramps.* This condition is often confused with PMS, but it is quite different. Dysmenorrhea involves pain on the first day or so of your period. Pain also can occur a few days before your period. PMS does not have pain as a major problem, and PMS occurs mostly in the week or so before the period begins. Women can have both PMS and dysmenorrhea.

▶ *Breast changes.* Many women may have painful breasts in the time before their period. Some may have fibrocystic breast changes. This is a benign (not cancer) condition in which lumpy, tender breasts become swollen and painful. This may be a problem if a woman mainly has premenstrual breast tenderness. Other women may have pain in their breasts, but no lumps. Women who have breast changes do not have other symptoms of PMS.

▶ *Endometriosis.* This is a condition in which tissue that looks and acts like the lining of the uterus is found outside the uterus in the pelvis. During menstruation, this tissue bleeds lightly and the blood irritates nearby tissue. This causes pain. In most cases, though, it does not have the other symptoms of PMS.

Keeping a Monthly Record

As yet, there are no tests that can help detect PMS. The only way to identify it is by keeping a daily record of your symptoms. This way, your doctor can see a pattern.

Be sure to make an entry each day. Your doctor will need to see the records of your symptoms for at least 2–3 months to determine if you have PMS.

PMDD and SSRIs

A small percentage of women (3–5%) may have a more severe form of PMS known as premenstrual dysphoric disorder (PMDD). PMDD is not the same as PMS because it causes severe strain in work, social, and relationship activities. Other symptoms of PMDD include:

▶ Feeling hopeless or sad

▶ Feeling tense or anxious

▶ Moodiness and crying frequently

▶ Constant irritability and anger that increase conflict with other people

▶ Lack of interest in things you used to enjoy

▶ Having problems concentrating

▶ Lacking energy

▶ Change in appetite

▶ Having trouble sleeping

▶ Feeling overwhelmed

Most of the time, symptoms begin the week before your period and end a few days after your period starts. If you have had these symptoms for most of the months of the last year, see your doctor. Recent studies have shown that selective serotonin reuptake inhibitors (SSRIs), a type of antidepressant, can help treat PMDD symptoms in some women.

American Psychiatric Association. Diagnostic and Statistical Manual of Mental Disorders, 4th ed. Washington, DC: APA, 1994. Reprinted with permission from the Diagnostic and Statistical Manual of Mental Disorders.

Your Menstrual Record

Keeping a record is simple. It can be done using only a calendar. If you use a calendar now to keep track of your cycle, you can use the same one to list any changes you feel during the month. This will make it easy to track symptoms that could be linked to PMS. Note the day of your cycle opposite the date, using day 1 as the day your period starts. Write down each symptom on the day it occurs. To know whether your symptoms improve or get worse, rate them on a scale of 0–10. Use "0" if a symptom is minimal or absent and "10" if it is severe.

You also can use this calendar to mark down when you get your period each month. After a few months, you should notice a pattern. This will help you know what days to expect your period to start.

Month	1	2	3	4	5	6	7	8	9	10	11	12	13	14	15	16	17	18	19	20	21	22	23	24	25	26	27	28	29	30	31
January																															
February																													▉	▉	
March																															
April																															▉
May																															▉
June																															▉
July																															
August																															
September																															▉
October																															
November																															▉
December																															

Keeping a daily record helps you to be aware of your body and your moods. Once a woman knows when to expect these changes and how long they last, she may be better able to manage them. Your records also will help the doctor decide what treatment is best for you.

Treatment

Treatment can help relieve certain symptoms of PMS. It usually consists of lifestyle changes or medical treatment, or both. To find the best treatment for your symptoms, you need to work closely with your doctor. You may have to try several types of treatment to find relief.

Lifestyle Changes

Some of the things that promote a healthy lifestyle may help improve symptoms. For instance, along with its other known benefits, exercise enhances well-being and improves ability to handle stress. Women who exercise regularly may have milder PMS symptoms.

When you can, adjust your schedule to avoid stress that may be harder to cope with when symptoms of PMS are at their worst. PMS can affect your relationships with others. Talk about what you are going through. If you share your feelings with your family, they may be more supportive when you are having symptoms. Being aware of symptoms also may help you avoid conflicts with your family and coworkers.

Medical Treatment

If your symptoms are not relieved through exercise or stress reduction, your doctor may suggest medical treatment. Many different kinds of over-the-counter products and nutritional supplements have been used for PMS, but most do not work well. A daily 1,000 milligram supplement of calcium is good for all women and may help relieve some of the symptoms of PMS. The treatment your doctor suggests will depend on your symptoms and how much they affect you.

Diuretics (or "water pills") are sometimes prescribed to help reduce fluid buildup. They help the body get rid of excess fluids through the kidneys. Your doctor may prescribe a drug to relieve the pain of headaches or cramps. In some women, the use of birth control pills has helped reduce the physical symptoms of PMS, such as pain, breast tenderness, or appetite changes. However, the birth control pill may not help the emotional symptoms of PMS.

For many women with severe PMS, certain medications that alter mood and are used to treat depression or anxiety have been shown to relieve symptoms. The drugs that seem to be most effective are those that increase the brain chemical "serotonin." Certain drugs that prevent ovulation—besides birth control pills—also may help. If the lifestyle changes don't help your symptoms, talk with your doctor to find out more about these other types of medications.

▶ PRENATAL CARE

Early and regular prenatal care (a program of care for a pregnant woman before the birth of her baby) can increase your chances of having a healthy baby. Prenatal care is more than just health care, though. It includes childbirth education and counseling, too.

You may be cared for by an obstetrician–gynecologist while you are pregnant. Often, you will receive care from a whole health care team that may include doctors, nurses, nurse–midwives, and childbirth educators. Feel free to ask any of them questions you may have. Together you can work toward having a healthy baby. Tell your doctor about any changes you have noticed since your last visit. If you have problems between visits, call your doctor.

If you have concerns about how to pay for care or how to get to an office or clinic, help is often available. Talk with your doctor, nurse, or local social service group.

Because pregnancy requires extra nutrients, your doctor may prescribe prenatal vitamin and mineral supplements for you. To be sure your body is absorbing the most vitamins and minerals, do not take these supplements with milk.

Your First Prenatal Visit

One of your first prenatal visits will be longer and more involved than other visits. It will include:

▶ History

▶ Physical exam

▶ Estimation of due date

▶ Tests

▶ A plan for the next visits and tests

History

One of the things you will be asked about is your history. This includes your health and lifestyle, the health of your family and the father's family, and your past pregnancies. This information can help your doctor to find problems that might come up. Your answers should be honest, complete, and accurate. Some questions you may be asked include:

▶ Do you take any medicines?

▶ Do you have any allergies or health problems?

▶ Have you been exposed to any infections?

▶ What are your periods like?

▶ When was your last menstrual period?

▶ What type of birth control have you used?

▶ Do you use alcohol, tobacco, or other drugs?

▶ Have you been pregnant before?

▶ Have you ever had a miscarriage?

▶ Have you ever had an induced abortion?

▶ If you have had a baby before:
   — What did the baby weigh at birth?
   — How long did labor last?
   — What type of delivery was it (vaginal or cesarean?)
   — Were there any problems?

▶ Is there a history of birth defects in your family?
   — Have you had a previous child with a birth defect?
   — What is your ethnic background?
   — What is the ethnic background of the father?

Physical Exam

During the physical exam, your height, weight, and blood pressure will be measured. Other parts of your body will be checked. Your pelvic organs—cervix, vagina, ovaries, fallopian tubes, and uterus—are checked during a pelvic exam. Your doctor also will check for changes in your cervix and the size of the uterus.

The Due Date

The due date is called the estimated date of delivery, or EDD. (The estimated date of confinement, or EDC, is a term that is also sometimes used.) An average pregnancy is 280 days, or 40 weeks, from the first day of the last menstrual period or 38 weeks from conception. However, a normal pregnancy can last between 37 and 42 weeks. Only about 5 of 100 babies are born on their due dates. Most women give birth within 2 weeks of this date.

The due date helps your doctor measure the growth of the fetus and the progress of your pregnancy. It also helps set the timing for some tests that are most accurate when they are done at certain times in pregnancy.

The 40 weeks of pregnancy are divided into three trimesters. These last about 12–13 weeks each (or about 3 months). The first trimester is from 0–13 weeks. The second trimester is from 14–28 weeks, and the third trimester is from 29–40 weeks (or delivery).

Tests

Several lab tests may be done early in your care. Blood tests check for:

▶ Blood type (A, B, AB, or O)

▶ Rh factor (positive or negative)

▶ Anemia

▶ Past German measles (rubella)

▶ Hepatitis B virus

Urine tests give information about levels of sugar and protein and find some infections. Pap tests check for changes of the cervix that could lead to cancer.

Some of these tests will be done more than once. Your doctor also may suggest other tests based on your history, family background, and race. Some women may be tested for diabetes. Your doctor may ask you if you wish to be tested for sexually transmitted diseases (STDs) including HIV (human immunodeficiency virus), the virus that causes AIDS (acquired immunodeficiency syndrome). Other tests to find birth defects may be offered.

Future Visits

After your first prenatal visit, the other visits are usually shorter. They are to find out how you are doing and how the fetus is growing.

The timing of your visits depends on your needs. You may follow a schedule like this:

▶ To 28 weeks: monthly

▶ 28–36 weeks: every 2 weeks

▶ 36 weeks to delivery (at about 40 weeks): weekly

Women with health or pregnancy problems may need more visits. Your doctor will watch for signs of problems throughout your pregnancy. At each visit, your doctor will check:

▶ Your weight

▶ Your blood pressure

▶ The growth and position of the fetus

▶ The fetal heartbeat

▶ Urine for protein and sugar

Some tests may be done. Lab tests and pelvic exams may not be done each time, though. Each visit will be noted on your medical record. The results of the first history, physical exam, and tests will be written there, too. Your doctor will discuss them with you. He or she also will give you advice on a healthy lifestyle.

Before you give your OK for a test or a treatment, be sure you know what it is and why it is needed. You also should be told about the risks, benefits, and options. This is called "informed consent."

▶ See also *Preconceptional Care, Prenatal Care*

▶ PRENATAL CLASSES

You and your partner can attend classes to prepare for having a baby. The doctor can direct you to a childbirth education class that's a good match for you and for the kind of birth you hope to have. These classes often meet over the course of a few weeks or months, so start looking into them as soon as you can. The class will inform you about the labor and delivery process and teach you how to help it go smoothly. You can't know how your labor will play out ahead of time. However, childbirth preparation will help ease your fears, teach you methods for coping with labor pain, and help you feel more in control.

The most common methods of preparation—Lamaze, Bradley, and Read—vary greatly, but each is based on the idea that pain is made worse by fear and tension. Classes aim to relieve labor pain through education, emotional support, relaxation techniques, and touch.

Some childbirth education classes will help you draft a birth plan. This is a written outline of what you'd like to happen during labor and delivery. It might include the setting you want to deliver in, the people you want to have with you, and the pain medications you want, if any. It also allows you to let your health care team know about the things you feel strongly about (such as episiotomy and circumcision). It is useful to make sure you and your doctor have the same ideas. Be sure to check your plan with the hospital in which you'll be delivering your baby, in case parts of it do not fit the hospital's policy.

Once you have drawn up your plan, go over it with your doctor. He or she will help you amend the plan based on your situation. The doctor also will let you know if your wishes conflict with hospital policies. Be sure to keep your birth plan both realistic and flexible. Each birth is unique, after all, and you won't know exactly what yours will be like until it happens.

Some classes are free. Others have set or flexible fees. Check with:

▶ Your doctor

▶ Hospitals or clinics

▶ Childbirth groups

▶ Community groups

▶ Health departments

Your doctor can tell you about childbirth classes near you. You also can call the International Childbirth Education Association at (612) 854-8660 (or check out www.icea.org) for information about certified childbirth educators in your area.

▶ See also *Labor*

▶ PRETERM LABOR

Preterm labor is labor that starts before the end of 37 weeks of pregnancy. It can lead to preterm birth. About 1 of every 10 babies born in the United States is born preterm.

Your baby can have problems if it is born too early. Serious illness or death can occur because the baby is not yet ready for life on his or her own.

What Is Preterm Labor?

In most pregnancies, labor starts between 38 and 42 weeks after the last menstrual period. Preterm labor starts before the end of the 37th week of pregnancy.

Labor starts with regular contractions of the uterus. The cervix thins out (effaces) and opens up (dilates) so the baby can enter the birth canal. It is not known for certain what causes labor to start. Hormones produced by both the woman and fetus play a role. Changes in the uterus, which may be caused by these hormones, may cause labor to start.

Preterm labor may be a normal process that starts early for some reason. Or, it may be started by some other problem, such as infection of the uterus or amniotic fluid. In most cases of preterm labor, the exact cause is not known.

Why the Concern?

Preterm birth accounts for about 75% of newborn deaths that are not related to birth defects. Growth and development in the last part of pregnancy is vital to the baby's health. The earlier the baby is born, the greater the risk of problems.

Preterm babies (also called premature babies or "preemies") tend to grow more slowly. They may have problems with their eyes, ears, breathing, and nervous system. School, learning, and behavior problems are more common in children who were preterm babies.

Signs of Preterm Labor

If preterm labor is found early enough, delivery can be prevented or postponed in some cases. This will give your baby extra time to grow and mature. Even a few more days may mean a healthier baby.

Sometimes the signs that preterm labor may be starting are fairly easy to detect. The box lists the early signs of preterm labor. If you have any of these signs, don't wait. Call your doctor or nurse or go to the hospital.

Diagnosing Preterm Labor

It can be hard to tell true and false labor apart. Preterm labor can be diagnosed only by finding changes in the cervix. This means your doctor will have to examine you.

It is common for women to have contractions before labor starts. This is called Braxton Hicks contractions or false labor. These may be painful and regular, but usually go away within an hour or with rest. If you have contractions more often than six times an hour that last for more than an hour, call your doctor or nurse right away.

Fetal monitoring tests are used to record the heartbeat of the fetus and contractions of your uterus. Ultrasound may be used to estimate the size and age of the fetus and to see where it is in the uterus. You may be watched for a time and then examined again to see whether your cervix changes.

Women at Risk

Some women are at greater risk for preterm labor than others. Women who have little or no prenatal care and those who have had preterm labor before are at increased risk. Preterm labor can happen to anyone, though, without warning.

A number of other factors also have been linked to preterm labor. There are also factors linked to the fetus that make preterm labor more likely. For instance,

---

The greater the number of fetuses within the uterus, the greater the risk for preterm delivery and problems after birth. Although multiple pregnancies account for only 1.1% of all pregnancies, they result in 10% of all preterm births.

Signs of Preterm Labor

Call your doctor or nurse right away if you notice any of these signs:

▶ Vaginal discharge

　—Change in type (watery, mucus, or bloody)

　—Increase in amount

▶ Pelvic or lower abdominal pressure

▶ Constant, low, dull backache

▶ Mild abdominal cramps, with or without diarrhea

▶ Regular or frequent contractions or uterine tightening, often painless

▶ Ruptured membranes (your water breaks)

too much fluid in the amniotic sac that surrounds the baby is a risk factor. Problems with the placenta or certain birth defects also increase the risk.

Despite what is known about these risk factors, much remains to be learned about preterm labor. Half of the women who go into preterm labor have no known risk factors.

If you are at risk for preterm labor, you may be advised to take certain steps to lower the risk of preterm birth. These steps may involve:

1. Changing your lifestyle

2. Having more frequent visits with your doctor or nurse

3. Learning how to time your contractions

If you are at risk for preterm labor, be sure to get early prenatal care, eat well, and get enough rest. You may need to see your doctor or nurse more often for exams and tests. You should not drink alcohol or smoke cigarettes.

In many cases, women at risk for preterm labor do not have to give up their jobs unless preterm labor has been diagnosed. You may be advised to avoid heavy lifting or other hard or tiring tasks during pregnancy.

If you take childbirth preparation classes, you should tell the teacher you are at risk for preterm labor. He or she may advise you to skip certain exercises. Women at risk also may be advised to cut down on travel. Ask your doctor or nurse about these and other changes you may need to make in your daily routine.

If you have a history of preterm labor or have signs of preterm labor, you may wonder about having sex during pregnancy. Many women worry that the uterine contractions that often follow sex and orgasm will lead to preterm labor. Although in most cases the contractions stop, these are natural and real concerns that should be discussed with both your partner and your doctor. You may be advised to restrict sexual activity or to monitor yourself for contractions after sex. Your doctor or nurse also may ask that your partner use a condom during sex to lower the risk of infection.

Risk Factors for Preterm Labor

You may be at risk for preterm labor if:

▶ You have warning signs of preterm labor.

▶ You have had preterm labor during this pregnancy.

▶ You had preterm labor or preterm birth in a previous pregnancy.

▶ You are carrying more than one baby (twins, triplets).

▶ You have had one or more second-trimester-induced abortions (the planned ending of a pregnancy).

▶ You have an abnormal cervix (due to surgery, for instance).

▶ You have an abnormal uterus.

▶ You have had abdominal surgery during this pregnancy.

▶ You have had a serious infection while pregnant.

▶ You have had bleeding in the second or third trimester of your pregnancy.

▶ You are underweight or you weigh less than 100 pounds.

▶ You were exposed to diethylstilbestrol (DES), a medication given to many pregnant women in the 1950s and 1960s) as a fetus.

▶ You smoke cigarettes or use cocaine.

▶ You have had little or no prenatal care.

Stopping Labor

Your doctor may try to stop preterm labor a number of ways. If your cervix begins to open earlier than it should, your doctor may suggest cerclage. This procedure places a stitch in the opening of the cervix to keep it closed. It is unclear how well it works to stop preterm labor.

Monitoring for Contractions

After about 20 weeks of pregnancy, you may be asked to monitor yourself for signs of uterine activity or tightening. To monitor yourself, lie down and gently feel the entire surface of your lower abdomen with your fingertips. This is called palpation. You are feeling for a firm tightening over the surface of your uterus. In most cases, these feelings of tightening are not painful.

If you feel contractions, turn onto your side and keep monitoring for an hour. Keep track of when each contraction starts and ends and the total number in 1 hour. If you have had very short labor before, you should call your doctor or nurse sooner—don't wait. Having some uterine activity before 37 weeks of pregnancy is normal. But, if your contractions occur more than once every 10 minutes (six or more per hour), you need to call your doctor or nurse right away. You may be in preterm labor.

Keep in mind, a diagnosis of preterm labor can be made only after a pelvic exam to see whether your cervix has begun to change. You should contact your doctor or nurse each time you have more than six contractions per hour, unless he or she has advised otherwise.

Treatment

Sometimes labor can be stopped. Other times, the baby must be delivered. Your doctor may try to stop labor if:

▶ It is detected early enough

▶ You or your baby are not in danger from infection, bleeding, or other complications

Sometimes bed rest and hydration—extra fluids given by mouth or through a

Corticosteroids

If preterm birth seems likely, your doctor will need to decide if the baby's lungs are mature enough to function outside the uterus. Amniocentesis may be used to check your baby's lungs. If the lungs are not mature, they are not coated with enough of a substance called surfactant. Without this coating, the baby may get respiratory distress syndrome. This means the baby has trouble breathing. It is the most common cause of death in preterm babies.

If it looks as though you may have the baby early, you may be given a medication called a corticosteroid. It will increase the amount of surfactant in the amniotic fluid. This helps the baby's lungs mature, reduces bleeding problems, and increases the baby's chance to live. Studies suggest that corticosteroids are most likely to work when preterm labor begins between 24 and 34 weeks of pregnancy.

tube inserted into a vein—are enough to stop contractions. You also may be given medications that stop contractions.

You may be able to go home if you are not really in preterm labor or if labor is stopped, or you may need to stay in the hospital for a while. This depends upon what the doctor's exam reveals and other factors.

You may need to take certain medicines after you have had signs of preterm labor. If you have been prescribed medication, ask about its side effects. If any symptoms persist or are strong, call your doctor. Your medicine may need to be changed.

Tocolytics

Many medications can be used to stop or slow preterm labor. These medications are called tocolytics. It is not always clear which, if any, of these medications should be used. As with all medications, tocolytics can have side effects. Each woman responds in her own way. Side effects can include:

- Fast pulse
- Chest pressure or pain
- Feeling dizzy
- Headache
- Feeling warm
- Feeling shaky or nervous

Limit Your Activity

If you have had preterm labor, your doctor may suggest limits on activity. If you have a job that requires heavy lifting or standing a lot, it may require some changes. You may have to stop working.

The kinds of limits advised can vary. It may be partial bed rest. This means you can get up, go to the bathroom, and have limited activity. It may mean staying off your feet and not doing certain activities, such as climbing stairs, or it may be total bed rest.

For most women, having to limit your activity week after week is very hard. You may feel moody, helpless, and depressed. Sometimes you may feel that the frustration and boredom just aren't worth it. You may be tempted to resume your activities. It can be hard for you to take care of your other children and spend time with your partner and friends.

If you must limit your activity, structure your life to help lessen your frustration. Arrange for help with housework, shopping, and older children. Don't be afraid to rely on others for support.

Because you will be less active, you may need to make changes in your diet so you take in fewer calories. High-fiber foods and plenty of fluids will help prevent constipation.

If bed rest is prescribed, plan your days to include a change into day clothes and tasks that you can do in bed. You may want to talk to your doctor about exercises you can do in bed to improve your circulation.

Preterm Delivery

Sometimes preterm labor may be too far along to be stopped, or there may be reasons that the baby is better off being born, even if it is early. These can include:

▶ Infection

▶ High blood pressure

▶ Bleeding

▶ Signs that the fetus may be having problems

Preterm labor, delivery, and care of the baby require care in a hospital with special facilities. You or your baby may be moved to a different hospital that can provide this expert care. Preterm babies may be delivered by cesarean birth, in which the baby is born through a cut made in the mother's abdomen and uterus.

Your Preterm Baby

Many preterm babies are tiny and fragile. The baby may need special medical care to breathe, eat, and keep warm. It depends on how early he or she is born. Preterm babies can have physical and mental disabilities that can be long term. Babies born before 32 weeks of pregnancy are most at risk.

Preterm babies may not be ready to live on their own. They may be cared for in a Neonatal Intensive Care Unit (NICU) for weeks and sometimes months. Preterm babies often are kept in an incubator to keep them warm. They are cared for by specially trained nurses and doctors. Today, with special NICU care, even very early, tiny babies have a much better chance of survival than in the past. In spite of the best medical care, though, not all babies survive.

Physical Features

Preterm babies often weigh less than 5½ pounds at birth (low birth weight). Babies born too early often have organs that are not developed enough to function as they should. For instance, the lungs of a preterm baby are often not fully developed, and the newborn may have trouble getting enough air. This condition is called respiratory distress syndrome (RDS).

Sometimes a woman in preterm labor is given medication to reduce the risks to the baby. Other drugs could be given to the baby after birth to improve breathing. Your baby may be placed on a respirator to help with breathing. Apnea, or interrupted breathing, often occurs in preterm and low-birth-weight babies in the first days or weeks of life.

Your preterm baby may not look like what you expected. Most preterm babies are red and skinny because they have less fat under their skin and their blood vessels are close to the surface. After a few days, your preterm baby may develop jaundice. This causes his or her skin to appear yellow for a short while.

A preterm baby also may have problems with swallowing. This means he or she may need to be fed through a tube. You may need to express or pump your breasts to provide breast milk for your baby. Preterm babies who are fed breast milk gain weight at a slower rate than those fed formula, but the benefits of breast milk outweigh the benefits of increased weight.

The rate of preterm births has not changed over the past 40 years. Despite a great deal of research and use of new methods of treatment, it is hard to prevent preterm labor.

Emotional Needs

Hospitals are often busy, crowded places. At first, you may feel that everyone else is taking care of your baby and there is no place for you. You may wish for privacy. You may feel frightened and awkward. These feelings are normal. Talk to the nurses and doctors caring for your baby. They will help you with any questions you may have and advise you on how often you should visit the baby.

Your baby needs to hear your voice and to feel your touch. Contact with the baby is important for the parents, too. As soon as you can, talk to your baby. Stroke him or her in the incubator. After a while, you may be able to hold and cuddle your baby for a longer time and help with the baby's care.

Care at Home

If you have a preterm delivery, you will be shown how to care for your new baby. Preterm babies often need special—and different—care. Preterm babies usually require more doctor visits in the first few months at home. This may include special eye and ear exams. You may have to give your baby special medicines, vitamins, or feeding supplements.

Some preterm babies can leave the hospital but need to take extra oxygen at home. You may need to watch for signs of breathing problems (such as wheezing or congestion). Sometimes monitors can be used to check the baby's breathing. You should be prepared to perform infant cardiopulmonary resuscitation (CPR) in case of an emergency.

A standard infant car seat may not be safe to use. It depends on the size of your baby. There are special car seats designed for smaller babies. Discuss this with your doctor.

Your preterm baby may be more irritable, more active, and more dependent on you than other children would be. Be patient and get support when you need it. There are many support services to help you. The hospital staff can discuss this with you.

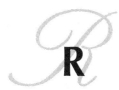

▎ RAPE

Rape means being forced to have sex against your will. Rape can range from touching your body to forced sexual intercourse. Rape is a crime, even if the attacker is a friend or family member. When a date or boyfriend assaults you sexually, the common term used is "date rape."

Rape can happen to anyone, even children and seniors. Women are the most common victims of rape, but men can be raped, too. Many rapists are driven by a need for power. They prey on women to gain a sense of control.

If you are raped, get to a safe place as soon as you can. Then go to the hospital emergency room. You can call the police from there. Do not wash your body or change your clothes before you go to the hospital.

The doctor will check you for injuries and do a blood test. You will be checked for pregnancy and for diseases that are passed on through sex. If you take birth control pills or have an intrauterine device (IUD), most likely you are not pregnant. If not, or just to be extra safe, you may want to take emergency contraception. There is a 5–10% chance of getting a sexually transmitted disease from rape. You also will be checked for evidence, such as hairs or semen, to help identify your attacker.

Being raped can have a major effect on your life. It can make you feel scared and depressed. Tell your doctor about any physical, emotional, or sexual problems you may have after the rape. Some women who are raped have trouble coping afterward. During the hours or sometimes even days after the rape, you may have "rape-trauma" syndrome. You may be anxious, angry, or scared. You may not be able to cope. You also may have body or pelvic pain, headaches, trouble sleeping, and loss of appetite. Later, you may have flashbacks and nightmares of the incident. There are many support services to help you, including social workers and rape crisis counselors.

Some safety tips to help prevent rape include the following:

▎ Replace locks when you move into a new home.

▎ Keep doors locked at all times and don't open them to anyone you don't know. Never admit that you are home alone.

▎ Ask all strangers to show an ID. If a repairman shows up uninvited, call his office to verify his reason for being there before letting him in.

There have been reports of a drug called flunitrazepam (sometimes called "roofies") being used to make women black out. During this time they may be raped or assaulted and cannot remember what happened to them when they wake up. This drug can be slipped into a drink without causing any odor or taste. It is banned in the United States, but is brought in illegally. Other drugs have been linked to rape and date rape as well. Always watch what you eat and drink when you are at parties or among strangers.

- Be aware of your surroundings and of the people around you.

- Lock your car doors and windows. Carry a flashlight, cellular phone or quarters for a phone call, and a small amount of cash for emergencies.

- Don't walk alone at night. If you are followed, go to the nearest police or fire station, or go to any well-lit place where you will find other people.

- If you sense you are in danger, run away. Yell or scream to attract attention.

- Use any available items, such as keys or your purse, as a weapon to resist your attacker.

If you are threatened or assaulted and need emergency help, call 911. You also can call the national 24-hour toll-free hotline numbers: 800-799-SAFE (7233) and 800-787-3224 (TDD).

▶ RH FACTOR

- See also *Anemia, Blood Types*

Just as there are different major blood groups, such as A and B type blood, there is also an Rh factor. The Rh factor is a type of protein on the surface of red blood cells. Most people have the Rh factor—they are Rh positive. Others do not have the Rh factor—they are Rh negative. A simple lab test can tell whether you are Rh positive or Rh negative.

More than 85% of people in the world are Rh positive. The Rh factor does not affect a person's general health. It can cause problems during pregnancy, though. Problems can arise when the fetus's blood has the Rh factor and the mother's blood does not. These problems can be prevented in most cases with the use of a special drug.

When Does the Rh Factor Cause Problems?

The Rh factor causes problems when an Rh-negative person's blood comes in contact with Rh-positive blood. If this occurs, the person with Rh-negative blood may become sensitized. This means he or she produces antibodies to fight the Rh factor as if it were a harmful substance.

An Rh-negative woman can become sensitized if she is pregnant with an Rh-positive fetus. If a pregnant woman's blood group is Rh negative, knowing whether the father is Rh positive or Rh negative will help find the risk of Rh sensitization. An Rh-negative mother and an Rh-positive father can conceive an Rh-positive child.

During pregnancy, mother and fetus do not share blood systems. Blood from the fetus can cross the placenta into the mother's system, though. When this occurs, a small number of pregnant women with Rh-negative blood who carry an Rh-pos-

The Rh Factor

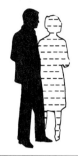

- Rh-negative
+ Rh-positive
⊕ Antibodies

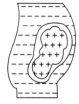

1st pregnancy: An Rh-negative woman may have an Rh-positive fetus.

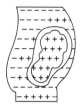

Cells from Rh-positive fetus enter the mother's bloodstream. Woman may become sensitized—antibodies form to fight Rh-positive cells.

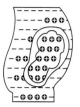

2nd pregnancy: In the next Rh-positive pregnancy, antibodies attack fetal blood cells.

itive fetus will react as if they were allergic to the fetal blood. They become sensitized by making antibodies. These antibodies go back to the fetus and attack the fetal blood. They break down the fetus's red blood cells and produce anemia (the blood has a low number of red blood cells). This condition is called hemolytic disease or hemolytic anemia. It can become severe enough to cause serious illness, brain damage, or even death in the fetus or newborn.

Once formed, these antibodies do not go away. In a first pregnancy with an Rh-positive fetus, the baby often is born before the mother's body develops many antibodies. A small number of these pregnancies start having problems during the last 3 months.

In a second pregnancy with an Rh-positive fetus, the antibodies are more likely to cause hemolytic disease in the fetus. In most cases, the condition becomes worse in later pregnancies.

Sensitization can occur any time the fetus's blood mixes with the mother's blood. It can occur if an Rh-negative woman has once had:

▶ A miscarriage

▶ An induced abortion or menstrual extraction

▶ An ectopic pregnancy

▶ Chorionic villus sampling

A woman also can become sensitized if she has ever had a blood transfusion.

How Can Problems Be Prevented?

A simple blood test can tell a woman's blood type and Rh factor. Another blood test, called an antibody screen, can show if an Rh-negative woman has developed antibodies to Rh-positive blood.

Hemolytic disease can be prevented if the Rh-negative woman has not made antibodies against the Rh factor. Rh immunoglobulin (RhIg) is a blood product that can prevent sensitization of an Rh-negative mother. It keeps her body from being able to respond to Rh-positive cells.

RhIg, first used in 1968, is safe and easily obtained. Its use can prevent sensitization in almost all cases. RhIg is not helpful if the mother is already sensitized, though.

If an Rh-negative woman is given RhIg, it likely will be injected into a muscle of the arm or buttocks. RhIg is safe for a pregnant woman to use. The only known side effects are a soreness where the drug was injected or a slight fever. Both side effects will go away.

When Is RhIg Used?

During Pregnancy and After Delivery

If a woman with Rh-negative blood has not been sensitized, her doctor may suggest that she receive RhIg around the 28th week of pregnancy to prevent sensitization for the rest of the pregnancy. This takes care of the small number of women who can become sensitized during the last 3 months of pregnancy.

Shortly after birth, if the child has Rh-positive blood, the mother should be given another dose of RhIg. In almost all cases, this treatment prevents the woman from making antibodies to the Rh-positive cells she may have received from her fetus before and during delivery. No treatment is needed if the father or baby is also Rh negative.

The treatment is good only for the pregnancy in which it is given. Each pregnancy and delivery of an Rh-positive child requires repeat doses of RhIg.

Rh-negative women also should receive treatment after any miscarriage, ectopic pregnancy, or induced abortion. This prevents any chance of the woman developing antibodies that would attack a future Rh-positive fetus.

Other Reasons RhIg May Be Given

Amniocentesis. Amniocentesis is a procedure in which a small amount of amniotic fluid (the fluid in the sac that surrounds the fetus) is withdrawn from the mother's uterus through a needle for testing. This can help detect certain birth defects in the fetus during pregnancy. If and when this is done, fetal Rh-positive red blood cells could mix with a mother's Rh-negative blood. This would cause her to produce antibodies. Thus, RhIg is given.

Postpartum Sterilization. An Rh-negative mother may receive RhIg after a birth even if she decides to have her fallopian tubes

Because RhIg's effects last only about 12 weeks, it is given again any time blood from the fetus and mother might mix.

tied and cut to prevent future pregnancies. Treatment might be given for three reasons:

1. The woman may decide later to try to have the sterilization reversed.

2. There is a slight chance that the sterilization may fail to prevent pregnancy.

3. The treatment prevents her from developing antibodies in case she ever needs to be given a blood transfusion in the future. The presence of antibodies makes matching blood types for transfusions harder.

RhIg is not always given in this instance. A woman should talk to her doctor about it.

What Happens if Antibodies Develop?

Once a woman develops antibodies, RhIg treatment does not help. Doctors are finding ways to save infants who get hemolytic disease. A mother who is Rh-sensitized will be checked during her pregnancy to see if the fetus is developing the disease.

In some cases of hemolytic disease, the doctor may suggest delivery at the normal time. Delivery may be followed by a type of transfusion for the baby that will replace the diseased blood cells with healthy blood. For more severe cases, the baby may be delivered early or given transfusions while still in the mother's uterus.

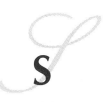

S

See also *Nutrition During Pregnancy*

▶ SEIZURE DISORDERS IN PREGNANCY

A woman who has a seizure disorder (also called epilepsy) may need to take medication to prevent seizures. Women with a seizure disorder who want to have a baby should work with their doctor to adjust their medication before and during pregnancy. Today, most women with a seizure disorder who become pregnant have healthy babies.

Seizure Disorders and Women

The nerve cells in the brain produce electrical impulses, which send messages throughout the body. These messages control the body's movements and functions. In a person with a seizure disorder, there is abnormal electrical activity in the brain. This causes the seizure.

Hormones can have an effect on seizure disorders. For women, this includes the sex hormones that control the reproductive system: estrogen and progesterone. Changes in these levels of hormones can make seizures more or less likely. Some women will have changes in seizure patterns when hormone levels shift, such as during pregnancy.

Treatment

Medications to treat seizure disorders are called antiepileptic drugs (AEDs), or "antiseizure" drugs. In most cases, AEDs will prevent seizures all or most of the time. You may have to try more than one AED before you find the right one for you.

Pregnancy can change your pattern of seizures and how your body reacts to AEDs. For this reason, women with seizure disorders should consult their obstetrician–gynecologist and neurologist if they are pregnant or planning pregnancy. They will need to receive special care before and during pregnancy.

Medications taken during pregnancy can affect a growing fetus. Seizures also can harm the fetus as well as the mother. If you are pregnant, it may be better to stay on AEDs than to risk having a seizure during pregnancy.

If a woman has not had a seizure in 2 or more years, she may be able to slowly stop taking her AED before she tries to become pregnant. Working closely with her doctor, the amount of AED may be reduced over several months. As many as half of women will need to go back on the AED after childbirth. You will need to discuss this with your neurologist.

AEDs affect the way the body uses folic acid. Not having enough folic acid has been linked to problems during pregnancy and to certain birth defects. Taking folic acid before and during the first weeks of pregnancy may decrease the risk of these problems.

Risks for the Mother

There is a chance that seizures will occur more often during pregnancy. This happens to as many as one third of women, even though they are taking an AED.

Because a pregnant woman who is taking AEDs for a seizure disorder is at an increased risk of having a child with neural tube defects, she should be sure to have 0.4 milligrams of folic acid a day.

The amount of medication you take may change during your pregnancy. This is because of hormone changes and changes in how the body processes AEDs during pregnancy. Levels of AEDs should be watched to keep them constant. If levels are too high, it can lead to side effects. If levels are too low, it can lead to seizures. You may have blood tests during pregnancy to check levels of the drug.

Women with seizure disorders are more likely to have other pregnancy problems. This includes high blood pressure as a result of pregnancy. Also, seizures can cause serious falls or other accidents, which may result in injury.

Risks for the Baby

Most babies are born healthy. In all women, the risk of having a baby with a birth defect is 2–3%. For women with a seizure disorder, the risk is slightly higher—6–8%. The risk may be related to the medication used, the disorder itself, or both. The direct cause often may not be known.

The medication needed to control seizures may cause birth defects. Such defects may include changes in the face, fingers, and nails. Other birth defects linked to seizure disorders include:

▶ Cleft lip or palate (the lip or roof of the mouth is not completely closed)

▶ Heart problems

▶ Neural tube defects (such as spine defects)

Babies born to women with a seizure disorder may be at higher risk for certain health problems:

▶ Low birth weight (small baby)

▶ Small head

▶ Delays in growth and development

▶ Bleeding (blood-clotting) problems

Children of women with a seizure disorder are at an increased risk for having a seizure disorder themselves. The reason for this is unclear.

After the Baby Is Born

After delivery, you may find the need to once again adjust your medication. You may wonder about the effects of AEDs on breastfeeding. For more information, see the box.

You also will want to choose a method of birth control. Many AEDs change hormone levels in your body. This can affect how well birth control methods work. The use of some AEDs may make birth control pills not work as well. You may need to change your method of hormonal birth control. Methods that do not use hormones are not affected by the use of AEDs.

You may want to use a barrier method (diaphragm, spermicide, or condoms) along with the hormonal method. Talk with your doctor about your AED and its effect on your birth control choices.

Breastfeeding

Most women with a seizure disorder can breastfeed their babies. AEDs are found in small amounts in breast milk, but in most cases this is not enough to affect the baby.

Some medications may make babies sleepy or cranky. If this happens, talk with your doctor and your baby's doctor. You may wish to use bottle feedings also. You may choose to pump and store your breast milk.

Breastfeeding may disrupt your sleep patterns. This can affect seizure activity. You may wish to have someone else—a partner, friend, or family member—bottle feed the baby at night with breast milk. Before you stop breastfeeding, discuss it with your doctor.

▶ SELECTIVE ESTROGEN RECEPTOR MODULATORS

▶ See also *Hormone Replacement Therapy, Menopause* in *"Women's Bodies,"* Osteoporosis

As a woman ages, her body makes less of the hormone estrogen and many changes occur. At menopause, the lack of estrogen may cause thinning of the bones (osteoporosis) and heart disease. Some women choose to take replacement estrogen to help prevent these problems. Women also can take selective estrogen receptor modulators (SERMs), which work like estrogen but have important differences.

What Are SERMs?

Selective estrogen receptor modulators are a type of medication that strengthen tissues of the heart and bones. Because SERMs target specific areas, they can treat only the areas that need to be treated. SERMs don't have an affect on the breast and uterus, the way hormone replacement therapy (HRT) does.

Some types of SERMs can be used for treating such conditions as breast cancer or infertility. SERMs also can help prevent bone loss that occurs during menopause. SERMs also decrease total cholesterol and "bad" cholesterol (LDL). They do not increase "good" cholesterol (HDL) levels, though. However, SERMs still may help reduce the risk of heart disease.

Tamoxifen may be a good treatment for women with breast cancer who do not have a uterus. Not having a uterus means there is no risk of endometrial cancer, one of the main risks of taking tamoxifen.

SERMs may be a good choice for women who need protection from osteoporosis or heart disease but can't or don't want to take HRT. This may include:

▶ Women at risk of breast or uterine cancer

▶ Women who can't tolerate the side effects of HRT

▶ Women who don't need relief from symptoms of menopause, such as hot flushes and vaginal dryness

Types of SERMs

Tamoxifen is one of the most widely known SERMs. Tamoxifen is used to prevent and treat breast cancer in women of all ages. Tamoxifen helps protect bones, but not as much as estrogen does. It also may protect the heart and blood vessels because it decreases total cholesterol levels. However, tamoxifen may increase the risk of endometrial cancer and polyps.

Raloxifene is a SERM used to prevent and treat osteoporosis. Raloxifene may reduce the risk of breast cancer, without increasing the risk of endometrial cancer. It helps build strong bones to protect against osteoporosis. Raloxifene also lowers total and LDL cholesterol levels. Side effects may include hot flushes and leg cramps. Like estrogen, in rare cases it may cause blood clots.

▶ See also *Pain During Sex, Sexuality* in *"Women's Bodies"*

▶ SEXUAL PROBLEMS

Many women have trouble with sex at some time in their lives. They often find it hard to talk about their sexual concerns—even with their partner, a trusted friend, or their doctor.

Sexual Problems

A woman's progress through the sexual response cycle varies greatly from one time to another. No one pattern is more "normal" than another. If any of the stages of the cycle do not occur, though, it may cause a sexual problem.

Sexual response depends on a complex interplay—physical and emotional—between two people. Because of this complex process, it's no surprise that problems with sex can happen. Sexual problems can be long-standing, or they can arise quickly. Some sexual problems are common among both women and men.

Sexual problems can be linked to a physical condition, such as pregnancy or an illness. They also can relate to daily stress, poor communication between partners, unrealistic ideas about sexual performance, or problems with trust and commitment.

Sildenafil and Women

In 1998, sildenafil (Viagra) was released on the market and became an overnight success among the many men seeking relief from erectile dysfunction (impotence). Studies have not shown it to be effective in women.

Conflicts can make it hard to have or enjoy sex. These conflicts can be within a woman herself or between her and her partner.

If problems in a relationship occur often, it's likely that they will lead to a sexual problem. Sometimes the problem is about sex only. The partner may not know what to do to please the woman or the woman does not respond. Talking between partners is the first step toward a healthy sex life.

Lack of Desire

Lack of interest in sex—or lack of desire—is the most common sexual problem in women. With a low level of sexual desire, a woman may have a hard time getting aroused.

Many women find that the stresses of daily living—such as concerns about work, family, and money—can create a lack of desire. A woman who has trouble having an orgasm may begin to think she cannot have one. This can cause her to lose interest in sex.

Women who have been abused or have had bad experiences with sex may find it hard to enjoy sex or to become aroused. Many women and men have a lack of desire at some point in their lives.

Lack of Orgasm

Most women are able to have an orgasm during sexual activity. Some may reach orgasm by masturbation or by having their partner arouse them with their hands or with oral sex.

Some women have a hard time reaching orgasm. This may result from not knowing what to do or how to tell their partners what they want. The woman and her partner may not know that orgasm can only happen with high levels of arousal, or the woman may have trouble talking with her partner about the best ways to touch and arouse her.

Problems with reaching orgasm can stem from negative feelings about sex learned in childhood. Women who have suffered a trauma related to sex, such as sexual abuse, may not be able to reach orgasm. Other causes may include:

▶ Fear of having pleasure or feeling "safe" with someone

▶ Anger

▶ Depression

▶ Use of medications, drugs, or alcohol

Some couples place too much importance on having an orgasm during sex. This focus on performance or technique—and not mutual pleasure—often lessens sexual excitement. The pressure to reach orgasm can create anxiety and distractions. This can cause lack of orgasm.

In a survey of sexual practices in the United States, 75% of men and 29% of women reported having an orgasm every time they had sex. About 1% of men and 4% of women reported rarely or never having an orgasm during sex. The survey also revealed that a person can feel sexually satisfied without having an orgasm.

Most women who do have orgasms don't always do so through sex alone. They need more stimulation to be aroused than sex alone provides. The stimulation may include kissing and caressing, as well as stroking and touching sensitive areas such as the breast and clitoris.

If a woman has no orgasm during sex, it does not mean it was a failure. Sharing love, closeness, warmth, and tenderness are often enough.

Painful Sex

Dyspareunia is a term for pain during sex. This may include pain during entry into the vagina, pain during deep thrusting, or pain after sex. The pain can be on the surface or deep, along the middle of the pelvis or on one or both sides.

Most sexually active women have had pain during sex at some point in their lives. The most common cause is that the vagina is not well lubricated. This can occur because of:

▶ Medication

▶ Illness

▶ Lack of arousal

▶ Infections

▶ Cysts or tumors

▶ Endometriosis

It also may occur because a woman lacks the hormone estrogen.

Vaginismus also can cause pain during sex. This is a spasm of the pubic muscles and lower vagina. It makes entering the vagina painful. In some cases, vaginismus is present the first time a woman has—or tries to have—sex. In some women, the pain is related only to sex. For others, the pain is so great that they cannot even have a pelvic exam by a doctor.

Vaginismus can have many medical causes. These include:

▶ Painful scars in the vaginal opening from injury, childbirth, or surgery

▶ Irritation from douches, spermicides, or the latex in condoms

▶ Pelvic infections

This condition also can be caused by a response to a fear of some kind, such as fear of losing control or fear of pregnancy. It also can stem from pain or trauma, such as rape or sexual abuse. In most cases, your doctor can treat this condition with success.

Conditions That Can Affect Sexual Function

Some conditions can have a big impact on sexuality. They may be short term, such as the flu or pregnancy, or may persist over time and require the couple to adjust.

Pregnancy

In most cases, sexual activity doesn't have to change during pregnancy. Sex does not harm the fetus unless certain conditions are present. Your doctor will discuss this with you. In the weeks after the baby's birth, a mixture of fatigue, changing hormone levels, and perhaps an episiotomy that is still healing may prevent couples from having sex. Couples can have sex again when the doctor says or when the woman feels ready.

If you are pregnant, you may worry that having sex will harm your baby. The fetus is safe in the uterus. Don't worry that a penis will poke or jab it.

Menopause

As women approach menopause, they may lose desire slowly, have a hard time getting aroused, and feel pain during sex. The lack of estrogen that occurs after menopause makes the vagina dry. Vaginal lubricants can help moisten the vagina and make sex more comfortable. Women may wish to take estrogen to help restore the vagina's flexibility and prevent other problems linked to low estrogen levels.

Cancer

Women with cancer often worry about how the disease will affect their sex life. Surgery, radiation, and chemotherapy can be painful and sap the woman's energy. She may struggle with fears of death, disfigurement, or the partner's rejection. The partner may be concerned that she may be injured during sex. Counseling before, during, and after treatment can help the couple deal with these problems.

Chronic Illness

Diseases that persist for a lifetime, such as diabetes, arthritis, or heart disease, can have a major impact on a woman's self-image and her ability to feel sexual. Some medications can affect her desire or make it hard to reach orgasm. A doctor may be able to switch medications or give advice to the woman and her partner.

Male Factor

If a male partner is having sexual problems, pleasure for both partners may be affected. Many men have trouble with impotence—not being able to achieve or keep an erection—at some time in their lives.

Impotence affects about 18 million men in the United States alone. Medication and lifestyle changes—such as stopping smoking, changing medications, or counseling—may improve symptoms in some men.

Impotence is usually caused by physical or medical factors. It often occurs as a side effect of some medications or alcohol and drug use. Stress, anger, or depression also can lead to impotence. In many cases, impotence comes and goes or can be reversed. Despite the cause, impotence can be a serious problem for couples and should be discussed with their doctors.

A doctor may suggest your partner take a medication called sildenafil. It causes more blood flow to the penis. This allows many men to achieve and maintain an erection. This medication treats the physical problem—it does not increase desire in men.

If your partner is prescribed sildenafil, you may want to use a lubricant when you have sex. This is even more true if you have not had sex for a while or are in or near menopause. Also, if your relationship has been nonsexual for a while, you and your partner may want to talk about how you feel before you have sex.

Men should not take sildenafil if it is not prescribed to them. It is not safe to use with some conditions and medications.

If You Think You Have a Problem

Nearly every couple has a problem with sex at some time in their lives. Some problems go away on their own or can be worked out with patience and a caring and informed partner. Others may take more effort and a change of approach.

If you think you may have a health condition that is stopping you from enjoying sex, see your doctor. Any pain in the pelvic, genital, or vaginal area is a sign that there may be a problem.

If your relationship or sexual problem is new, try an open, honest talk with your partner to relieve worries and clear up conflicts. Women who learn how to better tell their partners about their sexual needs and concerns have a better chance of having a good sex life. There are also many good books with useful tips to help you discuss problems in new ways.

If you suspect a sexual problem stems from feelings you don't understand or can't cope with—like shyness, fear, conflict, or guilt—there are many people with the skills and kindness to help.

Your doctor may be able to help you. Your doctor also can refer you to other experts. Sex counseling for individuals or couples is often short term and works well. The approach used in counseling depends on the problem. You may learn exercises to do at home alone or with your partner. The counselor may teach ways to help you relax, communicate better, and find out what gives you pleasure. You also may explore feelings that affect arousal or orgasm, such as anger or fear.

Your doctor or counselor also may refer you to a support group. Such groups can be helpful because they allow women and couples to talk about their concerns with others who have the same problems. It may help to know you are not alone.

▶ SEXUALLY TRANSMITTED DISEASES

▶ See also *Condoms*

Sexually transmitted diseases (STDs) are infections that are spread by sexual contact. Except for colds and flu, STDs are the most common contagious diseases in the United States, with about 12 million new cases of STDs each year. Some STDs can be cured. Others cannot.

Prevention is the key to fighting STDs. By knowing the facts, you can take steps to protect your health.

About STDs

Anyone who has sex with another person can get an STD. People with an STD may not know they have it. Often there are no symptoms. But that does not mean that it is not affecting your health.

STDs can cause severe damage to your body—even death. Even if there are no symptoms, a person with an STD can pass it to others by contact with skin, genitals, mouth, rectum, or body fluids.

Symptoms of an STD can range from mild irritation to severe pain. Often, symptoms occur only as the disease becomes more advanced. In most cases, the long-term health problems can be avoided by early treatment.

STDs are caused by being infected with tiny organisms. Those caused by bacteria are treated with antibiotics. Infections caused by viruses often cannot be cured, but symptoms can be treated.

If you suspect you may have been exposed to an STD, ask your doctor for advice. Even if there are no symptoms, a doctor can diagnose an STD. Tests can be done to detect infection. Anyone who is sexually active should know about these STDs and how to protect against them.

Gonorrhea and Chlamydia

Each year, about 800,000 people in the United States are infected with gonorrhea. About 4 million get chlamydia. These two diseases often occur at the same time.

Many women and men with gonorrhea and chlamydia have few or no symptoms. If symptoms do appear, however, they may appear from 2 days to 3 weeks after contact with an infected person. Symptoms may include:

▶ A discharge from a woman's vagina or a man's penis

▶ Painful or frequent urination

▶ Pain in the pelvis or abdomen

▶ Fever or chills

▶ Nausea or vomiting

▶ Burning or itching in the vaginal area

▶ Redness or swelling of the vulva

▶ Pain in the joints

▶ Sore throat

If not treated, both chlamydia and gonorrhea can cause pelvic inflammatory disease (PID) in women. PID is an infection of the uterus, fallopian tubes, and ovaries. It is the most common preventable cause of infertility in the United States. Symptoms of PID are fever, nausea and vomiting, and pain in the abdomen. PID can lead to long-term pelvic pain.

Human Papillomavirus

Human papillomavirus (HPV) is a virus that can cause genital warts. It is one of the most common STDs in the United States.

A person can be infected with HPV but have no warts. The virus can remain in the body for weeks or years without showing any symptoms.

Sometimes warts go away on their own. Several treatments for warts are available. But, even after the warts have cleared up, the virus may be present.

The HPV virus has been linked to some types of cancer, including those of the cervix and vulva. Regular Pap tests can help detect early signs of cervical cancer.

Syphilis

If not treated, syphilis can infect many parts of the body, causing major health problems—even death. Most people have no symptoms of syphilis. The first sign of syphilis may be a painless, smooth sore at the site of the infection. Syphilis is easily treated in this early stage.

Without treatment, the symptoms may go away, but the disease will remain. Years later, it can return in full force.

Genital Herpes

Genital herpes may be the most common STD of all. As many as 30 million Americans may now carry the herpes virus.

The most common symptom of herpes is sores on or around the genitals. These appear as red spots, bumps, or blisters. They last from a few days to a few weeks.

Are STDs Increasing or Decreasing in the United States?

It depends on the disease. Recent data show that chlamydia is decreasing in areas with screening and treatment programs, but infection rates remain high. Syphilis and gonorrhea have reached all-time lows and infection rates continue to decrease. Hepatitis B is decreasing and so is trichomoniasis. Herpes is believed to be increasing, with high rates recorded in the early 1990s. Human papillomavirus is widespread, but researchers are unsure if infection rates are increasing.

The symptoms go away by themselves, but the virus remains in your body. The sores may come back at any time, usually in the same place they first occurred. Treatment can help heal the sores, but it cannot kill the virus.

HIV Infection

The human immunodeficiency virus (HIV) is a virus that causes acquired immunodeficiency syndrome (AIDS). The rate of HIV infection is increasing most rapidly among women who have sex with men.

HIV enters the bloodstream by way of body fluids, usually blood or semen. Once in the blood, the virus invades and kills cells of the immune system—the body's natural defense against disease.

HIV weakens the immune system, leading to AIDS. With AIDS, a person's immune system is so weak that it can no longer fight off infections.

Treatment may decrease your risk of getting AIDS. The disease is most often fatal.

On average, it takes about 11 years from the time of HIV infection to develop AIDS. In some cases, though, it takes much less time. Because symptoms do not appear right away, a person may not know that he or she is infected with HIV. Someone who looks healthy can carry the virus for years without knowing it and can pass it to others.

Trichomonas Vaginitis

Trichomonas is a microscopic parasite that affects the vagina. It is spread through sex. Some women who have trichomonas vaginitis are at a higher risk of infection with other STDs. It can be cured.

Hepatitis B

Hepatitis B is a serious infection of the liver caused by the hepatitis B virus. The disease can be fatal. It is spread by direct contact with the body fluids (blood, semen, vaginal fluids) of an infected person. There is no cure.

How to Protect Yourself from STDs

The factors listed in the box increase the risk of an STD. If any apply to you, protect yourself.

The only sure way to prevent getting an STD is not to have sex. If you do have sex, you can reduce your risk:

▶ *Know and limit your sexual partners*—Your partner's sexual history is as important as your own. The more partners you or your partners have, the higher your risk of getting an STD.

▶ *Use a latex condom*—Using a latex condom every time you have sex lowers the chances of infection.

▶ See also: *Sexually Transmitted Diseases*

Are You at Risk?

You are at high risk for getting an STD if you:

▶ Are an adolescent who is sexually active

▶ Have many sexual partners

▶ Have a partner who has many sexual partners

▶ Have sexual intercourse with someone who has an STD

▶ Have a history of STDs

▶ *Use a spermicide*—Most birth control creams, jellies, and foams contain a chemical called nonoxynol 9 that may help guard against some STDs. Used with a condom, they may offer some protection.

▶ *Avoid risky sex practices*—Sexual acts that tear or break the skin carry a higher risk of STDs. Even small cuts that don't bleed let germs in and out. Anal sex poses a high risk because tissues in the rectum break easily.

▶ *Get immunized*—A vaccination is available that will help prevent hepatitis B.

▶ SEXUALLY TRANSMITTED DISEASES IN PREGNANCY

Sexually transmitted diseases (STDs) are infections that are passed from person to person during sex. All STDs can lead to serious problems. Some STDs are even more harmful during pregnancy (Table 23). For instance, if you have an STD, you are more likely to have preterm labor and an inflammation of the uterus called endometritis.

If you think you may have an STD, get tested and treated right away. Your partner also should be treated. Neither of you should have sex until you have finished treatment.

Chlamydia, Gonorrhea, and Pelvic Inflammatory Disease

Chlamydia and gonorrhea are the most common STDs in the United States. If you have these diseases, you can be treated with antibiotics, even during pregnancy.

Pregnant women who are infected have an increased chance of having their membranes break early and having the baby before it is fully mature. Some women may even have a miscarriage.

Chlamydia and gonorrhea can infect the fetus as it passes through the vagina during birth. They can cause eye infection and other problems. A newborn's eyes are an easy target for gonorrhea. To prevent damage, the eyes of all newborns are treated at birth whether or not the mother has gonorrhea.

Table 23. How Sexually Transmitted Diseases Can Affect You and Your Baby

Disease	Symptoms in Women	Effects on:	
		Mother	Fetus/Baby
AIDS*	May have no symptoms; appetite or weight loss, fatigue, swollen lymph nodes, night sweats, fever or chills, persistent diarrhea or cough	Immune system damage, leading to infections (such as pneumonia) or cancers; death	Immune system damage leading to death in as early as 3 years in some infants
Chlamydia	May have no symptoms; vaginal discharge, painful or frequent urination, pelvic pain	Endometritis or postpartum infection, preterm labor, pelvic inflammatory disease, ectopic pregnancy	Eye infection, pneumonia
Genital herpes	Flulike symptoms (fever, chills, muscle aches); small, painful, fluid-filled blisters on genitals or buttocks	Recurrent outbreaks	Severe skin infection, nervous system damage, blindness, mental retardation, death
Genital warts	Possible genital itching, irritation, or bleeding; warts may appear as small, cauliflower-shaped clusters	Warts grow in size and number; may have abnormal Pap test	Warts on the vocal cords in early adolescence
Gonorrhea	Most women have no symptoms; vaginal discharge, minor genital irritation, pain and fever	Pelvic inflammatory disease, arthritis	Eye infection if left untreated
Syphilis	A painless open sore called a chancre; later rash, sluggishness, or slight fever	Damage to heart, blood vessels, and nervous system; blindness, insanity, death	Miscarriage, stillbirth, syphilis in liveborn infant

*AIDS stands for acquired immunodeficiency syndrome.

Genital Herpes

Some people have only one outbreak of genital herpes. Others have many bouts during their lifetime. In rare cases, babies can become infected with the herpes virus during birth. This can cause severe skin infection, damage to the nervous system, blindness, mental retardation, or death. Infected infants are treated with medication (acyclovir, for instance).

If you have ever had genital herpes or have had sex with someone who has, tell your doctor or nurse. He or she will want to see if you have open lesions. If you have no herpes sores, the baby can be born vaginally. If there are signs of active infection when you are in labor, you may need to have your baby by cesarean birth. Cesarean birth lessens the chance that the baby will come in contact with the virus in the vagina. If the membranes have ruptured a number of hours before birth, the baby still may become infected.

Herpes is spread by direct contact with a person who has active sores. In some cases, the virus can be passed to others even when the sores have healed.

Human Papillomavirus

There is a very slight risk that babies born to mothers with human papillomavirus (HPV) may get the infection. Sometimes it is not found in these babies until adolescence. At that time it affects the larynx (voice box). This is not a reason for cesarean delivery, though.

Genital warts may go away on their own. If there are a lot of them or they are large, your doctor may suggest minor surgery to remove them. This treatment is safe to use during pregnancy in most cases. In some cases, your doctor may suggest you wait until after the baby is born to begin treatment. Your condition will be watched closely during your pregnancy.

Warts can grow in number and size during pregnancy. Rarely, warts can grow so large they block the birth canal or make it very narrow. If this occurs, cesarean birth is needed.

Trichomonas Vaginitis

Trichomonas vaginitis is an STD that affects the vagina. Women may have no symptoms, or they may have a vaginal discharge, burning, and irritation. There may be more problems with premature rupture of membranes and preterm delivery in women who are infected.

Pregnant women can be treated with an antibiotic that is safe to use during pregnancy. This will relieve symptoms, increase the chances of curing it, and make it less likely that the infection will be passed to others.

Syphilis

Syphilis can be hard to detect in women. The sore that marks the site of infection—called a chancre—may be in the vagina where it cannot be seen.

Syphilis can be passed from a pregnant woman's bloodstream to her fetus. This may cause miscarriage, stillbirth, or premature rupture of membranes. If the infant lives, it may be born with syphilis. Infants born with syphilis may have problems of the nervous system, skin, eyes, bones, liver, lungs, or spleen.

Treating an infected pregnant woman with antibiotics will halt further damage to her fetus, but it will not reverse any harm already done. If a woman is treated during the first 3–4 months of pregnancy, most likely the infant will not have any long-term damage. Treating an infected infant after birth will prevent more damage in many cases.

Human Immunodeficiency Virus Infection and Acquired Immunodeficiency Syndrome

Human immunodeficiency virus (HIV) infection and acquired immunodeficiency syndrome (AIDS) can be passed from mother to fetus. Breast milk also can pass the virus. Because with treatment the chance of the fetus being infected is greatly reduced, all pregnant women will be tested for the disease. Results will then be discussed with them.

If a pregnant woman is infected, she can transmit the virus to her fetus. The virus can attack the fetus as early as the eighth week of pregnancy. It also can occur during labor and delivery. Without treatment, about 1 in 4 pregnant women who are infected with HIV pass the virus to their fetuses.

For women who are treated with medication between weeks 14 and 34 of pregnancy, the risk of passing the virus to the fetus is greatly reduced. For best results, the medication should be taken during pregnancy, labor, and delivery, and the infant should take the drug during the first 6 weeks of life. Treatment with certain medications also helps prevent other common problems in the mother, such as infection, preterm labor, and giving birth to a very small baby.

After birth, a mother should take special care not to pass the infection to the baby in other ways. She should not breastfeed her baby. She should be careful not to cause contact of her body fluids with the baby's mucus membranes (the mouth, eyes, nose, and bottom). It is important for the mother to continue her treatment and not infect others. The best way to do this is to practice safe sex or not have sex.

▶ SKIN CANCER

Skin cancer is the most common form of cancer in the United States. Almost half of Americans who live to be 65 years old will develop some form of it. Fair-skinned people are more likely to get skin cancer than dark-skinned people. Too much exposure to ultraviolet light, such as from the sun or tanning lamps, increases your risk. Your risk is also increased if you have a family history of skin cancer.

Skin cancer ranges from basal cell and squamous cell cancer (which are usually curable after simple removal) to melanoma, which is the leading skin cancer killer. Basal cell and squamous cell cancers show up as pale, waxlike, pearly bumps or red, scaly patches.

Melanoma is more serious and needs care right away. It starts with small, molelike growths. The growths get bigger, change color, and get darker. They grow in an irregular—not round—shape and may bleed easily.

Warning signs for any type of skin cancer are:

▶ A change in the size or color of a mole

▶ Scaliness, oozing, or bleeding

▶ Itchiness, tenderness, or pain in or by a bump or mole

▶ A sore that does not heal

Cover Up!

Almost 80% of skin cancers could be prevented by protecting your skin from the sun's rays. Wear a hat, protective clothing, and plenty of sunscreen before you go out.

Taking antibiotics or other types of medicine may make your skin extra sensitive to the sun. Ask your doctor about any drugs you are taking and be sure to protect your skin.

Table 24. Which Sunscreen Is Best For You?

Sunburn and Tanning History	Recommended SPF
Always burns easily; rarely tans	20 to 30
Always burns easily; tans minimally	12 to under 20
Burns moderately; tans gradually	8 to under 12
Burns minimally; always tans well	4 to under 8
Rarely burns, tans easily	2 to under 4

U.S. Food and Drug Administration. Seven Steps to Safer Sunning. Washington, DC: FDA, 1997

To help prevent skin cancer, avoid being out in the sun without sun block, especially between 10 AM and 3 PM. This is when the sun's ultraviolet rays are strongest. Use sun block whenever you engage in outdoor activities and reapply it as needed, especially after swimming. Sun blocks are rated by SPFs (sun protection factors). The higher the SPF number, the more protection it gives. Be careful not to let yourself burn (Table 24). Even one instance of a burn that blisters increases the risk of cancer.

Regular self-exams are the best way to detect skin cancer early. Be sure to look at all parts of your body. Skin cancer can occur on parts not exposed to the sun. Tell your doctor about any changes in skin growths or any new growths. When skin cancer is treated before it spreads, the cure rate is almost 100%.

▸ SLEEPING DISORDERS

Almost 40 million people are affected by long-term sleep disorders each year, and another 20 million have had problems sleeping. Many times trouble falling or staying asleep can be caused by anxiety or stress. Lack of sleep is a problem for many women trying to balance the demands of work, home, and children. Pregnancy and menopause are other times in a woman's life when she may not be able to sleep regularly.

Snoring affects almost 44% of men and 28% of women. It becomes more common as you get older. Studies have shown that women who sleep with men who snore loudly lose about an hour of sleep each night. Sleep disorders not only affect the person who has it, but also their sleeping partner.

Some women may not get enough REM (rapid eye movement) sleep. REM sleep is when dreams occur. A key role of REM sleep is to rest the brain. Without REM sleep, you will not feel rested. When normal sleep rhythms are broken, a woman's moods, health, and ability to cope may be affected. She may have trouble concentrating or become depressed.

There are more than 70 sleep disorders. Most can be treated. The most common sleep disorders include insomnia, sleep apnea, restless legs syndrome, and narcolepsy.

Insomnia

At some point in life, almost everyone has short-term insomnia, the inability to fall or stay asleep. This lack of sleep can result from stress, diet, or many other factors. Insomnia almost always affects how you feel the next day and how well you can perform at your job. This problem is more common in women than men. Insomnia seems to occur more with age. It can sometimes be a symptom of another disorder.

You can often treat insomnia by practicing good sleep habits. Your doctor also may treat your symptoms by prescribing sleeping pills. However, you must be careful. Most sleeping pills stop working after several weeks of daily use. Long-term use of sleeping pills may even affect a good night's sleep.

Sleep Apnea

People who have sleep apnea have trouble breathing during sleep. It most often occurs in older people who are overweight or out of shape. This lack of muscle tone allows the windpipe to collapse while breathing during sleep (when muscles relax). This is called obstructive sleep apnea. People who have this disorder often snore loudly. But not everyone who snores has sleep apnea.

With obstructive sleep apnea, your windpipe collapses and blocks the air flow to the lungs and reduces the oxygen supply

---

Tips for a Good Night's Sleep

Set a schedule

Go to bed at a set time each night and get up at the same time each morning. Disrupting this schedule may lead to insomnia. "Sleeping in" on weekends also makes it harder to wake up early on Monday morning because it re-sets your sleep cycles for a later awakening.

Exercise

Try to exercise 20–30 minutes a day. Daily exercise often helps people sleep, although a workout soon before bedtime may interfere with sleep. For maximum benefit, try to get your exercise about 5–6 hours before going to bed.

Avoid caffeine, nicotine, and alcohol

Avoid drinks that contain caffeine, which acts as a stimulant and keeps people awake. Sources of caffeine include coffee, chocolate, soft drinks, non-herbal teas, diet drugs, and some pain relievers. Smokers tend to sleep very lightly and often wake up in the early morning due to nicotine withdrawal. Alcohol robs people of deep sleep and REM sleep and keeps them in the lighter stages of sleep.

Relax before bed

A warm bath, reading, or another relaxing routine can make it easier to fall asleep. You can train yourself to associate certain restful activities with sleep and make them part of your bedtime ritual.

Sleep until sunlight

If possible, wake up with the sun, or use very bright lights in the morning. Sunlight helps the body's internal biological clock to reset itself each day. Sleep experts recommend exposure to an hour of morning sunlight for people having problems falling asleep.

Don't lie in bed awake

If you can't get to sleep, don't just lie in bed. Do something else, like reading, watching television, or listening to music, until you feel tired. The anxiety of being unable to fall asleep can actually contribute to insomnia.

Control your room temperature

Maintain a comfortable temperature in the bedroom. Extreme temperatures may disrupt sleep or prevent you from falling asleep.

See a doctor if your sleeping problem continues

If you have trouble falling asleep night after night, or if you always feel tired the next day, then you may have a sleep disorder and should see a physician. Your doctor may be able to help you. If not, you likely can find a sleep specialist at a major hospital near you. Most sleep disorders can be treated effectively, so you can finally get that good night's sleep you need.

National Institute of Neurological Disorders and Stroke. Brain Basics: Understanding Sleep. Bethesda, MD: NIH, 1999

to the brain. This struggle to breathe may last anywhere from 10 seconds to a minute. When your oxygen level decreases, the brain sends you a signal to wake up and the windpipe is opened. Many times you just take a short breath and continue sleeping (and snoring). This may be repeated hundreds of times a night. This loss of sleep may cause you to be tired, irritable, or sometimes even depressed. The loss of oxygen can lead to headaches, high blood pressure, and increased risk of heart attacks and stroke. In rare cases, sleep apnea may cause a person to completely stop breathing and even lead to death during sleep.

It is hard for doctors to detect sleep apnea because most people only have symptoms when they are sleeping. Some patients may be referred to a sleep center. A sleep center treats sleeping disorders and has the equipment necessary to perform many tests to diagnose the symptoms. If sleep apnea is diagnosed, there are ways to treat it. Often, symptoms can be treated by losing weight or sleeping on your back. Sometimes surgery is needed to correct the problem. People who have sleep apnea should not use sleeping pills. They can prevent the person from waking up enough to breathe.

Restless Legs Syndrome

Restless legs syndrome (RLS) is a disorder that causes a prickling or tingling feeling in the legs and feet and an urge to move them for relief. This disorder is more common among older people, but it can affect people of all ages. RLS can lead to constant leg movement during the day and insomnia at night. It may also affect women who are pregnant, anemic, or diabetic. RLS often can be relieved by medication.

Narcolepsy

People with narcolepsy have sudden attacks of sleep. This may happen many times a day, even if they have had enough nighttime sleep. These attacks last from several seconds to 30 minutes or more. There are many side effects of narcolepsy including sudden loss of muscle control that causes the person to fall on the floor (cataplexy), hallucinations, and disrupted sleep. The symptoms of narcolepsy often appear during adolescence, but may not be diagnosed until later in life. The disorder often is inherited from the parents, but it also has been linked to brain damage from a head injury or neurological disease.

Once narcolepsy is diagnosed, stimulants, antidepressants, or other medications can help treat the symptoms and prevent falling asleep at irregular times. Taking naps also may reduce the daytime sleepiness.

▶ SPERMICIDES

▶ See also *Barrier Methods of Contraception*

Spermicides are a form of birth control. They are chemical barrier methods that include vaginal creams, gels, foams, films, and suppositories. Spermicides contain a chemical that kills sperm or makes them inactive. This keeps them from passing through the woman's cervix. Spermicides are easy to use and sold at low cost without a prescription.

Spermicides are inserted into the woman's vagina, close to the cervix, before each act of sex. Films (thin sheets that contain spermicide) and tablets should be placed in the vagina 10–30 minutes before sex—they require some time to melt and become active.

Be sure to follow the instructions supplied with the product. Use the applicator that comes with it. The best results are achieved when spermicides are used along with a physical barrier method, such as a condom, diaphragm, or cervical cap.

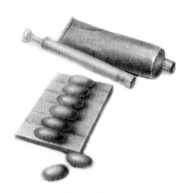

Spermicides

▶ STERILIZATION

▶ See also *Laparoscopy, Tubal Sterilization, Vasectomy*

Sterilization is an operation to prevent a woman from getting pregnant or a man from fathering a child. The sterilization procedure for women is called tubal sterilization. The procedure for men is called vasectomy. Sterilization is usually safe and free of problems. It is a permanent method of birth control and is a very effective way to prevent pregnancy.

Making the Decision

Sterilization is an important decision. Although there is a slight chance that pregnancy can occur after the procedure, it should be thought of as permanent. You and your partner must be certain that you do not want any more children—now or in the future.

People may choose sterilization for a number of reasons:

▶ They may feel they cannot support any more children.

▶ They may not want to worry about birth control any longer.

▶ They may fear that a health problem could pose a danger to the mother's or baby's life.

When thinking about sterilization, remember that it is meant to be permanent. Be aware that people may change their minds. If there is any chance that you may want to have children in the future, think about other forms of birth control. You also should avoid making this choice during times of stress,

Some women choose to get sterilized right after their babies are born, while they are still in the hospital. The surgery is easier then because the uterus is still enlarged and the fallopian tubes are pushed up in the abdomen. They can be grasped easily through a small cut near the navel, then tied or cut.

such as during a divorce or after a miscarriage, and never under pressure from a partner or others.

A number of temporary methods of birth control are available:

▶ Oral contraceptives (birth control pills)

▶ Intrauterine device (IUD)

▶ Barrier methods:
—Diaphragm
—Cervical cap
—Condom (male and female)
—Spermicides (cream, jelly, or foam)

▶ Contraceptive implant

▶ Contraceptive injection

▶ Natural family planning/periodic abstinence

Looking toward the future, if you are certain that you never want to become pregnant or father a child under any circumstances, you may wish to choose sterilization as a means of permanent birth control.

What If I Change My Mind?

Sterilization is an elective procedure. This means that it is your choice whether to have it done. If you have doubts at any time—even after you've signed papers giving consent—let your doctor know so that your doubts can be discussed. If you wish, the operation can be canceled.

If you change your mind after the operation, attempts to reverse it may not work. The success of reversal depends on the type of procedure used. After tubal sterilization is reversed, rates of pregnancy vary widely. Also, the risk of problems such as ectopic pregnancy is increased. In men, the chances that a vasectomy can be successfully reversed also vary widely. Reversing any sterilization operation for women or men requires major surgery.

Factors Affecting Choice

As with any surgery, sterilization has some risks. Problems occur in about 1 in 1,000 women who have the operation. Most of the time, these problems can be treated and corrected.

The method of sterilization a man or a woman chooses will depend on physical factors, medical history, and personal choice. Sometimes previous surgery, obesity, or other conditions may affect which method can be used. The person should be fully aware of the risks, benefits, and other options before making a choice. Overall, vasectomy is easier and has less risk than female sterilization.

The decision should be carefully discussed with your partner. The final choice is yours and the consent of others is not needed. The decision should be made with full knowledge of the procedure and the feelings of those close to you.

Sterilization can be done at any time. There may be waiting periods after consent forms are signed, or certain age requirements. Discuss the rules and laws that apply in your situation with your doctor before surgery.

Afterward

Most women and men are able to return to their normal routine after a short period of rest. Side effects are minor and should go away in a few days.

The surgery does not affect either partner's ability to have or enjoy sex. It only prevents pregnancy. If a man and woman had a good relationship before the surgery, it should remain good. Many couples say that sex improves after sterilization because sex is more spontaneous without the need to use birth control.

▶ STROKE

▶ See also *High Blood Pressure*

A stroke is a sudden interruption of blood flow to all or part of the brain, caused by blockage or bursting of a blood vessel in the brain. A stroke that continues for a few minutes can cause permanent brain damage or death. Depending on the part of the brain affected, signals from the brain to the body can be disrupted and can affect speech, movement, and other bodily functions.

Strokes are one of the leading causes of death in women. After menopause, a women's risk of heart disease and stroke increases. Hormone replacement therapy helps protect against heart disease and stroke.

Risk Factors

Many strokes can be prevented by treating risk factors. You may be at risk if you have any of the following conditions:

▶ High blood pressure

▶ High cholesterol levels

▶ Heart disease

▶ Diabetes

Strokes are more common in older people. Almost 75% of all strokes occur in people 65 years of age or older. However, a person of any age can have a stroke.

You also may be at risk if you smoke. If you have any of these risk factors, see your doctor for ways to manage them.

Symptoms

If you have any of these symptoms, call your doctor right away. It is best to be treated as soon as possible.

▶ Sudden numbness or weakness of face, arm, or leg on one side of the body

▶ Sudden confusion or trouble speaking

▶ Sudden trouble seeing

▶ Sudden trouble walking, dizziness, or loss of balance

▶ Sudden severe headache with unknown cause

▶ See also *Condoms, Sexually Transmitted Diseases, Sexually Transmitted Diseases* in *Pregnancy*

▶ SYPHILIS

Infection with syphilis, a sexually transmitted disease (STD), is rare, but can be serious if it is not treated. All STDs are passed by vaginal, anal, or oral sex.

Syphilis occurs in stages. It is more easily spread in some stages than in others. If not treated, syphilis may affect your heart, blood vessels, and nervous system. It can cause brain damage, blindness, paralysis, and even death. If syphilis is treated early, it will cause less damage.

Symptoms

Syphilis first appears as a painless sore called a chancre. It lasts 10 days to 6 weeks after contact with the disease. You also may have swollen lymph glands in the groin area.

If not treated, the next stage begins a week to 3 months later when a rash may appear. In most cases, the rash is on the soles of the feet and palms of the hands. Flat warts also may be seen on the vulva, outside the vagina. During this stage, you may feel like you have the flu. This stage is highly contagious.

The rash goes away in a few weeks or months, but that does not mean the disease is gone. It is still in your body. This is called the latent period. Years later, the disease may return.

Each year, almost 12 million new STD infections are diagnosed in the United States. These include over 110,000 new cases of syphilis.

How Syphilis Is Spread

Syphilis is spread by contact with a chancre. It also can be spread by touching the rash, warts, or infected blood during the second stage. It enters the body through a cut in the skin or mucus membrane.

Diagnosis

In the early stages, your doctor can examine discharge from open sores to see if you have syphilis. A blood test also may be done. It may need to be done more than once. If you have other STDs, you also may be given a blood test for syphilis.

Treatment

Syphilis is treated with antibiotics. If it is caught and treated early, long-term problems can be prevented. Antibiotics should clear up the infection. Because it is easy to spread the disease in the first and second stages, you should avoid sexual contact until your and your partner's treatment is finished.

Problems During Pregnancy

If you are pregnant when you get syphilis, problems can occur—for both you and your baby. The infection can be passed from mother to baby and cause these problems:

 ▶ Preterm birth (birth before 37 weeks)

 ▶ Premature rupture of membranes, when the sac that surrounds the baby breaks before labor begins

 ▶ Miscarriage

 ▶ Eye infection in the baby, called conjunctivitis, which can lead to blindness. This is treated routinely with eye drops at birth to prevent problems.

 ▶ Pneumonia

Because of these risks, many pregnant women are tested for syphilis if they are at risk for the disease. The mother then can be treated during pregnancy. There is less risk to the baby that way.

Treating a pregnant woman with syphilis with antibiotics will halt further damage to her fetus, but it will not reverse any harm already done. If a woman is treated during the first 3–4 months of pregnancy, most likely the infant will not have any long-term damage.

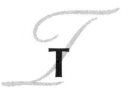

▶ See also *Stroke*

▶ THROMBOEMBOLISM

Thromboembolism occurs when blood clots are formed in the veins or arteries. When an embolism (a blood vessel blocked by a clot) occurs, tissues fail to get key nutrients and start to die. This can happen anywhere in the body, such as the legs, lungs, or brain.

Blood clots tend to affect people who are overweight or do not get enough exercise. They also are more common in women older than age 35 who smoke and take birth control pills. Sometimes blood clots form after surgery or a serious injury.

When blood clots are diagnosed and treated early, there is less chance of major problems. The most common symptoms are pain and swelling. For instance, if a clot lodges in your lung, you may feel sudden pain, be short of breath, or develop a cough. Massive clots can cause a sudden blackout or death.

The main treatment of thromboembolism is drugs that thin the blood and reduce clotting. You may be told to rest in bed and keep your legs raised. Heating pads and pain medicine may provide short-term relief. Wearing elastic support stockings also may be helpful.

Although blood clots affect less than 0.5% of pregnant women, they are one of the most common causes of death during pregnancy. If you develop a blood clot during pregnancy, you may be injected with blood-thinning drugs (through an intravenous tube) during labor and delivery.

If you have a family history of blood clots, tell your doctor. There are tests to see if you are at risk of problems.

▶ THYROID DISEASE

An underactive thyroid can cause changes in the menstrual cycle. In some cases, this may be a cause of infertility.

The thyroid is a gland that controls key functions of your body. Disease of the thyroid gland can affect nearly every organ in your body and harm your health. Thyroid disease is eight times more likely to occur in women than in men. In most cases, treatment of thyroid disease is safe and simple.

The Thyroid Gland

The thyroid gland is located at the base of your neck in front of your trachea (or windpipe). It has two sides and is shaped like a butterfly.

The thyroid gland makes, stores, and releases two hormones—T_4 (thyroxine) and T_3 (triiodothyronine). Thyroid hormones control the rate at which every part of your body works. This is called your metabolism. Your metabolism controls whether you feel hot or cold or tired or rested. When your thyroid gland is working the way it should, your metabolism stays at a steady pace—not too fast or too slow.

The thyroid gland is controlled by the pituitary gland (a gland in your brain). The pituitary gland makes thyroid-stimulating hormone (TSH). TSH tells the thyroid gland to make more hormone if needed.

If there is not enough thyroid hormone in the bloodstream, the body's metabolism slows down. This is called hypothyroidism (underactive). If there is too much thyroid hormone, your metabolism speeds up. This is called hyperthyroidism (overactive). Certain disorders can cause the thyroid gland to make too much or too little hormone.

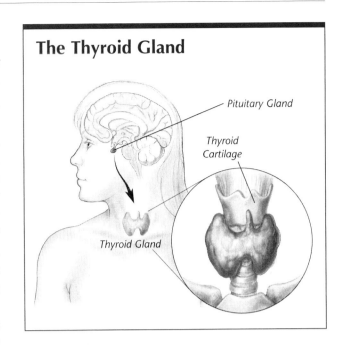

The Thyroid Gland

Pituitary Gland

Thyroid Cartilage

Thyroid Gland

Diagnosing Thyroid Disease

To diagnose thyroid disease, your doctor will do an exam and tests and ask questions about your symptoms. Any woman age 19 years or older who has a strong family history of thyroid disease or autoimmune disease (a disease in which your body produces antibodies to destroy its own tissues and cells) should have a TSH test. Symptoms of thyroid disease can be much like symptoms of other health problems.

Your doctor will examine your neck while you swallow. The thyroid gland moves when you swallow. This makes it easier to feel. Your doctor also may examine your skin and eyes and check your weight and temperature.

Your doctor will use lab tests to help find the exact cause of the problem. You may have a(n):

) Blood test

) Thyroid scan

) Ultrasound

During a thyroid scan, you must drink a small amount of radioactive iodine. A special camera then detects the areas of thyroid gland that absorb the radioactive iodine. These are the problem areas. This will not be done if you are pregnant.

Hypothyroidism

Hypothyroidism occurs when the thyroid gland is not working hard enough (it's underactive). It is not making enough of the thyroid hormones to maintain your normal body metabolism.

Causes

The most common cause of hypothyroidism is a disorder known as thyroiditis—an inflammation of the thyroid gland. This is also called Hashimoto's disease. It causes the immune system—your body's natural defense against disease—to mistake cells in the thyroid gland for harmful invaders. Your body sends out white blood cells to destroy them. The pituitary gland then releases TSH to tell the thyroid gland to make more thyroid hormone. This demand on the thyroid gland can cause it to enlarge. This enlargement is called a goiter.

Hypothyroidism also can result from a diet that does not have enough iodine. The diet of most Americans is thought to have enough iodine because of the use of iodized salt. Other food sources of iodine include:

▶ Spinach

▶ Shrimp

▶ Oysters

▶ Lobster

Taking too high a dosage of medication to treat hyperthyroidism can lead to hypothyroidism, too.

Symptoms

The symptoms of hypothyroidism are slow to develop. You may have the condition but not have any symptoms for months or years. Common symptoms of hypothyroidism are:

▶ Fatigue or weakness

▶ Weight gain

▶ Decreased appetite

▶ Change in menstrual periods

▶ Loss of sex drive

▶ Feeling cold when others don't

▶ Constipation

Thyroid disease in pregnant women has been linked to a greater risk of repeated miscarriage. Sometimes treatment of the illness can improve the chances for a successful pregnancy. This is even more true if it is under control before a woman becomes pregnant.

◗ Muscle aches

◗ Puffiness around the eyes

◗ Brittle nails

◗ Hair loss

If your lab tests show that the hormone levels are normal, some other condition may be causing your symptoms.

Treatment

In most cases, hypothyroidism is treated with medication that contains thyroid hormone. The dose of the medication is increased slowly until a normal level has been reached in the blood.

Most people with hypothyroidism have to take the hormone for the rest of their lives. The dose may need to be changed from time to time. The level of the hormone in the blood is checked regularly.

Hyperthyroidism

Hyperthyroidism results when the thyroid gland is making too much thyroid hormone (it's overactive). This causes your metabolism to speed up.

Causes

The most common cause of hyperthyroidism is a disorder known as Graves' disease. It most often affects women between the ages of 20 and 40 years. Women with Graves' disease make a substance that causes the thyroid gland to make too much thyroid hormone. A late sign of Graves' disease is often a wide-eyed stare or bulging eyes.

Hyperthyroidism also may result from medication. Taking too much of thyroid hormone when being treated for hypothyroidism can lead to symptoms of an overactive thyroid. Another cause is lumps in the thyroid called hot nodules. These lumps produce too much thyroid hormone.

Any woman age 19 or older who has a strong family history of thyroid disease or autoimmune disease should have a thyroid-stimulating hormone test.

Symptoms

The more common symptoms of hyperthyroidism are:

◗ Fatigue

◗ Weight loss

◗ Nervousness

◗ Rapid heartbeat

◗ Increased sweating

◗ Feeling hot when others don't

◗ Changes in menstrual periods

▶ More frequent bowel movements

▶ Tremors

Treatment

Treatment for hyperthyroidism will lower the amount of thyroid hormone and relieve your symptoms. Antithyroid medication can be used to reduce the amount of thyroid hormone your body is making. Medications known as beta blockers control rapid heartbeat.

If these medications don't help, your doctor may suggest treatment with radioactive iodine to destroy parts of the thyroid gland. In some cases, surgery may be needed to remove the thyroid gland.

Thyroid Nodules

A nodule is a lump in the thyroid gland. You may notice the lump on your own, or your doctor may detect the lump during a routine exam. When a thyroid nodule is found, it will be checked to see if it is benign (not cancer) or malignant (cancer).

Your doctor also may use ultrasound to examine the nodule. Nodules may be further examined by a procedure known as fine needle aspiration or biopsy.

If no cancer cells are found, your doctor may prescribe a thyroid hormone to decrease the size of your nodule, or your doctor may suggest surgery to remove it. If cancer cells are found, further treatment will be needed. Thyroid cancer usually can be treated with success.

▶ See also *Menstrual Hygiene Products*

Super absorbent Rely brand tampons were found to be used by many of the woman diagnosed with TSS during the outbreak in 1980 (about 800 cases were reported to the Centers of Disease Control). These tampons are no longer available for sale. Only five menstrually related cases of TSS were reported in 1997.

▶ TOXIC SHOCK SYNDROME

Toxic shock syndrome (TSS) is a rare, but serious, condition caused by the bacteria *Staphylococcus aureus*. These bacteria sometimes can be found in the nose, skin, or vagina and, in most cases, do not cause a problem. However, sometimes they can lead to infection after surgery or in relation to tampon use.

The symptoms of TSS are a high fever, chills, vomiting, diarrhea, dizziness, fainting, and a rash that looks like a sunburn. If you have symptoms of TSS while using a tampon, remove it and see a doctor right away. TSS usually can be treated with antibiotics.

The risk of TSS increases with higher-absorbency tampons. To lower your risk of TSS, choose a tampon with the lowest absorbency to meet your needs. And be sure not to wear the same tampon for more than 24 hours.

▶ TUBAL STERILIZATION

▶ See also *Sterilization, Vasectomy*

Tubal sterilization is an operation to prevent a woman from getting pregnant. Almost half of the women who choose sterilization have it performed postpartum—while still in the hospital after the birth of their babies. Because the woman is already in the hospital and the new baby can be cared for in the nursery, this is a convenient time to have the procedure done. It usually does not prolong the hospital stay.

In a sterilization procedure, both fallopian tubes are closed by being tied or sealed with a ring, clip, or electric current. This prevents the egg from moving down the tube and keeps the sperm from reaching the egg.

There are different ways in which tubal sterilization can be done. If you are planning to be sterilized, you and your doctor will decide which method is best for you. The two methods used most often are laparoscopy and minilaparotomy. Both methods have similar success rates and risks. Both can be done as outpatient procedures, which means you can go home the same day.

Tubal sterilization may be performed under general or local anesthesia. The type of anesthesia used depends on your medical history, the type of procedure used, personal choice, and the experience and advice of your gynecologist or anesthesiologist.

Tubal sterilization does not cause your menstrual periods to stop. However, if you use birth control pills before you have the surgery, it may take a while to return to your normal cycle.

Types of Tubal Sterilization

Postpartum

In general, postpartum sterilization is done within 1–2 days of the birth of a woman's last baby. Many factors affect the exact time to perform a postpartum tubal sterilization:

▶ Health of the mother just after birth

▶ Health of the baby

▶ Time and personnel available for the procedure

In some cases, the procedure can be done a few minutes after the birth, with the same anesthesia used for the delivery. If no anesthesia is used for birth, your doctor will often wait a while before giving anesthesia and performing the operation.

The Uterus After Delivery

Just after birth, the uterus is still enlarged and the ovaries and fallopian tubes are pushed up just under the surface of the abdomen (left). This gives the doctor easier access to the tubes than it would several weeks after delivery (right).

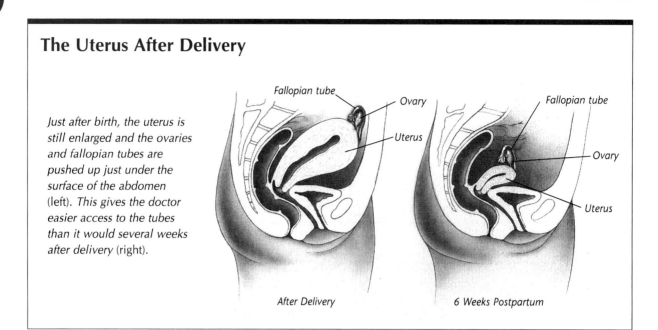

Fallopian tube   *Ovary*   *Uterus*

Fallopian tube   *Ovary*   *Uterus*

After Delivery   *6 Weeks Postpartum*

There may be waiting periods after consent forms are signed. Discuss the rules and laws that apply in your situation with your doctor during your pregnancy.

After a woman gives birth, the still-enlarged uterus pushes the fallopian tubes up, just under the abdominal wall below the navel. In most cases, a small, ½- to 1-inch incision through the relaxed abdominal wall is all that is needed to bring the tubes into the doctor's view for the operation. If you have had a cesarean birth, sterilization may be performed through the incision already made.

The type of anesthesia used for postpartum sterilization depends on your medical history, personal choice, and the advice of your obstetrician or anesthesiologist. The surgery is often performed under a general anesthetic. This means you will not be awake during the operation. When general anesthesia is used, a tube may be placed down the throat to aid breathing during the operation. With epidural or spinal block anesthesia, an injection is given in the lower back, and the lower half of the body is numbed. You may be awake during the operation but will not feel any pain. Sometimes a local anesthetic may be used.

The doctor brings the fallopian tubes through a small incision made just below the navel. Each fallopian tube is then tied (or cut) to keep the egg from joining with the sperm. This is done by closing off (tying) a section of each tube with surgical threads and cutting out the section between the ties. After the tubes are "tied" and the section between the ties is removed, the incision below the navel is closed with stitches and a bandage.

The operation takes about 30 minutes. Having it done right after childbirth usually does not make your hospital stay any longer.

Laparoscopy

First anesthesia is given. The surgery then follows these steps:

1. A small incision (cut) is made in or near the navel.

2. A gas (usually carbon dioxide) may be passed into the abdomen to inflate it slightly. This moves the abdominal wall away from the organs next to it and allows the doctor to see the reproductive organs more easily.

3. The laparoscope (a slender, light-transmitting telescope) is inserted into the abdomen, allowing the doctor to see the pelvic organs.

4. A smaller device is inserted to move and hold the tubes. The device may be inserted either through the laparoscope or through a second tiny incision made just above the pubic hairline.

5. The tubes are sealed by using one of various methods.

6. The gas (if any was used) in the abdomen is withdrawn. The incisions are then closed, usually with one or two stitches, and covered with a small bandage.

Although the risk of failure is low, the procedure does not guarantee sterility. That is, sometimes the sterilization does not work, and a woman can get pregnant. If you get pregnant after sterilization, it is more likely to be an ectopic pregnancy. See your doctor if you miss a menstrual period after the procedure and think you might be pregnant.

No surgery is without some degree of risk, but serious problems are rare with sterilization. Problems such as infections, bleeding, burns, or complications from anesthesia occur in only about 1 out of every 1,000 women who have the operation.

Minilaparotomy

A minilaparotomy is an incision made in the abdomen that may be only 1–2 inches long. Through this incision, the tubes are closed.

1. After an anesthetic is given, a small incision is made in the abdomen just above the pubic hairline.

2. The doctor may remove sections of the tubes and use surgical thread to tie the new openings shut, or the tubes may be closed with electric current, bands, or clips.

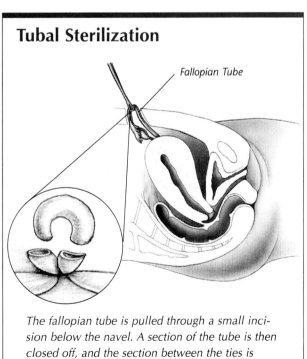

Tubal Sterilization

Fallopian Tube

The fallopian tube is pulled through a small incision below the navel. A section of the tube is then closed off, and the section between the ties is removed.

Sterilization by Laparoscopy

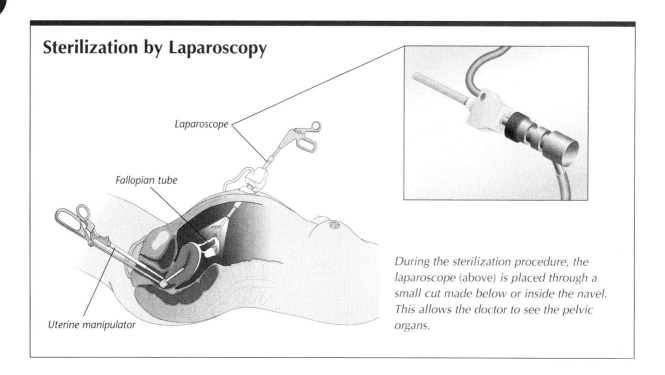

Laparoscope

Fallopian tube

Uterine manipulator

During the sterilization procedure, the laparoscope (above) is placed through a small cut made below or inside the navel. This allows the doctor to see the pelvic organs.

3. A few stitches are used to close the incision, which is then covered by a small bandage.

The rate of pregnancies that occur after this procedure is about 1%. Major problems, such as infection, bleeding, or complications from anesthesia, are uncommon. You may have some discomfort after minilaparotomy. Also, this procedure may require a hospital stay.

After the Surgery

Side effects after surgery depend on how you tolerate pain, the type of anesthesia used, and your overall healing ability. You may have slight abdominal pain and tiredness. Less often, you may feel dizzy or nauseous or have shoulder pain, abdominal cramps, a gassy or bloated feeling, or general fatigue. If you had general anesthesia, you may have a sore throat.

Most or all of these symptoms usually go away within 1–3 days, and most women return to their usual routines a couple of days after surgery. After that time you may feel tired later in the day, have slight soreness over the incision, and have minor changes in bowel movements. Your discomfort can usually be relieved with mild pain medication.

Sterilization in women is effective right away. Birth control is no longer needed. However, sterilization does not prevent STDs (sexually transmitted diseases). Condoms should be used to protect against STDs. The procedure does not affect the menstrual cycle or your ability to enjoy sex.

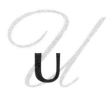

▶ ULTRASOUND EXAM

Ultrasound, which creates pictures of the internal organs from sound waves, can be found today in every major hospital and in many doctors' offices. This technology is useful for the general health care of women. It is especially valuable during pregnancy and childbirth.

What Is Ultrasound?

Ultrasound is energy in the form of sound waves produced by a small crystal. The sound waves move at a frequency too high to be heard by the human ear. They are directed into a specific area of the body through a device called a transducer. The transducer is moved across the skin, or it can be used inside different parts of the body, such as the vagina. The sound waves bounce off tissues inside the body, like echoes. They are changed into pictures of the internal organs and—during pregnancy—the fetus. The pictures appear on a screen similar to a television. The type of ultrasound that is most often used, called real-time, combines still pictures one after another to show movement, somewhat like the single frames that make a motion picture.

Ultrasound is not designed to take pictures of the fetus for mementos. Ultrasound should not be done only to try to detect the baby's sex, although the images sometimes show if the fetus is male or female.

Ways Ultrasound Is Used

Ultrasound is not necessary for every woman or in every pregnancy. Your doctor will discuss with you whether ultrasound will be used. Ultrasound is often used to help find a possible problem or check a known condition. It is an important diagnostic tool that gives information other tests do not.

Obstetrics

Ultrasound is used in obstetrics to examine the growing fetus inside the mother's uterus. Being able to evaluate the pregnancy this way is especially important if the doctor suspects that the fetus is grow-

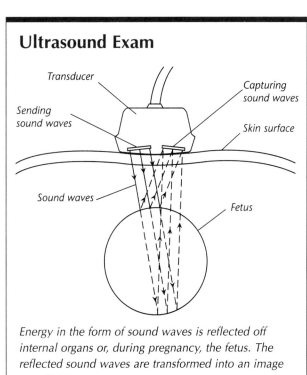

Ultrasound Exam

Transducer

Sending sound waves

Capturing sound waves

Skin surface

Sound waves

Fetus

Energy in the form of sound waves is reflected off internal organs or, during pregnancy, the fetus. The reflected sound waves are transformed into an image on a TV-type screen.

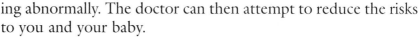
ing abnormally. The doctor can then attempt to reduce the risks to you and your baby.

Ultrasound can provide valuable information about the fetus's health and well-being, including:

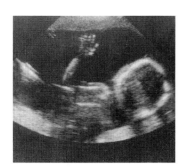

Sonogram of a fetus in the mother's uterus.

▶ Age of the fetus

▶ Rate of growth of the fetus

▶ Placement of the placenta

▶ Fetal position, movement, breathing, and heart rate

▶ Amount of amniotic fluid in the uterus

▶ Number of fetuses

▶ Some birth defects

Ultrasound can be used to monitor the fetal heart rate before and during labor. The fetal heart rate can indicate the well-being of the baby. Ultrasound is used to measure the flow of blood within vessels of the uterus, fetus, and umbilical cord, which connects the fetus and the placenta. In this case, the ultrasound does not create a picture. It records the sound of the heartbeat.

Ultrasound is used during pregnancy to find the cause of bleeding or pain. It also can be used to diagnose an ectopic pregnancy.

Gynecology

Ultrasound is used in gynecology to examine the pelvic organs and—along with mammography—the breasts. Ultrasound can help:

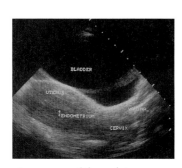

Sonogram of the pelvic organs.

▶ Identify a pelvic or breast mass

▶ Show the location and characteristics of a mass

▶ Detect problems causing pelvic pain

▶ Locate the position of an intrauterine device (IUD)

▶ Monitor ovulation in treating infertility

Ultrasound also is useful in infertile couples. It can be used to retrieve eggs for in vitro fertilization, a process in which an egg is fertilized in a dish in a laboratory and then placed inside the woman to grow into a fetus. It can also be used to check the number and size of eggs when ovulation is induced.

The Exam

Ultrasound exams are done in doctors' offices or hospitals by a doctor or a specially trained technician. To prepare for an ultrasound exam, wear clothes that allow your abdomen to be exposed easily. Some hospitals may ask you to wear a hospital gown.

You may need a full bladder for your exam. This will require drinking several glasses of water an hour before the exam and not urinating until after the procedure. A full bladder helps to locate and view the pelvic organs.

As you lie on the table with your abdomen exposed from the lower part of the ribs to the hips, mineral oil or a gel is applied to the surface of the abdomen. This improves contact of the transducer with the skin surface. The transducer is then moved along the abdomen.

When vaginal ultrasound is used, a condom, or some other protective cover, is placed over a transducer before insertion into the vagina. Ultrasound with a vaginal probe is a painless exam that may feel like the exam you have for a Pap test.

To further study the wall and lining of the uterus, a procedure called sono-hysterography (hysterosonography) may be done along with vaginal ultrasound.

Vaginal Ultrasound Exam

The vaginal transducer can be inserted in the vagina to help view pelvic organs. Ultrasound with a vaginal probe may feel like the exam you have for a Pap test. This exam is being done more often to detect disorders during pregnancy, such as placenta previa.

With sonohysterography, a small amount of sterile fluid is inserted into the cavity of the uterus through a thin plastic tube. The fluid can be seen on the same screen used for the vaginal ultrasound to highlight what may be a problem (such as polyps or fibroids) in the uterus.

▶ URINARY INCONTINENCE

▶ See also *Kegel Exercises*

Many women leak small amounts of urine from time to time. Leakage of urine can happen with certain movements, during pregnancy, or during other stress, such as coughing. Some women find that they lose urine when they hear the sound of running water or when they have their hands in water. Others find that, at times, they feel the urge to urinate and are unable to control it. When leakage of urine becomes frequent or severe enough to become a social or hygiene problem, it is called urinary incontinence.

Urinary incontinence is more common in women than men. It affects 10–25% of women younger than age 65 and 15–30% of women older than 60 who do not live in nursing homes. Incontinence is even more common in nursing home residents— over half may be affected.

Almost 13 million Americans have urinary incontinence and 11 million of them are women, according to the National Institute of Diabetes and Digestive and Kidney Diseases. Incontinence also is more common in older people.

Incontinence does not always mean that a woman leaks often. For an active woman or a woman who loses a large amount of urine each time, even one time a week or less may be too much.

Women are sometimes reluctant to tell their doctor about their symptoms of urinary incontinence. Less than one half of women seek medical care. Instead, they rely on absorbent pads or changes in lifestyle to deal with this condition. They may feel embarrassed and may even avoid certain social or work situations. Some women have the false belief that urinary incontinence is a normal part of aging and that nothing can be done to correct it. However, urinary incontinence often can be treated.

Tell your doctor if you have any leakage of urine. Proper diagnosis and treatment may correct your problem and ease your symptoms.

Normal Voiding

The urinary tract is made up of kidneys, which produce urine; tubes called ureters that carry urine to the bladder, a saclike, muscular organ, where it is stored; and the urethra, a small, muscular tube about 2 inches long that carries urine from the bladder to the outside of the body.

Normal urination, or voiding, occurs when a woman is able to empty her bladder whenever she has a natural desire to do so. In normal voiding, the muscles around the urethra relax, the bladder contracts, and urine flows from the bladder to the urethra and out of the body. When the bladder is almost empty, the muscles around the urethra contract, the bladder relaxes, and the stream of urine stops flowing.

Types of Incontinence

There are three types of incontinence: urge, stress, and overflow. The most common type is urge incontinence. It is due to the detrusor muscle—the muscle wall of the bladder—being overactive. This leads to loss of leakage of urine.

Stress incontinence occurs when the pressure inside the bladder, which moves urine out, is greater than the pressure in the urethra, which keeps urine in. It causes involuntary loss of urine during coughing, laughing, sneezing, or physical activity. Its most important cause is the weakening of the tissues that surround and support the urethra and bladder.

In overflow incontinence, the bladder fails to empty during voiding. This results in a steady leakage of small amounts of urine. Overflow incontinence is less common than urge incontinence and is due to the detrusor muscle being underactive.

Symptoms

Women who have urinary incontinence may leak urine often. They may have to wear a pad to keep from wetting their clothes. Some women with incontinence feel such a strong desire to urinate that they cannot control it. This results in a loss of urine.

A woman with urinary incontinence may also have other symptoms:

▶ *Urgency:* A strong desire to urinate, whether or not the bladder is full. This often occurs along with pelvic discomfort or pressure, as well as the fear of leakage or fear of pain.

▶ *Frequency:* Urinating more than every 2 hours or more than 7 times a day

▶ *Nocturia:* The need to urinate two or more times during hours of sleep

▶ *Dysuria:* Painful urination

▶ *Enuresis:* Bed-wetting or wetting while sleeping

Causes

There are many possible causes of urinary incontinence. These include infection, damage to organs, and muscular disorders.

Urinary Tract Infection

Urinary incontinence may be due to an infection of the urinary tract. Often such an infection occurs along with pain, frequency, and blood in the urine. Infections of the bladder (cystitis) and of the urethra (urethritis) are very common in women.

Incontinence may be the first and only symptom of a urinary tract infection. Treating the infection may relieve or cure the problem.

Pelvic Support Problems

Pelvic support problems happen when the tissues that support the pelvic organs are stretched and damaged. This allows the organs that they support to sag out of place. If the tissues that normally support the urethra, bladder, uterus, and rectum are weakened, these organs may drop and lead to urinary incontinence or difficulty in passing urine.

Two types of pelvic support problems are the cystocele and the cystourethrocele. When the bladder drops from its normal place into the vagina, it is called a cystocele. The place where the bladder joins the urethra is called the bladder neck. When tissues that support the bladder neck are damaged, it may drop and push against the vaginal wall. A dropped bladder neck is called a cystourethrocele.

The main causes of pelvic support problems are childbirth and aging. As the baby passes through the vagina during childbirth, the vaginal wall and ligaments may be damaged. They may become weak. In later years, when a woman goes through menopause, the loss of the female hormone estrogen may make these problems worse.

Urinary Tract Abnormalities

Fistulas are abnormal openings between the urinary tract (urethra, bladder, or ureters) and the vagina. These openings can allow urine to leak out through the vagina. Fistulas may result from pelvic surgery, childbirth, radiation treatment, or advanced cancer of the pelvis.

Urinary incontinence can also be caused by a urethral diverticulum, a small pocket that bulges out of the wall of the urethra. Urine can collect in this pocket and then spill out later.

Abnormal growths in the urinary tract also can cause incontinence. Sometimes, a small bladder size may cause problems as well.

Neuromuscular Disorders

Neuromuscular disorders are problems with the nerves that control the function of the bladder and urethra. Bladder spasms—uncontrolled contractions—may occur. If the nerves do not control the contractions of the bladder muscle, the bladder may expel urine. The bladder also may become too full, and urine may leak. Most of the time it is not known why the nerves lose control of the bladder muscle. It could be linked to other medical conditions, such as diabetes.

Water pills (diuretics) take fluid from swollen areas of your body and send it to the bladder. This may cause the bladder to leak because it fills more quickly than usual. Caffeine drinks such as coffee and cola have the same effect.

Drug Therapy

Urinary incontinence may be a side effect of medications taken for some other condition. For example, diuretics, sedatives, tranquilizers, or even antihistamines may cause some women to leak urine. Your doctor may only have to change the dosage or type of medication in order to ease your symptoms.

Physical Limitations

Some women have nothing wrong with their bladder or urethra. They have conditions, such as arthritis, that prevent them from moving quickly. They may lose urine before they can get to the bathroom. Such limits are a real problem for many older women.

Diagnosis

There may be a number of steps involved in finding the cause of urinary incontinence. These steps may vary depending on the nature of the problem.

The first step often is to provide a detailed medical history. You will be asked questions about factors that may affect your voiding habits. One of the most important methods used to diagnose incontinence is the voiding diary. The doctor may ask you to record the time and amount of urine leakage over 24–72 hours. You may also be asked to record how much water or other fluids you drank and any activity that might have caused the leakage.

Secondly, a pelvic exam will be done. It can detect physical conditions that might be linked to incontinence. Other exams and tests used may include:

> *Some women may feel ashamed about loss of bladder control. They should not fear talking about it. Millions of other women have the same problem. Nearly everyone with a bladder control problem can be helped.*

- ◗ Lab tests to detect urinary tract infection

- ◗ Stress test (patient must cough repeatedly with a full bladder, and any loss of urine is recorded)

- ◗ Pad test (patient wears a preweighed pad for 1 hour while doing a series of movements; if pad weighs more at end of hour, there was a loss of urine)

- ◗ Dye test (patient wears a pad while a nontoxic dye is put into the bladder; if pad is stained with the dye, there was a loss of urine)

- ◗ Cystometry (measurement of the pressure and volume of the bladder as it is filled with fluid)

These tests can help detect the cause of the problem. Some patients may have more than one cause. Knowing the cause helps your doctor select the best treatment for you.

Treatment

Many women delay seeking medical care until their symptoms are so severe that they need surgery. In the meantime, they use pads for protection. Pads or adult diapers may offer security, but they have drawbacks. They can irritate the skin. These products should not be the first—or only—treatment tried for incontinence. They should only be used to make other treatments work better or when other treatments have failed.

There is a wide variety of treatments available, depending on the cause of your problem. They include behavior modification, medication, special devices, or surgery.

Behavioral Treatments

The goal of behavioral treatment is to help a woman understand why leakage occurs and how to avoid it. It often may include bladder retraining and pelvic muscle exercises.

With bladder retraining, you will be taught about normal and abnormal voiding patterns. You will be instructed to void on a regular schedule, whether or not you have the urge. You will be told about ways to help you ignore any urges to pass urine. One is distraction—thinking about other things. After a few weeks you should have fewer instances of leaking urine. Success with this method can be quite good.

Pelvic muscle exercises such as Kegel exercises improve urine control in 40–75% of women who use them. Biofeedback might be used with this or other treatments to improve your response. Biofeedback is a process that gives you information about your body functions, which helps you to gain control of these same functions.

Medication

Medications that help control muscle spasms can help prevent leakage. Your doctor also may suggest collagen injections. These injections and other drugs strengthen the smooth muscle of the urethra and improve symptoms. These medications may cause dry mouth, constipation, nausea, blurred vision, or sleeplessness.

If you have gone through menopause, your doctor may prescribe estrogen replacement therapy. This improves the elasticity of the muscles and surrounding tissues. Treatment can be with a cream that is placed in the vagina, pills, or a patch applied to the skin. Although it may take a while for the medications to take effect, they must be continued. Symptoms improve in many patients with this therapy.

If you have a urinary tract infection, you will be given antibiotics. Leakage may stop once the infection is cured.

Special Devices

One device that may be used is a pessary. A pessary is a stiff ring that fits into the vagina to hold the pelvic organs in place. Its main purpose is to prevent the bladder from leaking urine.

Pessaries tend to be used if other treatments fail or your health is too poor for surgery. There are many different types of pessaries. Your doctor will fit you with the right one for you. If you use a pessary, it must be removed, cleaned, and reinserted often. If not, it might cause a bad-smelling discharge or ulcers in the vagina. Women who use pessaries should watch for infections of the vagina or urinary tract. Regular doctor visits are important, too.

Sometimes devices can be used to strengthen the pelvic muscles. Weighted cones are devices like a tampon that a woman places in her vagina twice a day. When she contracts her pelvic muscles to keep the cone in place, the muscles are strengthened.

The pelvic muscles also can be made to contract by using electrical stimulation. This may help women who were not aided by other treatments.

For more information on urinary incontinence and the available treatments contact:

National Association for Continence
PO Box 8310
Spartanburg, SC 29305
Phone: 800-BLADDER or (803) 579-7900

Surgical Treatment

Surgery has different risks of complications than drug or behavioral therapy. If you are thinking about surgery, you should understand the chances of success as well as the possible complications.

Factors that put extra pressure on the pelvic muscles contribute to the problem of urinary incontinence. Making the following changes in your lifestyle, before and after your operation, can increase your chances for a successful surgery:

◗ Stop smoking

◗ Get treatment for lung diseases

◗ Lose weight

◗ Avoid constipation

◗ Avoid heavy lifting

There are many different types of operations used to correct urinary incontinence. Your doctor's evaluation will help determine if your incontinence is due to lack of support at the bladder neck or from weakness of the bladder neck itself.

The most common cause of incontinence in women is lack of support at the bladder neck. This type of incontinence can be treated with three basic procedures: with an abdominal incision, through vaginal surgery, or with a more minor procedure (a needle suspension). The abdominal incision has the highest long-term success rates, but it is also more serious surgery. You and your doctor will need to consider many factors before choosing the surgery that is right for you, including:

◗ Your age

◗ Your lifestyle

◗ Need for hysterectomy or correction of pelvic prolapse

◗ Whether you've had radiation or prior operations for incontinence

◗ Your general health

Some of the possible complications after surgery are:

◗ Difficulty emptying your bladder

◗ Bladder spasms

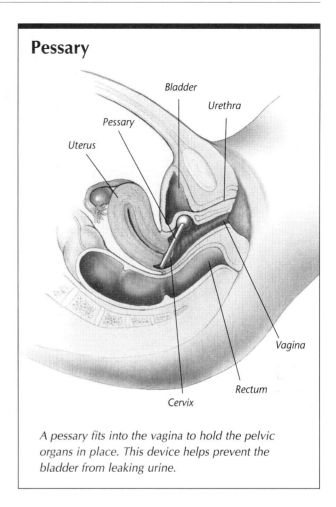

Pessary

A pessary fits into the vagina to hold the pelvic organs in place. This device helps prevent the bladder from leaking urine.

> Bladder infection

> Injury to the bladder during surgery

> Recurrence of incontinence

Bladder spasms are usually temporary. They last while the bladder is going through the healing process and can be controlled with medication. If you are unable to empty your bladder after surgery, this too, is usually temporary. You may need to wear a catheter for a few weeks, or you may be taught to empty your own bladder with a small disposable catheter.

> # URINARY TRACT INFECTIONS

About 1 of every 5 women will have a urinary tract infection (UTI) during her life. Some women will have more than one or get them often. Most UTIs are not serious. They are easy to treat with antibiotics. Symptoms are relieved quickly.

A Woman's Urinary Tract

The urinary tract includes:

> The kidneys, which make urine

> Tubes called ureters that carry urine to the bladder where it is stored

> The urethra, a short, narrow tube that urine passes through on its way out of the body

The urinary tract in women has a lower part and an upper part. The lower urinary tract is made up of the urethra and the bladder. Most infections occur in the lower urinary tract where it is easy for bacteria to enter. Infections of the bladder or urethra rarely cause problems unless a woman is pregnant.

The upper urinary tract consists of the kidneys and ureters. An infection in the upper tract may cause a more severe illness.

How Urine Is Made

The kidneys are organs located in the lower back. The kidneys produce urine. Each has many nephrons—units that filter the blood in a two-step process.

In the first step, the nephrons remove wastes, water, and salts from the blood as it enters the kidneys. In the second step, the nephrons screen the liquid removed from the blood. This allows most of the water and salts in this liquid to be reabsorbed by the blood. Whatever is left after this process is urine.

Storage and Release

The ureters transport urine from the kidneys to the bladder (where urine is stored). To prevent urine from leaking out of the bladder, there is a muscle along the urethra that can tighten. As it fills with urine, the bladder expands.

When the bladder is stretched to a certain limit, the urge to urinate is felt. Urine will not be released until the urethra muscle relaxes and the bladder muscle contracts. The urine then passes out of the body through the urethra.

Types of Urinary Tract Infections

Most UTIs start in the lower urinary tract. Bacteria can enter through the urethra and spread upward to the bladder. This causes cystitis, a bladder infection. In most cases, urethritis occurs at the same time.

Bacteria that have infected the bladder may travel up the ureters to the kidneys. This may cause pyelonephritis, a kidney infection.

Causes

Urinary tract infections often are caused by bacteria from the bowel that live on the skin near the rectum or in the vagina. These bacteria can spread and enter the urinary tract through the urethra. They then travel up the urethra. They may cause infections in the bladder and, sometimes, in other parts of the urinary tract.

Sex is one of the causes of UTIs. Because of their anatomy, women are prone to UTIs after having sex. In front of the vagina is the opening of the urethra. During sex, bacteria in the vaginal area could be massaged into the urethra by the back and forth motion of the penis.

Urinary tract infections also tend to occur in women who change sexual partners or begin having sex more often. Some women get an infection each time they have sex. This is rare, though.

The Female Urinary Tract System

Kidneys

Upper Tract

Ureters

Lower Tract

Uterus

Bladder

Urethra

The female urinary tract system is divided into a lower tract and an upper tract.

Pregnant women are no more likely to get a UTI than other women. However, 2–4% of pregnant women develop a UTI. When a UTI occurs during pregnancy, it may be easier for the bacteria to travel to the kidneys because of shifts in the position of the urinary tract.

Waiting too long to urinate also can result in UTIs. The bladder is a muscle that stretches to hold urine and contracts to expel it. If you go for hours without urinating, the bladder muscle is stretched too much. This weakens the muscle so that it can't contract with enough force to expel all of the urine it holds. Some urine remains in the bladder after urination. Any time this happens, the risk of a UTI increases.

Certain other factors increase your chances of having a UTI. You are more likely to have an infection if you:

▶ Are pregnant

▶ Had UTIs as a child

▶ Are past menopause

▶ Have diabetes

Symptoms

Symptoms of UTIs can come on quickly. The first sign of a UTI is a strong urge to urinate (urgency) that cannot be delayed. As urine is released, a sharp pain or burning (dysuria) will be felt in the urethra. Very little urine is released. The urine may be tinged with blood. The need to urinate returns minutes later (frequency). Soreness may occur in the lower abdomen, in the back, or in the sides.

This cycle may repeat itself many times during the day or at night (nocturia). It is normal to urinate about six times a day. If you are urinating more often, you may have a UTI.

If the bacteria enter the ureters and spreads to the kidneys, symptoms also may include:

▶ Back pain

▶ Chills

▶ Fever

▶ Nausea

▶ Vomiting

Symptoms linked with a UTI, such as painful urination, can be caused by other problems (such as an infection of the vagina or vulva). Only your doctor can make the correct diagnosis. It is up to you to let your doctor know when you are aware of any of these changes.

Diagnosis

Urinary tract infections are diagnosed on the basis of the number of bacteria and white blood cells found in a urine sample. To detect the presence of bacteria and white blood cells, a sample of your urine will be studied under a microscope. It also will be cultured in a substance that promotes the growth of bacteria. A pelvic exam may be needed as well.

Treatment

Antibiotics are used to treat UTIs. Most patients with UTIs have to take antibiotics for up to 10 days. But with some infections, only a single dose of an antibiotic is needed.

Be sure you take all of the medication you are given even though your symptoms may go away before you finish your prescription. If you stop treatment early, the infection may still be present or it could come back after a short time. About a week after you finish treatment, another urine test may be done to see whether the infection is cured.

Repeated Infections

Urinary tract infections may recur a few weeks after treatment. These are recurrent infections. They can be frustrating, stressful, time consuming, and hard to treat.

Repeated UTIs may cause severe health problems. A kidney infection may occur if bacteria go up the ureters to the kidneys. It only rarely results in severe damage to the kidneys leading to kidney failure, the point at which the kidneys stop making urine.

If you have only two or three repeated infections, your doctor likely will treat these simply as if they were normal infections. When infections occur more often, a week or two apart, the doctor may prescribe a low dose of an antibiotic to be taken each day or after sex. It is hoped that this newer approach to treating this type of UTI will prevent it completely.

Often the cause of repeated UTIs is never found. Doctors may look for some blockage in the urinary tract that would trap urine and aid bacteria in starting an infection. One of these problems may cause repeated infections:

▶ Kidney stones lodged in some part of the urinary tract

▶ One of the tubes narrows in the urinary tract

▶ Diverticula—small pockets that bulge out of the bladder wall or out of the urethra and hold urine

▶ Cystocele—a condition in which the supports that hold the bladder in place become weakened, allowing the bladder to protrude into the vagina

About 4 out of 5 women who have a UTI get another in 18 months. Many women have them even more often.

Testing

Your doctor may refer you to a urologist if infections recur or resist treatment. A urologist is a doctor who specializes in problems of the urinary tract. The urologist will do some tests to find out whether there are any defects in the urinary tract that could be causing your infections.

Intravenous pyelography, or IVP, is a test that helps find defects or abnormal structures in the urinary tract. The test is performed by injecting a chemical into the body that shows up on an X-ray. As this chemical enters the kidneys, ureters, and bladder, X-rays are taken. If there is a blockage or abnormal structure in the urinary tract, it will show on the X-ray.

In a similar test, cystourethrography, a chemical is inserted into a woman's bladder. X-rays are taken as she urinates. This detects any urine that might be backing up in the urinary tract instead of flowing downward. This problem, called reflux, often results in UTIs.

Another test, cystoscopy, is often done to examine the urethra and the inside of the bladder. A cystoscope is a slender metal tube like a telescope with a light. During the exam, it is inserted through the urethra into the bladder. Samples of urine and small bits of tissue can be removed through the cystoscope for further testing.

Most cases of recurrent infection cannot be cured with surgery. If these tests do not reveal a problem that can be treated with surgery, some other treatment must be found.

How You Can Prevent Urinary Tract Infections

There are a number of ways to try to prevent UTIs. Some of them work some of the time or in only some women. It is likely you will find one that works for you:

▶ Practice good hygiene. This is the best and easiest thing you can do to avoid infections. After a bowel movement or after urinating, wipe from front to back. Each day, wash the skin around the rectum, the vagina, and the area in between. Before and after you have sex, wash these areas again.

▶ Drink plenty of fluids to flush bacteria out of your urinary system.

▶ Empty your bladder as soon as you feel the urge or about every 2–3 hours.

▶ Get enough vitamin C in your diet. It makes the urine acidic. This helps keep the number of harmful bacteria in check.

▶ Wear underwear with a cotton crotch. Cotton breathes. Other fabrics can trap moisture.

▶ During sex, you may want to try different positions that cause less friction to your urethra. Your doctor may suggest taking an antibiotic pill right after sex if you tend to have repeated UTIs.

To avoid UTIs, some doctors suggest drinking cranberry juice. In large amounts, this juice prevents the growth of some bacteria by acidifying the urine.

UTERINE BLEEDING

See also *Biopsy, Dilation and Curettage, Hysterosalpingography, Hysteroscopy, Polycystic Ovary Syndrome*

The menstrual period is the time during a woman's cycle when bleeding occurs. Bleeding may last up to 7 days. When the menstrual cycle is not regular, bleeding lasts longer or is heavier than normal, or bleeding occurs between periods, it is known as abnormal uterine bleeding.

Causes of Abnormal Uterine Bleeding

It is normal for menstrual periods to be irregular at certain times of life. For the first few years after a girl begins to have periods (around 9–16 years of age), they are often irregular. As women approach menopause (around 50 years of age), their periods once again may become irregular. Periods may become lighter or heavier because women at this age ovulate less often. If you have gone through menopause and are not taking hormones, any uterine bleeding is abnormal. Increased bleeding as a woman approaches menopause is also abnormal.

Menstrual cycles that are longer than every 35 days (bleeding too seldom) or shorter than every 21 days (bleeding too often) are not normal. Women with such cycles should be checked by a doctor.

Abnormal or heavy uterine bleeding may occur because of hormonal problems, or it can occur as a result of other conditions.

A hormone imbalance occurs when the body makes too much or not enough of a certain hormone. It can be caused by:

- Weight loss or gain
- Heavy exercise
- Stress
- Illness
- Use of some medications

The most common result of a hormone imbalance is anovulation—when the ovaries do not release an egg and a woman does not have a period. Chronic anovulation can cause endometrial hyperplasia. This is a condition in which the lining of the uterus grows too much. It occurs when the balance between progesterone and estrogen in the woman's body is disturbed. Over a long period, endometrial hyperplasia may turn into cancer.

Anovulation may occur if the ovaries produce too much androgen—a male hormone. Often, when anovulation

What Bleeding is Abnormal?

Abnormal uterine bleeding may include:

- Absence of menstrual periods
- Bleeding between periods
- Bleeding after sex
- Spotting
- Any change in normal flow

occurs, the ovaries develop many cysts. This condition is known as polycystic ovary syndrome.

Symptoms of polycystic ovary syndrome include:

) Irregular uterine bleeding

) Irregular periods from an early age

) Infertility

) Acne

) Excessive facial hair or hair on the abdomen or chest

If you have more than one of these symptoms, you should see your doctor.

Diagnosis

To diagnose abnormal uterine bleeding, your doctor will obtain a history of your health. This includes information about any past illness and your use of medications and birth control. You will be asked about any change in your weight, eating and exercise habits, and level of stress. Your doctor also will ask about your menstrual periods. It is helpful for you to keep track of the dates and length of your periods by marking them on a calendar. You also may be asked to keep a daily record of your temperature. This can help show if you are ovulating.

Your doctor also will do a physical exam. You may have blood tests to check your blood count and hormone levels and to see if you are pregnant. Other tests may be needed based on your symptoms:

) Endometrial biopsy

) Ultrasound

) Hysteroscopy

) Laparoscopy

) Dilation and curettage (D&C)

) Hysterosalpingography

Some of these tests can be done in the doctor's office. Others may be done in a day surgery center with pain relief.

Treatment

Treatment for abnormal uterine bleeding will depend on the cause. You may be given hormones or other medications, or surgery may be needed.

Causes of Abnormal Uterine Bleeding

Other causes of abnormal uterine bleeding include:

) Pregnancy

—Miscarriage

—Ectopic pregnancy

) Problems linked to some birth control methods, such as an intrauterine device (IUD) or birth control pills

) Infection of the uterus or cervix

) Uterine fibroids

) Problems with blood clotting

) Certain types of cancer, such as cancer of the uterus, cervix, or vagina

) Chronic medical conditions (for instance, hyperthyroidism and diabetes)

Hormone Therapy

Your doctor may prescribe hormones, such as birth control pills, progesterone, or thyroid medication. These hormones will cause your periods to be more regular and may improve other symptoms. Progesterone also can help prevent and treat endometrial hyperplasia. It may take a few months for hormones to control abnormal bleeding. The type of hormone given to you will depend on whether you want to become pregnant.

After a few menstrual cycles, your doctor should be able to judge how well treatment is working. You may need to be tested again. If you think you might be pregnant, let your doctor know before you start any hormone therapy.

Other Medications

Some medications, such as antiinflammatory drugs (for instance, ibuprofen), may be helpful for heavy bleeding. They also may be used to relieve menstrual cramps. If you have an infection, you will be given antibiotics.

Surgery

Some women with abnormal uterine bleeding will have surgery to remove growths (such as polyps or fibroids) that are causing the bleeding. This may be done with hysteroscopy.

Endometrial ablation is another method for treating abnormal uterine bleeding. Endometrial ablation is intended to stop or reduce bleeding permanently. It uses a form of energy to destroy the lining of the uterus.

Hysterectomy—removal of the uterus—also may be used to treat abnormal uterine bleeding. This may be done when other forms of treatments have failed or are not an option.

Hysterectomy and endometrial ablation are both major surgeries. After these procedures, a woman likely will no longer have periods or be able to get pregnant. Before you decide on treatment, think about all of your options.

See your doctor if you notice that your cycles have become irregular. There is no way of telling why bleeding is abnormal until your doctor examines you. Once the cause is found, abnormal uterine bleeding often can be treated with success.

▶ UTERINE CANCER

▶ See also *Cancer, Dilation and Curettage*

Cancer of the uterus most often affects the lining of the uterus (endometrium). If it is found and treated early, the cure rate is very good. It can be better than 90% when the disease is in an early stage. The more advanced the disease is, the lower the cure rate. This is why finding it early is best.

What Is Cancer?

Normally, healthy cells that make up the body's tissues grow, divide, and replace themselves on a regular basis. This keeps the

Sarcoma of the uterus most often occurs after menopause. Women who have received treatment with high-dose X-rays to their pelvis are at a higher risk of sarcoma of the uterus. These X-rays are sometimes given to women to stop bleeding from the uterus.

body in good repair. Sometimes, however, certain cells develop abnormally and begin to grow out of control. Too much tissue is made, and growths or tumors begin to form. Tumors can be benign (not cancer) or malignant (cancer).

Most types of uterine cancer are adenocarcinomas. Adenocarcinomas involve cells in the lining of the uterus.

Sarcomas are another type of uterine cancer. They arise from muscle and other tissue. Sarcomas are rare, though.

Who Is at Risk?

Cancer of the uterus is rare in women younger than 40 years. It most often occurs in women between the ages of 60–75 years.

Women are at a higher risk of uterine cancer if they:

▶ Are obese

▶ Do not ovulate regularly and often miss periods

▶ Have late menopause

▶ Have polycystic ovary syndrome

▶ Have endometrial hyperplasia

▶ Have had cancer of the ovary, breast, or colon

▶ Have a close family member with uterine cancer

Some women take estrogen after menopause to replace the hormone that is no longer produced by the ovaries. These women may be at risk for cancer of the uterus. If estrogen is combined with another hormone—progesterone—the risk of uterine cancer may be reduced.

The most common type of birth control pills is the combination (estrogen plus progesterone) pill. Women who have used these pills have a lower risk of uterine cancer. This lower risk lasts for at least 10 years after a woman stops taking the pill.

Even if a woman has some or all of the risk factors described here, she may never have uterine cancer. But women at risk should be aware of the symptoms of uterine cancer. They should discuss their concerns with their doctor and have routine checkups that include pelvic exams.

Symptoms

At present, there is no simple way to detect uterine cancer at an early stage in women with no symptoms. The key to finding the disease early is being alert to its symptoms.

The main symptoms of uterine cancer are abnormal bleeding, spotting, or discharge from your vagina. It may be steady or off and on. A watery discharge that has an odor may occur before abnormal bleeding begins. The discharge may be the first sign of a problem. The cause of any abnormal bleeding or discharge needs to be looked into by your doctor. Except when combination hormone therapy is being taken, any bleeding or spotting after menopause is not normal. Ask your doctor about any bleeding or spotting you have after menopause.

Diagnosis

Most of the methods used to diagnose cancer of the uterus can be done in the doctor's office. Methods that may be used include ultrasound or endometrial biopsy. Sometimes hysteroscopy may be done in the doctor's office with local anesthesia. The patient may have dilation and curettage (D&C) done in the hospital.

Although the Pap test should be part of a regular checkup, it is not a good test for uterine cancer. It can detect cancer or pre-cancer of the cervix, but it is less likely to detect uterine cancer.

Treatment

If cancer of the uterus is found, surgery will be done to decide the stage of the disease and how it should be treated. Staging helps your doctor decide what treatment has the best chance for success.

About 75% of the women with uterine cancer have stage I disease. Of these women, 85–90% will have no sign of cancer 5 years or more after treatment. The chance for a cure decreases as the cancer becomes more advanced.

To treat uterine cancer, most patients have both hysterectomy (removal of the uterus) and salpingo-oophorectomy (removal of the ovaries and fallopian tubes). Tissue from lymph nodes in the pelvic region may be tested to find out if the cancer has spread. Some cases of uterine cancer also may require radiation therapy after surgery.

If tests show that the cancer has spread or come back after surgery or radiation, your doctor may advise more drug therapy. Chemotherapy or progestin (a hormone) therapy may be used to treat uterine cancer that has spread to other organs.

When cancer spreads to another part of the body, the new cancer has the same kind of abnormal cells and the same name as the original cancer. For instance, if uterine cancer spreads to the lungs, the cancer cells in the new tumor are uterine cancer cells.

Prevention

There are things you can do to lower your risk of uterine cancer and improve the chance of finding it early:

▶ Report any abnormal vaginal bleeding promptly to your doctor. Most bleeding is not caused by cancer. Only your doctor can perform the tests needed to find the cause of the problem.

> Get a yearly pelvic exam.

> Eat foods that are low in fat and cholesterol and high in fiber. This includes fruits, vegetables, and whole-grain breads and cereals.

> Maintain a normal body weight

> See also
> *Diethylstilbestrol,
> Hysteroscopy, Magnetic
> Resonance Imaging,
> Ultrasound Exam*

> # UTERINE DEFECTS

Some women are born without a uterus. Others have a uterus with an odd shape. One out of every 200–600 women is born with an odd-shaped uterus. The most common types are:

> *Double uterus*—a uterus with two cervixes (openings) and a wide vagina.

> *Bicornuate uterus*—the uterus is partly divided into two sections.

> *Arcuate*—heart-shaped; the top of the uterus is indented.

> *Septate*—the uterus is divided into two sections by a thin wall of tissue.

> *Unicornuate uterus*—the uterus curves to one side. Sometimes a small piece of uterine tissue extends out of the other side.

One cause of uterine defects is fetal exposure to the drug diethylstilbestrol (DES). Diethylstilbestrol is a man-made estrogen that doctors prescribed until 1971 to help prevent miscarriage in pregnant women. Other causes may be genetic.

Some women with uterine defects have trouble getting pregnant. Often times, this is how the problem is first detected. Many times, they can be seen more clearly during a magnetic resonance image of the uterus or a transvaginal ultrasound exam.

Many women with these defects can conceive a baby, but they may face problems carrying it to term. Uterine defects may result in miscarriages or preterm births. Often times this does not need to be treated unless you have had problems with other pregnancies. Sometimes uterine defects can be treated by surgery. This technique is called hysteroscopy, which can be done with local, regional, or general anesthesia. You doctor may dilate your cervix before inserting the hysteroscope through the vagina and cervix into your uterus. Small instruments will then be inserted through the hysteroscope to complete the surgery. After this procedure, a woman can have many normal pregnancies.

In the disorder called müllerian dysgenesis, a woman does not have a uterus, cervix, or upper vagina. About 1 of every 5,000 females is born with this problem. Some of them also have defects of the urinary system and lower spine. These women often have ovaries that work normally, but their vagina is a small pouch. Often, the problem isn't found until the woman realizes she is not getting periods.

Women with this disorder cannot get pregnant. Many can stretch (dilate) their vaginas with a special device given to them by their doctor called a dilator. This allows them to have sex normally. Others can have a vagina built surgically with skin grafts.

▶ UTERINE FIBROIDS

Uterine fibroids are benign (not cancer) growths in the uterus. They are the most common type of growth found in a woman's pelvis. They occur in about 20–25% of all women. Many women who have fibroids are not aware of them because the growths can remain small and not cause symptoms. Fibroids can cause problems because of their size, number, and location. Like any growth, fibroids should be checked by a doctor.

▶ See also
*Hysterosalpingography,
Hysteroscopy, Laparoscopy,
Ultrasound Exam*

Types of Fibroids

Uterine fibroids are growths that develop from the cells that make up the muscle of the uterus. They also are called leiomyomas or myomas.

The size, shape, and location of fibroids can vary greatly. They may appear inside the uterus, on its outer surface, within its wall, or attached to it by a stemlike structure.

Fibroids can range in size from small, pea-sized growths to large, round ones that may be more than 5–6 inches wide. As they grow, they can distort the inside as well as the outside of the uterus. Sometimes fibroids grow large enough to completely fill the pelvis or abdomen.

A woman may have only one fibroid or many of varying sizes. Whether they will occur singly or in groups is hard to predict. They may remain very small for a long time, suddenly grow rapidly, or grow slowly over a number of years. Because it is hard to predict their growth, fibroids can be hard to treat.

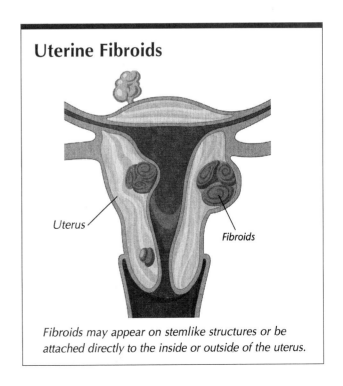

Uterine Fibroids

Uterus

Fibroids

Fibroids may appear on stemlike structures or be attached directly to the inside or outside of the uterus.

Fibroids may be a cause of infertility in some women. However, only 2–3% of infertile women are unable to conceive because of uterine fibroids.

Causes

Fibroids are most common in women aged 30–40 years, but they can occur at any age. Fibroids occur more often in black women than in white women. They also seem to occur at a younger age in black women and to grow more quickly.

Although fibroids are quite common, little is known about what causes them. The female hormone estrogen seems to increase their growth. The levels of estrogen in the body can increase or decrease based on natural events. For instance, pregnancy causes an increase in estrogen and menopause causes a decrease. Medications also may cause a change in estrogen levels.

Symptoms

Most fibroids, even large ones, produce no symptoms at all. When symptoms occur, they often include:

▶ Changes in menstruation
—More bleeding
—Longer or more frequent periods
—Menstrual pain (cramps)
—Vaginal bleeding at times other than menstruation
—Anemia (from blood loss)

▶ Pain
—In the abdomen or lower back (often dull, heavy and aching, but may be sharp)
—During sex

▶ Pressure
—Difficulty urinating or frequent urination
—Constipation, rectal pain, or difficult bowel movements
—Abdominal cramps

▶ Miscarriages and infertility

These symptoms also may be signs of other problems. Therefore, you should see your doctor if you have any symptoms.

Diagnosis

During a routine pelvic exam, the first signs of fibroids can be found. There are a number of tests that may show more information about fibroids:

▶ Ultrasound uses sound waves to create a picture of the uterus or of the pelvic organs.

▶ Hysteroscopy uses a slender device (the hysteroscope) to help the doctor see the inside of the uterus. It is inserted through the vagina and cervix (opening of the uterus). This permits the doctor to see some fibroids inside the uterine cavity.

▶ Hysterosalpingography (HSG) is a special X-ray test. It may detect abnormal changes in the size and shape of the uterus and fallopian tubes.

▶ Laparoscopy uses a slender device (the laparoscope) to help the doctor see the inside of the abdomen. It is inserted through a small cut just below or through the navel. The doctor can see fibroids on the outside of the uterus and some inside the uterine wall with the laparoscope.

Imaging tests, such as magnetic resonance imaging (MRI) and computed tomography (CT) scans, may be used but are rarely needed. Sometimes fibroids are found when these or other procedures are used to check some other medical problem or symptoms. Some of these tests may be helpful in checking on the growth of the fibroid over time.

Complications

Although most fibroids do not cause problems, there can be complications. Fibroids that are attached to the uterus by a stem may twist. This can cause pain, nausea, or fever. Fibroids may become infected. In most cases, this happens only when there is an infection already in the area. In very rare cases, very rapid growth of the fibroid and other symptoms may signal cancer.

A very large fibroid may cause swelling of the abdomen. This can make it hard to perform a thorough pelvic exam.

Fibroids also may cause infertility by preventing conception or causing miscarriage. Other factors should be explored before fibroids are called the cause of a couple's infertility. When fibroids are thought to be a cause, many women are able to become pregnant after they are treated.

Large fibroids that press against the bladder may result in urinary tract infections. Pressure on the ureters may cause urinary obstruction and possibly kidney damage.

Treatment

Fibroids that do not cause symptoms, are small, or occur in a woman nearing menopause often do not require treatment. Certain signs and symptoms, though, may signal the need for treatment:

▶ Heavy or painful menstrual periods

▶ Bleeding between periods

▶ Uncertainty whether the growth is a fibroid or another type of tumor, such as an ovarian tumor

▶ Rapid increase in growth of the fibroid

▶ Infertility

▶ Pelvic pain

If you have fibroids or have had them in the past, make sure to have regular checkups. If you have symptoms of fibroids, see your doctor right away. There is no need to limit your sexual activity unless the fibroids cause pain during sex.

Fibroids may be treated by removing them with surgery. Drugs, such as gonadotropin-releasing hormone (GnRH) agonists, may be used to shrink fibroids temporarily and to control bleeding to prepare for surgery.

The fibroids may be removed with myomectomy or hysterectomy. The choice of treatment depends on factors such as your own wishes and medical advice about the size and location of the fibroids.

Myomectomy

Myomectomy removes the fibroids, leaving the uterus in place. Because a woman keeps her uterus, she may still be able to have children. If a woman does become pregnant after a myomectomy, she may need to have a cesarean delivery (the baby is born through a surgical cut made in the mother's abdomen and uterus). Sometimes, though, a myomectomy causes internal scarring that can lead to infertility.

Fibroids may develop again, even after the procedure. If they do, more surgery is needed in 20–40% of cases.

Myomectomy may be done in a number of ways:

▶ Laparotomy

▶ Laparoscopy

▶ Hysteroscopy

The method used depends on the location and size of the fibroids. For a laparotomy, an incision (cut) is made in the abdomen. The fibroids then are removed through the incision. Fibroids also can be removed through the laparoscope that is used to view the inside of the abdomen.

Hysteroscopy can be used to remove fibroids that protrude into the cavity of the uterus. The fibroids may be removed with a resectoscope, a tiny wire loop that uses electric power, or with a laser. Either of these instruments can be inserted through the hysteroscope. While it cannot remove fibroids deep in the walls of the uterus, it often can control the bleeding these fibroids cause. This type of treatment is often done with pain relief, but you may not need to stay in the hospital.

Hysterectomy

Hysterectomy is the removal of the uterus. The ovaries may or may not be removed. It depends on other factors. Hyster–ectomy may be needed if:

▶ Pain or abnormal bleeding persists

▶ Fibroids are very large

▶ Other treatments are not possible

▶ A woman no longer wants children

If your doctor thinks you need a hysterectomy, he or she will first rule out other problems with the uterus, such as dis-eases of the endometrium (the lining of the uterus).

Uterine Fibroids and Pregnancy

A small number of pregnant women have uterine fibroids. If you are pregnant and have fibroids, they likely won't cause problems for you or your baby.

During pregnancy, fibroids may increase in size. Most of this growth occurs from blood flowing to the uterus. Coupled with the extra burden placed on the body by pregnancy, growth of fibroids may cause discomfort, feelings of pressure, or pain. Fibroids decrease in size after pregnancy in most cases.

Fibroids can increase the risk of:

▶ Miscarriage (in which the pregnancy ends before 20 weeks)

▶ Preterm birth

▶ Breech birth (in which the baby is in a position other than head down)

Rarely, a large fibroid can block the opening of the uterus or keep the baby from passing into the birth canal. In this case, a cesarean delivery is done. In most cases, even a large fibroid will move out of the fetus's way as the uterus expands during pregnancy. Women with large fibroids may have more blood loss after delivery.

Often no treatment of fibroids is needed during pregnancy. If you are having symptoms such as pain or discomfort, your doctor may prescribe rest. Sometimes a pregnant woman with fibroids will need to stay in the hospital for a time because of pain, bleeding, or threatened preterm labor. Very rarely, myomectomy may be performed in a pregnant woman. Cesarean birth may be needed after myomectomy.

Every fibroid is different. The type of treatment suggested depends on the number, size, location, and rate of growth of the fibroids. It also depends on the severity of the symptoms.

V

▶ See also *Forceps*

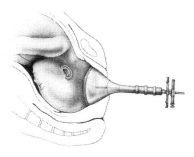

Vacuum Extraction

▶ See Also *Cesarean Birth, Labor, Placental Disorders*

▶ VACUUM EXTRACTION

In some cases, a doctor may need to help delivery of a baby along by using vacuum extraction. Vacuum extraction is much like forceps delivery. A plastic cup is inserted into the vagina and applied to the baby's head. Suction holds the cup in place. A handle on the cup allows the doctor to pull the baby through the birth canal.

In most cases, using vacuum extraction to help delivery causes no major problems. Still, it can bruise the baby's head or tear the vagina or cervix.

▶ VAGINAL BIRTH AFTER CESAREAN DELIVERY

A cesarean birth is the delivery of a baby through an incision (cut) made in the mother's abdomen and uterus. It was once thought that if a woman had one cesarean birth, all other children she had should be born the same way. Today, many women who have had a cesarean delivery can safely give birth through the vagina. This is called vaginal birth after cesarean (VBAC) delivery. VBAC is an option for many women. There are some risks, though.

Reasons to Try VBAC

Of women who try VBAC, about 60–80% succeed and are able to deliver vaginally. Other women may try VBAC but need to switch to a cesarean birth.

There are some good reasons to try VBAC. Advantages to a vaginal birth include:

▶ No abdominal surgery

▶ Shorter hospital stay

▶ Lower risk of infection

▶ Less need for blood transfusions

▶ Faster recovery

Is VBAC Right for You?

In deciding if you can try VBAC, a key factor is the type of incision you had in your uterus for your previous cesarean birth. For cesarean birth, one incision is made in your abdomen and another in your uterus. Any incision makes a scar. Certain types of incisions have a higher risk of the scar tearing during the next birth.

You can't tell what type of scar you have in your uterus by looking at the scar on your skin. Your medical records should show which type of incision was used. There are three types of incisions:

1. *Low transverse*—A side-to-side cut made across the lower, thinner part of the uterus

2. *Low vertical*—An up-and-down cut made in the lower, thinner part of the uterus

3. *High vertical (or classical)*—An up-and-down cut made in the upper part of the uterus

Women with high vertical (classical) scars on the uterus have a higher risk of rupture. Women who have had more than one cesarean delivery also may have an increased risk of rupture. Although it does not occur often, a rupture of the uterus may be harmful to you or your baby. If your doctor thinks you are at high risk for rupture of the uterus, VBAC should not be tried.

Having a vaginal birth after a cesarean delivery can be a safe option for many women. Depending on your needs, VBAC may be a good choice for you.

Other Factors to Consider

Other factors may affect whether VBAC is an option for you. It may not be a good choice in some cases:

▶ *Small pelvis/large baby*—the baby is too large to pass safely through your pelvis during delivery

▶ *Problems for the baby*—there are signs that the baby may have problems during labor or vaginal delivery

▶ *Problems with the placenta*—includes placental abruption (when the placenta separates from the wall of the uterus before the baby is born) or placenta previa (when the placenta covers or partly covers the opening of the uterus)

▶ *Certain conditions*—includes certain serious medical or obstetric conditions, including multiple pregnancy, more than two prior cesarean births, and breech birth

If problems arise or worsen during labor, or if labor is taking too long to progress, cesarean delivery may be needed. The facility where you deliver your baby should be equipped to handle an emergency cesarean delivery. There is a higher risk for infection in the mother and baby in women who try VBAC and then give birth by cesarean.

No labor or delivery is risk free. When considering VBAC, know the risks. Before deciding, a woman should weigh those risks against the benefits.

▶ See also *Cancer, Cervical Cancer*

▶ Vaginal Cancer

Cancer of the vagina is rare. This cancer occurs most often in older women. A common warning sign is bleeding after sex. Women who smoke or are at high risk for cervical cancer often are at a high risk for vaginal cancer.

Any unexplained vaginal bleeding should be checked by a doctor at once. Vaginal cancer may be diagnosed during a pelvic exam or with a Pap test. Often a biopsy is done to find the cause of the problem. If it is found early, vaginal cancer can be treated with success.

▶ Vaginitis

Vaginitis is an inflammation of a woman's vagina. As many as one third of women will have symptoms of vaginitis sometime during their lives. Vaginitis affects women of all ages. There are many possible causes, and the type of treatment depends on the cause.

The Vagina

The vagina has a normal discharge—fluid that passes out of the vagina—that is clear or cloudy and whitish. A healthy vagina keeps a balance of many organisms, such as bacteria and yeast.

Many factors can affect the normal balance of the vagina:

▶ Antibiotics

▶ Changes in the body's normal hormone levels, such as those that occur with pregnancy, breastfeeding, or menopause

▶ Douches

▶ Spermicides

▶ Sexual intercourse

▶ Sexually transmitted diseases (STDs)

A change in the normal balance can allow either yeast or bacteria to increase and result in vaginitis. Vaginitis can result from irritation, from growth of organisms in the vagina, or from infection.

There are things you can do to lower the risk of getting vaginitis. Some of these include:

▶ Do not use feminine hygiene sprays or scented, deodorant tampons. You should not try to cover up a bad odor. It could be a sign of infection that should prompt you to see your doctor.

- Do not douche. It is better to let the vagina cleanse itself.

- Thoroughly clean diaphragms, cervical caps, and spermicide applicators after each use.

- Use condoms during sex.

- Check with your doctor about preventing yeast infections if you are prescribed antibiotics for another type of infection.

Diagnosis and Treatment

To diagnose vaginitis, your doctor will take a sample of the discharge from your vagina and look at it under a microscope. Your doctor also may suggest other tests. To ensure the results of the test are accurate, do not douche or use any vaginal medications or spermicide before you see your doctor.

Treatment may depend on the cause of the vaginitis, as well as on your special needs. For instance, some medications may not be used during pregnancy. Treatment may be either with a pill or by applying a cream or gel to the vagina.

Follow your doctor's instructions exactly, even if the discharge or other symptoms go away before you finish the medication. Even though the symptoms disappear, the infection could still be present. Stopping the treatment may cause symptoms to come back. If symptoms recur after the treatment is finished, see your doctor again—a different treatment may be needed.

Vaginitis can sometimes be a sign of other health problems. Knowing more about the signs and symptoms of this condition will help women get the right treatment.

Types of Vaginitis

Yeast Infection

Yeast infection also is known as candidiasis. It is one of the most common types of vaginal infection.

Cause. Yeast infection is caused by a fungus called Candida. It is found in small numbers in the normal vagina. However, when the balance of the vagina is changed, the yeast may overgrow and cause infection.

Many women who take antibiotics will get yeast infections. The antibiotics kill normal vaginal bacteria, and the yeast then has a chance to overgrow. A woman is more likely to get yeast infections if she is pregnant or has diabetes. Overgrowth of yeast can also occur if the body's immune system, which protects the body from disease, isn't working well. For example, in women infected with HIV (human immunodeficiency virus), yeast infections may be severe. They may not go away, even with treatment, or may recur often. In many cases, the cause of a yeast infection is not known.

Symptoms. The most common symptoms of a yeast infection are itching and burning of the vagina and vulva. The burning may be worse with urination or sex. The vulva may be red and swollen. The vaginal discharge is usually white and has no odor. It may look like cottage cheese. Some women with yeast infections notice an increase or change in discharge. Others do not notice a discharge at all. Some women may have no symptoms.

Treatment. Yeast infections are usually treated by placing medication into the vagina. Some doctors may prescribe a single dose you take by mouth. In most cases, treatment of male sex partners is not necessary. You can buy over-the-counter yeast medication, but be sure to see your doctor if:

▶ This is the first time you've had a vaginal infection

▶ Your symptoms do not go away after treatment

▶ Your vaginal discharge is yellow or green or has a bad odor

▶ There is a chance that you have an STD

Sometimes a woman thinks she has a yeast infection when she actually has another problem. The medication may mask another cause for vaginitis. If there is another cause, it may be harder to find if a woman is taking medication for a yeast infection.

Bacterial Vaginosis

Causes. The bacteria that cause bacterial vaginosis occur naturally in the vagina. Bacterial vaginosis is caused by overgrowth of several of these bacteria. It is not clear whether it can be passed through sex.

Symptoms. The main symptom is increased discharge with a strong fishy odor. The odor is stronger during your menstrual period or after sex. The discharge is thin and dark or dull gray. Itching is not common, but may be present if there is a lot of discharge. Some women may have no symptoms.

Treatment. Two antibiotics are used to treat bacterial vaginosis. One is a drug called metronidazole. It can be taken by mouth or applied to the vagina as a gel. The other drug is called clindamycin. It also can be taken by mouth or applied to the vagina as a cream.

When metronidazole is taken by mouth, it can cause side effects in some patients. These include nausea, vomiting, and darkening of urine. Do not drink alcohol when taking metronidazole. The combination can cause severe nausea and vomiting.

Usually there is no need to treat a woman's sex partner. But if the woman has repeated infections, treatment of the partner may be helpful. Some doctors may suggest that the couple not have sex or that they use a condom during treatment.

Pregnant women may have a greater risk of preterm birth, premature rupture of membranes, and endometritis if they have this infection.

Bacterial vaginosis often comes back. It may require long-term or repeated treatment. In most cases, treatment eventually works in time. Sometimes when bacterial vaginosis keeps coming back it may mean that you have another STD. Your doctor may test you for other infections.

It is not always easy to diagnose vaginitis because different types can have the same symptoms. Do not douche before your visit with your doctor. This may make accurate testing difficult or impossible.

Trichomonas Vaginitis

Causes. Trichomonas is a parasite that is spread through sex. Women who have trichomonas vaginitis are at higher risk for infection with other STDs.

Symptoms. Signs of trichomoniasis may include a yellow-gray or green vaginal discharge. The discharge may have a fishy odor. There may be burning, irritation, redness, and swelling of the vulva and vagina. Sometimes there is pain during urination.

Treatment. Trichomoniasis usually is treated with a single dose of metronidazole by mouth. Do not drink alcohol for 24 hours when taking this drug because it causes nausea and vomiting. Sexual partners must be treated at the same time for treatment to work.

Atrophic Vaginitis

This type of vaginitis is linked with not having enough estrogen. It can occur during breastfeeding and after menopause. Symptoms include vaginal dryness and burning. Atrophic vaginitis is treated with estrogen, either taken by mouth or applied as a vaginal cream. If for some reason a woman cannot take estrogen, she may find a water-soluble lubricant helpful.

▶ VARICOSE VEINS

Varicose veins are bulging veins that become enlarged with pools of blood. They are very common, especially in women of childbearing age and older. Varicose veins appear most often in the legs and thighs. They look like swollen, twisted blue lines. They may make your legs feel heavy and achy. Sometimes your feet and ankles may swell.

Over 25 million Americans have varicose veins. For some, they are simply a cosmetic problem. For others, varicose veins can cause pain and discomfort.

Varicose veins tend to run in families and are more likely to occur as you get older. Varicose veins may be caused by poor circulation that occurs when valves in the veins are weak or missing. Weak vein walls may cause blood to pool resulting in varicose veins. In severe cases, varicose veins may rupture or cause open sores on the skin.

Spider veins are a related problem. They look like a cluster of short, fine lines or starbursts. The most common problem of spider veins and varicose veins is the way they look. Varicose veins are rarely harmful. Some of the main treatments for varicose veins are:

▶ Wearing elastic support stockings

▶ Walking regularly to maintain good circulation

▶ Avoiding being on your feet for long periods

▶ Propping your feet up when you are sitting.

There are many ways varicose veins can be removed. Problem veins can be "stripped" out during surgery and removed through a small cut in the groin. Another approach is sclerotherapy. Using a fine needle, the doctor injects a liquid into the vein that makes it swell. The blood inside it clots, and then the vein turns into scar tissue that fades from view. Both surgery and sclerotherapy work on spider veins, as well.

Your doctor will help select the best treatment for you. The best approach depends on the size of the veins, your age, your health history, and other factors.

▶ See also *Sterilization*

▶ VASECTOMY

A vasectomy is an operation to prevent a man from fathering a child. In a vasectomy, the tubes that carry the sperm to the urethra (vas deferens) are clamped, cut, and sealed to prevent the release of sperm. The egg cannot be fertilized without sperm. This method of birth control is permanent and is a very effective way to prevent pregnancy.

The Procedure

A vasectomy may be done on an outpatient basis in a doctor's office, clinic, or hospital. The procedure is simple and effective, and there are rarely any side effects. Most men are surprised at how easily it is done.

After cleaning the scrotum with antiseptic, the doctor locates each vas in the scrotum. Next, each side of the scrotum is numbed with an injection of local anesthetic. Then, one or two small openings are made into the skin of the scrotum. Each vas is pulled through the opening until it forms a loop. A small section is cut out of the loop and removed. The two ends are tied and may be sealed with heat so scar tissue will grow to block the tubes. Each vas is then placed back in the scrotum.

After the Surgery

After the surgery, the man should rest, apply ice packs, and wear an athletic supporter ("jock strap"). For 2–3 days after the operation, there may be some swelling and discomfort in the scrotum. If these symptoms last for more than a few days, or if there is a fever, severe pain, or other symptoms, the man should call the doctor.

A man can have sexual intercourse again as soon as he feels comfortable. Unlike tubal sterilization in women, though, a vasectomy is not effective right away. Some sperm may still be in the tubes. For this reason, a couple must still use a method of birth control until the man has returned to the doctor or clinic for a final sperm count (in which the number of sperm in a semen sample are counted). It usually takes about 1–3 months for the semen to become totally free of sperm.

After a vasectomy, a man's sexual function does not change. He can still have an erection and ejaculate. Because sperm normally make up only 5% of semen, there will be little difference in the amount of fluid ejaculated.

Vasectomy is highly effective—well under 1% of vasectomies fail to prevent pregnancy. For men who change their minds and want to father a child again, it may be possible to rejoin the tubes. This does not always work, however, so vasectomy should be considered permanent. As with sterilization of women, vasectomy does not guarantee sterility or protect against sexually transmitted diseases.

An issue of some concern to men is whether vasectomy increases the risk of prostate cancer. Current research shows no increased risk.

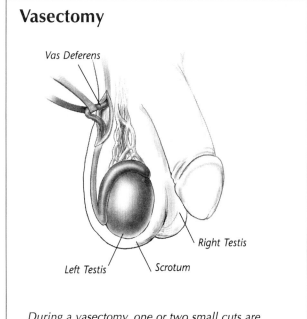

Vasectomy

Vas Deferens

Right Testis

Left Testis

Scrotum

During a vasectomy, one or two small cuts are made in the skin of the scrotum. Each vas is pulled through the opening until it forms a loop. A small section is cut out of the loop and removed.

See also *Cancer,
Vulvar Disorders*

VULVAR CANCER

Invasive cancer of the vulva is most common in women older than 60 years, although it is becoming more frequent in young women. It is more common in smokers than in nonsmokers. History of some sexually transmitted diseases also can be a risk factor. It occurs most often in areas of the vulva where there is chronic inflammation or vulvar intraepithelial neoplasia. Symptoms include itching, discomfort, and abnormal bleeding. Sometimes a lump or sore is present, and the lymph nodes in the groin may be enlarged.

Invasive cancer of the vulva is diagnosed by biopsy. Surgery usually is needed to remove all cancerous tissue. Some nearby normal tissue also is removed to help treat the cancer. In most cases, lymph node tissue also is removed from the groin. Radiation (X-ray treatment) and chemotherapy (drug treatment) also may be used at the same time.

The outlook for invasive vulvar cancer depends on the extent of the disease when it is treated. In general, the earlier the cancer, the better the chances for a full recovery. This is a good reason to do a self-exam.

See also *Vulvodynia*

VULVAR DISORDERS

The vulva, the outer part of the female genital area, can be the site of certain diseases. Some may annoy you and cause discomfort. Others, such as cancer, can be more severe if not treated early.

The Vulvar Self-Exam

Just as you would examine your breasts or skin for changes that could mean cancer, you should examine your vulva. Many diseases of the vulva have symptoms that are alike. The vulvar self-exam will help you to be aware of any changes in the vulvar area that could mean an infection or other problem. This is especially important if you have ever had any vulvar disease before.

Some changes in the vulva may mean cancer. Often cancer won't occur if changes in the vulva are caught early enough.

Tell your doctor if you see any changes or have symptoms that don't go away. These symptoms include itching, bleeding, or discomfort. If a problem does occur, your chances of catching it at an early stage—when treatment is most successful—are best if you have examined yourself regularly.

Types of Vulvar Disease

To diagnose your vulvar condition, your doctor will ask questions about your symptoms. He or she also will examine you. A number of tests may be performed.

Contact Dermatitis

Contact dermatitis is caused by chemical irritation of the skin of the vulva. It may be caused by:

▶ Perfumed or dyed toilet tissue

▶ Underwear or bathing suits

▶ Soaps, detergents, or fabric softeners

▶ Talcum powder

▶ Feminine hygiene sprays

▶ Deodorant pads

▶ Spermicidal foams, creams, and jellies

▶ Rubber products, such as diaphragms or condoms

▶ Poison ivy or similar plants

The chief symptoms of contact dermatitis are redness and itching. (Insect bites or stings can cause the same symptoms.) Your doctor may diagnose it after examining the vulvar area and asking you about the substances that come in contact with your vulva.

Getting rid of the source of the irritation is the first step in treating this condition. If the dermatitis is severe, your doctor may prescribe a cream. Applying cool compresses also may relieve the itching.

To avoid having this problem again, stay away from what caused it in the first place. Always wash your hands before you touch your genital area.

Yeast Infections

Yeast infections are the most common type of vulvar infections. The condition seen most often is called Candida vulvitis. The vagina often is infected, too. Some women are at greater risk of yeast infection:

▶ Women with diabetes

▶ Pregnant women

▶ Women taking antibiotics

The Vulvar Self-Exam

1. Wash your hands before you begin. Lie or sit up in a comfortable position in a good, strong light with a hand mirror—a magnifying mirror may work best. It may help to prop up your back with a pillow, or you can squat or kneel. The key thing is to find a position in which you can clearly see the vulvar area, perineum, and anus.

2. Gently separate the outer lips of the vulva. Look for any redness, swelling, dark or light spots, blisters, bumps, or other unusual signs.

3. Next, separate the inner lips and look at the area between them, as well as the entrance to the vagina.

4. Gently pull back the hood of the clitoris and examine the area under the hood and the tip of the clitoris.

5. Be sure to inspect the area around the urethra, the perineum, the anus, the outside of the labia majora, and the mons.

Symptoms of yeast infection can include redness, itching, and a whitish, clumpy discharge. Sometimes women have burning with urination. Other vaginal infections also produce vulvar irritation and itching.

To diagnose this infection, the discharge on the skin of the vulva or in the vagina may be taken and examined under a microscope. Antifungal drugs and good hygiene are the treatment. A cream or tablet (or both) can be inserted into the vagina and applied to the vulvar skin. These drugs can be bought over the counter. If you have not had a yeast infection before or if your symptoms do not go away after self-treatment, you should see your doctor.

Sexually Transmitted Diseases

The most common sexually transmitted diseases (STDs) affecting the vulva are viruses. The best way to prevent getting or passing these viruses is to use barrier methods of contraception. Condoms are the best choice.

Genital Warts. Genital warts (condyloma) are caused by human papillomavirus (HPV). They often are spread through sexual contact. The warts appear on the vulva as raised and sometimes reddened patches that may hurt or itch. Sometimes there may be a cluster of warts that look like tiny cauliflowers.

There are a number of ways to treat genital warts:

- Solutions, such as trichloroacetic acid (TCA), applied to the warts
- Podophyllin, a drug that is painted on the warts
- Interferon, a drug that is injected into the warts or into a muscle
- Laser treatment
- Cryotherapy (cold cautery), which destroys the warts by freezing
- Hot cautery, which burns off the warts with an electrical device
- Surgery

These treatments do not get rid of the virus, though. The warts may come back.

Genital warts also can appear on the cervix. Certain types of viruses that cause cervical warts have been linked to the growth of cancer of the vulva and the cervix. See your doctor right away if you notice anything that looks like a wart on your genital area.

Herpes. Genital herpes infection is caused by herpes simplex virus. It can be spread through sexual contact. The infection is marked by sores or ulcers that appear on the vulva. They may last from a few days to a few weeks, then may go away and come back. They

There is no vaccine to protect against HPV, and there is no cure for it. Help prevent it by lowering your risk—limit your number of sexual partners and use a condom every time you have vaginal, anal, or oral sex. The virus may be found in semen even if no warts are present.

can cause severe pain and discomfort, especially during a first outbreak. Later outbreaks often are less severe.

There is no treatment for genital herpes that will kill the virus. A drug called acyclovir, though, can help relieve symptoms during an outbreak. The drug is available as an ointment or pill. It also can make the sores go away faster and help prevent recurrences.

Systemic Diseases

Systemic diseases—those that arise in other parts of the body—also may affect the vulva. Psoriasis, for instance, is a skin disease that appears as red, thick, scaly patches that may itch. Crohn disease, in which ulcers form in the digestive system, may show up on the vulva before it appears elsewhere. Infection of the sweat glands also may appear on the vulva.

If the systemic disease can be treated, then vulvar symptoms often go away as well. If not, the vulvar symptoms are treated with creams or ointments.

Vulvar Dystrophies

A dystrophy is abnormal growth of the skin of the vulva. It can be too thin, too thick, or a mixture of both. When it is too thin, it may look like thin, wrinkled paper, and the vaginal opening may shrink. When it is too thick, white, hardened patches on the vulvar area may appear.

A biopsy may be done to diagnose this problem (especially when the skin is too thick). Lumpy sores may be a sign of cancer. Vulvar dystrophies often are chronic. They require long-term treatment with creams or ointments. These are rubbed into the vulvar tissue. Your doctor also may suggest keeping your vulva dry. The aim is to control, rather than cure, the disease. In some cases, surgery may be needed.

Vulvar Intraepithelial Neoplasia

Vulvar intraepithelial neoplasia (VIN) is a noninvasive growth confined to the skin of the vulva. Its most severe form is called carcinoma in situ of the vulva. It is caused by changes in the cells of the vulvar tissue that cause them to grow abnormally.

Genital warts caused by HPV infection have been linked to VIN. Rarely, high-grade VIN (VIN 3) can progress to invasive cancer. This happens in only 1–2% of cases and often progresses slowly. Sometimes it clears up by itself, especially after a woman has had a baby.

Care of the Vulva

To help clear up certain vulvar diseases or prevent them from coming back, your doctor may ask you to do the following:

- Keep the vulva clean and dry.
- Don't wear tight-fitting pants or underwear.
- Don't wear pantyhose unless they have a cotton crotch.
- Don't use pads or tampons with deodorant.
- Don't use perfumed soap or scented toilet paper.
- Don't douche or use feminine sprays or talcs.
- Don't sleep in tight-fitting garments.

Symptoms of VIN include itching and raised lesions of various colors (brown, red, pink, white, or gray). The disease also can occur without any symptoms. Tests to diagnose VIN include colposcopy and biopsy.

VIN often can be treated with success by using simple treatments, such as minor surgical or laser removal. For this reason, and because VIN may not produce any symptoms, you should have regular checkups by your doctor. This is even more true if you have a history of genital warts or if you smoke.

Paget Disease of the Vulva

Paget disease is another type of intraepithelial neoplasia. It may mean that a form of skin cancer is present in the same area.

The symptoms of Paget disease are soreness and severe itching that keeps coming back. There also may be sharp-bordered, red, velvety lesions or white patches on the vulva, perineum, anus, or vagina. Symptoms often are long lasting.

The cause of Paget disease is unknown. It is diagnosed by biopsy and is treated with surgery in most cases.

Invasive Cancer

Invasive cancer of the vulva is most common in women older than 60 years. It is more common in smokers than in nonsmokers. History of some STDs also can be a risk factor. It occurs most often in areas of the vulva where there is chronic inflammation or VIN.

Symptoms include itching, discomfort, and bleeding. Sometimes a tumor or ulcer is present. The lymph nodes in the groin also may be enlarged.

Vulvar cancer accounts for about 500 deaths a year in the United States. Because the disease has symptoms that can be seen easily, it can be found in its early stages—when it is easiest to treat.

Any lump or sore that does not heal should be checked by a doctor at once. Often a biopsy is done to find the cause of the problem. The outlook for invasive vulvar cancer depends on the extent of the disease when it is treated. If it is found early, vulvar cancer can be treated with success. This is a good reason to do a self-exam.

Melanoma

Melanoma is a rare form of skin cancer. It occurs most often after puberty on any area of the skin. Melanoma on the vulva can be found during a vulvar self-exam. Look for changing moles or those that are red or have uneven borders.

Treatment for vulvar melanoma is surgery to remove the cancer as well as some normal tissue around it. If the disease has spread to the lymph nodes in the groin, they may be removed, too. The outlook for recovery depends on the depth of invasion of the cancer and whether it has spread to other parts of the body.

▶ Vulvodynia

▶ See also *Pain During Sex, Vulvar Disorders*

Some women have chronic pain in the vulva. This condition is called vulvodynia. At least 200,000 women in the United States have vulvodynia. A woman of any age can have it. No one knows what causes vulvodynia. But treatment can help relieve some of the pain.

What Is Vulvodynia?

Vulvodynia is chronic pain of the vulva. Chronic means that the pain occurs again and again or never goes away. The pain caused by vulvodynia can affect your health and your sex life.

One kind of vulvodynia—vestibulitis—causes pain of the vestibule. The pain may occur when you urinate, insert a tampon, or have sex. Vestibulitis may last for months or years if not treated.

If you have chronic pain, you may become afraid to have sex. This fear may lead to vaginismus. This is a spasm of the muscles around the vagina. You can't control these spasms, and they make it hard for your partner to enter you. Problems with sex can frustrate both of you.

Vulvodynia can disrupt your daily life. Chronic pain can make it hard to work or be active. Dealing with pain on a long-term basis may lead to problems with your self-image. It also may cause depression to develop or worsen.

Your emotions can play a role in how you feel pain and cope with it. Stress can make the pain worse.

Symptoms

With vulvodynia, you may have some of these symptoms around your vulva:

▶ Burning

▶ Stinging

▶ Rawness

▶ Itching

▶ Aching

▶ Soreness

▶ Throbbing

The pain may be constant, or it may come and go. Symptoms may be felt during exercise or even while sitting or resting.

Causes

No one is sure what causes vulvodynia. It may be the result of more than one cause, such as:

▶ Infections

▶ Irritation of the gland openings

▶ Spasms of the muscles that support the pelvic organs

▶ Allergies to certain chemicals or substances

▶ Hormonal changes

▶ Sensitive nerves of the vulva

▶ Sexual contact or history of sexual abuse

Vulvodynia can be a symptom of many conditions that, if diagnosed, can be treated. Certain skin diseases or infections can cause the pain. Often, no exact cause can be found for the symptom. This doesn't mean that there is no cause, just that one can't be found.

How Is Vulvodynia Diagnosed?

To diagnose vulvodynia, your doctor will do an exam and tests. You may be asked questions about:

▶ Your symptoms—what they feel like, how long they last, what brings them on, what makes them feel better, what makes them feel worse

▶ Your sexual practices

▶ Your lifestyle—diet, exercise, clothing, products used on your skin

▶ Your medical history—whether you have had any kind of infections or skin problems

▶ What medications you are taking or have taken in the past (including over the counter)

During the exam, your doctor will examine your vulva and vagina carefully. A sample of discharge from your vagina may be taken and examined. Your doctor also may suggest other tests, such as colposcopy and biopsy.

One form of vulvodynia, called chronic vestibulitis, has no known cause. Because it is hard to diagnose, it also is hard to treat. In fact, there are at least a dozen different treatments for this disorder in use in the United States. Some treatments take a number of months or even years before symptoms are relieved.

How Is It Treated?

There are many kinds of treatment that may relieve your symptoms. No one method works all the time. Some women find relief from a mixture of methods. In most cases, the simplest method is used first. If it doesn't work, your doctor may suggest something else. Some treatments take a few months before you get any relief.

Your symptoms may be treated with medications, including:

▶ Antibiotics or anti-yeast medications

▶ Antiinflammatories

▶ Steroids

▶ Estrogen creams

▶ Local anesthetics

▶ Antidepressants or anticonvulsants

Some medications have side effects and make vulvodynia worse. Treatment may relieve symptoms for a while, but symptoms may come back later. If treatment does not work and pain is severe, surgery may help some patients.

Other things may help you cope with the pain. One of them is to make changes in your diet. Certain foods, like greens, chocolate, berries, beans, and nuts, may produce urine that is irritating. Eating less of these foods may help.

Some women may try physical therapy or biofeedback. Physical therapy treats muscle spasms and teaches exercises that strengthen the pelvic muscles. Biofeedback trains you to control the muscles in the vagina. Control of these muscles may help lessen your pain. Women with vaginismus also can learn exercises that will help with muscle control during sex.

Coping with the Pain

Chronic pain can affect your daily life. If you have vulvodynia, get as much information about it as you can. Support groups can be a good way to do this. Sometimes a therapist who counsels people with chronic illnesses can be helpful.

You should take special care of your vulva:

▶ Keep the vulva clean and dry.

▶ Don't wear tight-fitting pants or underwear

▶ Don't wear pantyhose.

▶ Don't use pads or tampons with deodorants.

▶ Don't use perfumed soap or scented toilet paper.

▶ Don't douche or use feminine sprays or talcs.

▶ Be sure your partner uses lubricated condoms when you have sex.

▶ Use ice packs. They also may provide some relief. Your doctor may suggest other forms of relief.

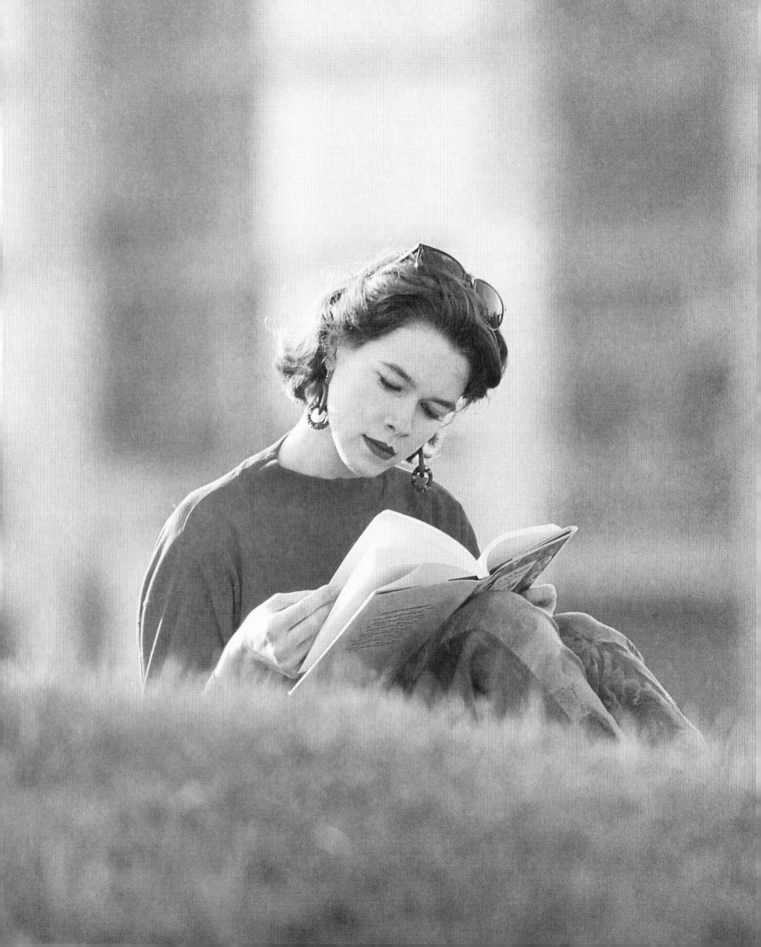

RESOURCES

Finding quality information is the first step to learning more about your health care. Your doctor should be your first resource for health information. He or she understands your needs and can help you find information that works for you. To make the best use of your time and your doctor's time, be informed. This includes using other sources of health information, such as books, the Internet, and health associations to gather information about your health. This section is designed to provide women with the resources to allow them to take an active role in their health care.

KEYS TO GOOD INFORMATION ABOUT YOUR HEALTH

With the explosion of health care information available today, how can a woman know what's best for herself and her family? How can she find the best information and ensure it is accurate? One way is to go to the right sources. Another way is to know how to judge quality information. Both traditional printed materials and the Internet are important ways to keep informed. If you know how to find high-quality printed materials, you can apply the same principles to finding and evaluating materials on the Internet.

Finding Information

Your first source of health information should be your own doctor. He or she is familiar with the details of your situation and can direct you to materials that are relevant to you and to local practices. If you do obtain medical information from other resources, it's a good idea to discuss it with your doctor to ensure that they apply to your care.

Another source of information is your local library. The librarian can recommend books, journal articles, and Internet sites and help you obtain these materials through the library. If you live in or near a city, you may have access to information through a medical school library, public library, or government library. You can call the National Network of Libraries of Medicine, the U.S. regional library network, for referral to your closest medical library (800-338-7657).

For this book, the librarians from the ACOG Resource Center have prepared a reading list entitled Additional Resources. Tips for searching MEDLINE to find articles in medical journals also are provided.

Searching MEDLINE (PubMed) on the World Wide Web

MEDLINE is the National Library of Medicine's (NLM) database of more than 9 million abstracts of articles in more than 3,800 medical journals. PubMed <www.ncbi.nlm.nih.gov/pubmed> is the National Library of Medicine's free version of MEDLINE. Help for PubMed is found on the main page on the left-hand side of the screen. You also may wish to check out the Overview and Frequently Asked Questions (FAQs).

Basic Searching

To search by subject in PubMed, just type the word or words that describe your topic into the search box. You can enter more than one search term. PubMed will automatically combine the terms and look for them in the title, abstract, and subject headings of the record. A listing of the articles about your search item will be displayed. Click on titles that interest you. An abstract of the full article will display the content of the study or research as well as the study's result. Also, the citation of the article will be listed so you can find the full article at the library.

To narrow your search to fewer articles, use some of PubMed's shortcuts:

▶ **Title Words:** Narrows the topic so that your term will be in the title of the article. To find an article with infertility in the title, type: infertility [ti].

▶ **MeSH Terms or MeSH Major Term:** These are the NLMs Medical Subject Headings (how an article is indexed on MEDLINE). To find all articles under the subject heading infertility, type: infertility [mh] or infertility [majr].

▶ **Text Words:** All the words in the title and abstract as well as MeSH terms are searched. To find an article with infertility anywhere in the record, type: infertility [tw].

▶ **Date of Publication:** Narrows the search to a specific year, month, or date. To find an article that was published on July 6, 1999, type: 1999/07/06 [dp].

▶ **Language:** Narrows the search to articles written in a certain language. To find an article in English, type: english [la].

▶ **Exclusion of a Topic:** Narrows the search to a leave out a certain subject within a topic. To find an article on infertility that does not include erectile dysfunction, type: infertility NOT erectile dysfunction.

Ways to Find More Articles:

▶ Remove terms from your search.

▶ Use broader concepts. (Example: Instead of using "thinprep" (a type of Pap test), use "Pap test").

▶ Use OR with synonyms (words that are very close in meaning). For instance, antenatal OR prenatal OR antepartum.

▶ Use Boolean Operators. The terms AND, OR, NOT (they must be capitalized) can be used to make your search broader, narrower, or more complex. For example, Pregnancy [mh] AND smith jb [au] NOT Labor [mh] OR Delivery [majr].

Author Searching

Enter an author's last name and initials with no punctuation (smith ja). You also can use the field designation when searching for a specific author: Author Name [au] (smith jb [au]).

How to Get a Document

You should be able to obtain items through your local public library (although they may not be free of charge). Ask your local librarian to help you search. You can also call 800-338-7657 to find the nearest medical library that may be able to help you. To find other information, you also can search the National Library of Medicine's site MEDLINEplus <www.nlm.nih.gov/medlineplus/>, which has information on clearinghouses, directories, and other consumer information.

Medical associations, the federal government, and health groups often are great resources. Many of these resources are mentioned in this book; others can be found through the Internet or through your public library.

You also may have bookstores in your area that include health sections and well-informed staff. If you do not have such a bookstore close to you, try finding health materials through a bookstore Internet site, such as <www.amazon.com>, <www.bordersbooks.com>, and <www.bn.com>.

The Internet

The Internet is full of information on health. You just need to know how to find it. There are many ways to search for information on the Internet. Terms that may be helpful to you during your search are defined in the box.

1. Use search engines. Some web sites, such as Yahoo, Excite, Alta Vista, and HotBot can search for information on other web sites. Try several search engines to see what gives you the most useful results. Go to <www.allonesearch.com> to gain access to several engines. Learn how to use at least one search engine well so you can do more advanced searches. Bookmark your favorite search engines. Because general search engines are not specific to medicine and some may be corrupted (biased in favor of finding certain web sites, depending on the sponsors), evaluate your results carefully.

If you have limited experience on the Internet, you may want to get a copy of the "Parents Guide to the Internet," published by the U.S. Department of Education, November, 1997. This document walks you through the entire process of using the Internet, from finding or buying a computer, selecting your Internet service provider, to using specific search engines. Several organizations, including the American Academy of Pediatrics and the American Library Association, provided input. You can print a copy through <www.ed.gov/pubs/parents/internet/> or call 800-USA-Learn.

2. Try metasearch engines, such as Meta Crawler and DogPile, to search multiple search engines in one search. Using metasearch engines saves you time, but you may not find as much through a metasearch as through advanced searches in individual search engines.

3. Go directly to the home page of the best source of the information you need. For instance, if you are looking for information on birth defects, go directly to the March of Dimes home page <www.modimes.org>.

4. Go directly to a metasite (a gateway). A gateway or metasite has lots of subject-related links. You may be able to find all of the information you need through the links from the metasite. A good metasite is run by a well-known organization, such as the federal government. It includes carefully selected materials and links and has easy-to-use search features. Some good health-related sites are shown in the box "Metasites for Women's Health Information."

5. Join newsgroups, mailing lists, and web-based forums, but use them with caution because they may be biased or present one-sided or incorrect views. Support groups that focus on your specific disease may be a rich source for information as well. To find support groups on specific health topics, visit the American Self-Help Clearinghouse web site <www.mentalhelp.net/selfhelp/>.

Internet Terms

Address: The unique location of an information site on the Internet, a specific file (for example, a web page), or an E-mail user.

Bookmark: A saved link to a web site that has been added to a list of saved links so that you can simply click on it rather than having to retype the address when visiting the site again.

CD-ROM (Compact Disc Read-Only Memory): A compact disc that can store large amounts of information and generally is used on computers with CD-ROM drives.

Chat Room: A location on an online service that allows users to communicate with each other about an agreed-upon topic in "real time" (or "live"), as opposed to delayed time as with e-mail.

Download: To copy a file from one computer system to another. From the Internet user's point of view, to download a file is to request it from another computer (or from a web page on another computer) and to receive it.

E-mail (Electronic Mail): A way of sending messages electronically from one computer to another, generally through a modem and telephone line connected to a computer.

Freenet: A community network that provides free online access, usually to local residents, and often includes its own forums and news.

Hardware: A term for the nuts, bolts, and wires of computer equipment and the actual computer and related machines.

Homepage: The site that is the starting point on the World Wide Web for a particular group or organization.

Hypertext Link: An easy method for retrieving information by choosing highlighted words or icons on the screen. The link will take you to related documents or sites.

Hypertext Transfer Protocol: A standard used by World Wide Web servers to provide rules for moving text, images, sound, video, and other multimedia files across the Internet.

Icon: A small picture on a web page that represents the topic or information category of another web page. Frequently, the icon is a hypertext link to that page.

Internet: A worldwide collection of computer networks that allows people to find and use information and communicate with others.

ISP (Internet Service Provider): A generic term for any company that can connect you directly to the Internet.

Modem: A device that allows computers to communicate with each other over telephone lines or other delivery systems by changing digital signals to telephone signals for transmission and then back to digital signals. Modems come in different speeds: the higher the speed, the faster the data is transmitted.

Mouse: A small device attached to the computer by a cord that lets you give commands to the computer. The mouse controls an arrow on the computer screen and allows you to point and click to make selections.

Netiquette: Rules or manners for interacting courteously with others online (such as not typing a message in all capital letters, which is equivalent to shouting).

Online Service: A company such as America Online or Prodigy that provides its members access to the Internet through its own special user interface as well as additional services such as chat rooms, children's areas, travel planning, and financial management.

Search Engine: A program that performs keyword searches for information on the Internet.

Software: A computer program or set of instructions. System software operates on the machine itself and is invisible to you. Application software allows you to carry out certain activities, such as word processing, games, and spreadsheets.

URL (Uniform Resource Locator): The World Wide Web address of a site on the Internet. For example, the URL for the White House is www.whitehouse.gov.

Usenet Newsgroups: A system of thousands of special interest groups to which readers can send or "post" messages; these messages are then distributed to other computers on the network. Usenet registers newsgroups, which are available through Internet Service Providers.

Virus: A piece of programming code inserted into other programming to cause some unexpected and usually undesirable event, such as lost or damaged files. Viruses can be transmitted by downloading programming from other sites or be present on a diskette. The source of the file you're downloading or of a diskette you've received often is unaware of the virus. The virus lies dormant until circumstances cause its code to be executed by the computer.

Web Browser: A software program that lets you find, see, and hear material on the World Wide Web, including text, graphics, sound, and video. Popular browsers are Netscape and AltaVista. Most online services have their own browsers.

World Wide Web (Web or WWW): A hypertext-based system that allows you to browse through a variety of linked Internet resources organized by colorful, graphics-oriented home pages.

U.S. Department of Education. Parents Guide to the Internet. Washington, DC: 1997

Evaluating Information

Whether you are reviewing printed materials or Internet sites, you need to ask two questions: Can I trust the information? and Does it help me? Here are some things to consider.

DISCERN <www.discern. org.uk> is designed to help users of consumer health information judge the quality of print and web information about treatment choices. It was developed by the British Library and the University of Oxford for the National Health Services (U.K.).

Trust

The main aspects of trust are the authority of the web site, the objectivity of the information, and its basis on evidence. You also may want to consider whether advertising and promotion affect the content and the users' privacy.

Authority. You should be able to tell who is in charge of the site, the webmaster, the content provider(s), the parent organization, and the sponsoring organization. You should be able to contact the webmaster by e-mail and find information about the parent organization and how to contact it. Health care web site content should be developed by experts and should clearly state that these contents do not substitute for consultation with your own doctor. Examples of good web sites are those sponsored by the federal government and national nonprofit health care groups. University sites are often very good, but watch out for academic URLs with ~ (tilde), which indicate that the site may be written by students or faculty members and may not represent official policy.

Objectivity. Contents should be accurate, complete, unbiased, and balanced. There should be mention of why certain informa-

Metasites for Women's Health Information

healthfinder (www.healthfinder.gov). healthfinder is a free gateway to consumer health and human services information developed by the U.S. Department of Health and Human Services. It can lead you to selected online publications, clearinghouses, databases, web sites, and support and self-help groups, as well as the government agencies and not-for-profit organizations that produce reliable information for the public. You can select topics from a list or search the text.

Medem (www.medem.com). Seven national medical organizations have jointly formed Medem, which provides consumer health materials and other services. Members of these organizations can host a web page to provide personalized information to their patients. ACOG is participating in Medem, and more than 130 current ACOG consumer pamphlets are included in Medem.

MEDLINEplus (www.nlm.nih.gov/medlineplus/). MEDLINEplus provides up-to-date, quality health care information from the U.S. National Library of Medicine, part of the National Institutes of Health. MEDLINEplus provides access to extensive information about specific diseases and conditions and also has links to consumer health information from the NIH, clearinghouses, dictionaries, lists of hospitals and physicians, and clinical trials. You can choose a topic by letter, select from a list, or go directly to full-text searching.

National Women's Health Information Center (www. 4woman.gov). The National Women's Health Information Center (NWHIC), a service of the Office on Women's Health of the U.S. Department of Health and Human Services, provides a gateway to the vast array of federal and other women's health information resources.

tion was used or left out, and the review process should be described. The resources upon which the information is based should be cited and linked to the site if possible. Cited resources should be based on scientific studies. Health care sites should discuss alternative therapies, as well as outcome without treatment. Watch out for publications by special interest groups, personal opinion, and anything that is misleading or inaccurate (information not substantiated by real data or studies).

Promotion and Advertising. Advertising and promotion on a web site should not keep you from getting the unbiased information you need. Be aware of the relationships between advertising, sponsorship, and contents on a site. Be careful about giving out personal information on the Internet. One way for a site to gather personal information is to say that they will send you information matched to your health care needs. The first step is online profiling, which is gathering confidential information about you. For your own protection, find out what the site will do with this information before giving it to them. Will they protect the confidentiality of your information?

Helpfulness

Whether or not information is helpful to you depends upon the design and content of a site, as well as your specific information needs. A well-designed site is easy to use and understand, has a consistent format and command system throughout the site, is well-organized, provides a good "road map" to the organization of the site, and is well-written and edited. Pages are attractive and legible. Each page includes the URL, host organization name, and date of last update. All links work and allow easy return to the main home page. The site should include a search engine for full-text searching, as well as a subject index. Search results should be ranked according to how closely they relate to the topic. Graphics should be small to save online time. A thesaurus to show related terms and online support are useful features.

The contents of a site should be current, reliable, stable, and detailed enough to meet your information needs. A good site will state clearly the scope of the information and the purpose of the site. Copyright should be indicated and respected throughout the site. Any links to outside groups are to high-quality sites, and information on how these links are selected is presented.

Finally, only you can decide if the information is right for you. A site could be authoritative, well-designed, and full of information, but still not meet your specific needs. It may not be in the right language, presented at the right level, aimed at the right age group, sensitive to gender and ethnic issues important to you, or accessible by you if you are disabled or have limited access to technology.

IQ Tool <hitiweb.mitretek. org/iq/default.asp> is sponsored in part by the Health Information Technology Institute of Mitretek Systems, a nonprofit organization that seeks to find ways to use technology for public benefit. The IQ user responds to yes-or-no questions about the quality and content of a medical Internet site. IQ computes a score and comments about the strengths and weaknesses of the site.

ADDITIONAL RESOURCES

American College of Obstetricians and Gynecologists. Planning Your Pregnancy and Birth. Washington, DC: ACOG, 2000

American Medical Association. Complete Guide to Women's Health. New York: Random House, 1996

Bell, Ruth. Changing Bodies, Changing Lives: A Book for Teens on Sex and Relationships. New York: Times Books, 1998

Boston Women's Health Book Collective. Our Bodies, Ourselves for the New Century: A Book by and for Women. New York: Simon & Schuster, 1998

Bullough, Vern L. Contraception: A Guide to Birth Control Methods. Amherst, New York: Prometheus Books, 1997

Carlson, Karen J. The Harvard Guide to Women's Health. Cambridge, Massachusetts: Harvard University Press, 1996

Carlson, Karen J. The Women's Concise Guide to a Healthier Heart. Cambridge, Massachusetts: Harvard University Press, 1997

Chism, Denise M. The High-Risk Pregnancy Sourcebook. Los Angeles: Lowell House, 1997

Clayman, Charles B. American Medical Association Family Medical Guide. New York: Random House, 1994

Curtis, Glade B. Your Pregnancy Week-by-Week. Tucson, Arizona: Fisher Books, 1997

Dennerstein, Lorraine. Hysterectomy: New Options and Advances. New York: Oxford University, 1995

Doress-Worters, Paula B. Midlife and Older Women Book Project. The New Ourselves, Growing Older: Women Aging with Knowledge and Power. New York: Simon & Schuster, 1994

Epps, Roselyn Payne. American Medical Women's Association. The Women's Complete Healthbook. New York: Delacorte, 1995

Froemming, Paul. The Best Guide to Alternative Medicine. Los Angeles: Renaissance, 1998

Fromer, Margot Joan. The Endometriosis Survival Guide: Your Guide to the Latest Treatment Options and Best Coping Strategies. Oakland, California: New Harbinger, 1998

Hoshiko, Sumi. Our Choices: Women's Personal Decisions about Abortion. Binghamton, New York: Haworth Press, 1993

Hutcherson, Hilda. Having Your Baby: A Guide for African-American Women. New York: One World/Ballantine, 1997

Jones, Maggie. Motherhood After 35: Choices, Decisions, Options. Tucson, Arizona: Fisher Books, 1998

Kelly, Robert B. American Academy of Family Physicians. Family Health and Medical Guide. Dallas: Word Publishing, 1996

La Leche League International. The Womanly Art of Breastfeeding. New York: Plume, 1997

Murphy, Gerald P. American Cancer Society. Informed Decisions: The Complete Book of Cancer Diagnosis, Treatment, and Recovery. New York: Viking, 1997

Reader's Digest. Foods That Harm, Foods That Heal: An A–Z Guide to Safe and Healthy Eating. Pleasantville, New York: Reader's Digest, 1997

Schiff, Isaac. Massachusetts General Hospital. Menopause: The Most Comprehensive, Up-to-Date Information Available To Help You Understand This Stage of Life, Make the Right Choices, and Cope Effectively. New York: Times Books/ Random House, 1996

Villarosa, Linda. National Black Women's Health Project. Body & Soul: The Black Women's Guide to Physical Health and Emotional Well-Being. New York: Harper Perennial, 1994

White, Evelyn C. The Black Women's Health Book: Speaking for Ourselves. Seattle: Seal Press, 1994

White, Jocelyn. The Lesbian Health Book: Caring for Ourselves. Seattle: Seal Press, 1997

HEALTH ASSOCIATIONS

Alcoholics Anonymous
PO Box 459
Grand Central Station
New York, NY 10163
Phone: (212) 870-3400
Fax: (212) 870-3003
Web Address: www.aa.org

Alzheimer's Association
919 N Michigan Ave
Suite 1100
Chicago, IL 60611-1676
Phone: 800-272-3900
Web Address: www.alz.org

**American Academy of
Allergy, Asthma &
Immunology**
611 East Wells Street
Milwaukee, WI 53202
Phone: (414) 272-6071
Fax: (414) 272-6070
Web Address: www.aaaai.org

**American Academy of
Dermatology**
930 N Meacham Rd
Schaumburg, IL 60173
Phone: 888-462-DERM
Web Address: www.aad.org

**American Academy of Family
Physicians**
11400 Tomahawk Creek Pkwy
Leawood, KS 66211-2672
Phone: 800-274-2237
Fax: (913) 906-6975
Web Address: www.aafp.org

**American Academy of
Pediatrics**
141 Northwest Point Blvd
Elk Grove Village, IL 60007-
1098
Phone: (847) 228-5005
Fax: (847) 434-8000
Web Address: www.aap.org

**American Academy of
Physical Medicine and
Rehabilitation**
One IBM Plaza
Suite 2500
Chicago, IL 60611-3604
Phone: (312) 464-9700
Fax: (312) 464-0227
Web Address: www.aapmr.org

**American Anorexia Bulimia
Association, Inc.**
165 W 46th St
Suite 1108
New York, NY 10036
Phone: (212) 575-6200
Fax: (212) 278-0698
Web Address: www.aabainc.org

**American Association of
Gynecologic Laparoscopists**
13021 E Florence Ave
Santa Fe Springs, CA 90670-
4505
Phone: 800-554-AAGL
Fax: (562) 946-0073
Web Address: www.aagl.com

American Association of Sex Educators, Counselors, and Therapists
PO Box 238
Mount Vernon, IA 52314
Fax: (319) 895-6203
Web Address: www.aasect.org

American Cancer Society
1599 Clifton Road, NE
Atlanta, GA 30329
Phone: 800-ACS-2345
Web Address: www.cancer.org

American College of Medical Genetics
9650 Rockville Pike
Bethesda, MD 20814-3998
Phone: (301) 530-7127
Fax: (301) 571-1895
Web Address: www.faseb.org/
genetics/acmg

American College of Obstetricians and Gynecologists
409 12th Street, SW
PO Box 96920
Washington, DC 20090-6920
Phone: (202) 638-5577
Fax: (202) 484-5107
Web Address: www.acog.org

American Council for Drug Education
164 W 74th St
New York, NY 10023
Phone: 800-488-DRUG
Fax: (212) 595-2553
Web Address: www.acde.org

American Diabetes Association, Inc.
National Office
1701 N Beauregard St
Alexandria, VA 22311
Phone: 800-342-2383
Web Address: www.diabetes.org

American Dietetic Association
216 W Jackson Blvd
Chicago, IL 60606-6995
Phone: 800-877-1600
Fax: (312) 899-4758
Web Address: www.eatright.org

American Heart Association National Center
7272 Greenville Ave
Dallas, TX 75231
Web Address: www.amhrt.org

American Institute of Stress
124 Park Ave
Yonkers, NY 10703
Phone: (914) 963-1200
Fax: (914) 965-6267
Web Address: www.stress.org

American Liver Foundation
75 Maiden Lane, Suite 603
New York, NY 10038
Phone: 800-GO-LIVER
Web Address: www.liverfoun
dation.org

American Lung Association
1740 Broadway
New York, NY 10019
Phone: 800-LUNG-USA
Fax: (212) 265-7374
Web Address: www.lungusa.org

American Medical Association
515 N State St
Chicago, IL 60610
Phone: (312) 464-5000
Web Address: www.ama-assn.org

American Psychiatric Association
1400 K St, NW
Washington, DC 20005
Phone: 888-357-2721
Fax: (202) 682-6850
Web Address: www.psych.org

American Psychological Association
750 First St, NE
Washington, DC 20002-4242
Phone: 800-374-2721
Web Address: www.apa.org

American Social Health Association
PO Box 13827
Research Triangle Park, NC 27709
Phone: (919) 361-8400
Fax: (919) 361-8425
Web Address: www.ashastd.org

American Society for Colposcopy and Cervical Pathology
20 W Washington St, Suite 1
Hagerstown, MD 21740
Phone: 800-787-7227
Fax: (301) 733-5775
Web Address: www.asccp.org

American Society for Reproductive Medicine
1209 Montgomery Highway
Birmingham, AL 35216-2809
Phone: (205) 978-5000
Fax: (205) 978-5005
Web Address: www.asrm.org

American Urogynecologic Society
2025 M St, NW
Suite 800
Washington, DC 20036
Phone: (202) 367-1167
Fax: (202) 367-2167
Web Address: www.augs.org

Anxiety Disorders Association of America
11900 Parklawn Dr, Suite 100
Rockville, MD 20852
Phone: (301) 231-9350
Fax: (301) 231-7392
Web Address: www.adaa.org

AVSC International
440 Ninth Ave
New York, NY 10001
Phone: 800-564-AVSC
Web Address: www.avsc.org

Centers for Disease Control and Prevention
1600 Clifton Rd, NE
Atlanta, GA 30333
Phone: 800-311-3435
Web Address: www.cdc.gov

Compassionate Friends
PO Box 3696
Oak Brook, IL 60522-3696
Phone: (630) 990-0010
Fax: (630) 990-0246
Web Address: www.compassion atefriends.org

DES Action USA
Phone: 800-DES-9288
Web Address: www.desaction.org

Endometriosis Association
8585 N 76th Place
Milwaukee, WI 53223
Phone: 800-992-3636
Fax: (414) 355-6065
Web Address: www.endometrio sisassn.org

Health Education Resource Services
353 S 5th St
Coos Bay, OR 97420
Phone: 503-267-3134
Fax: 510-841-6641
E-mail: larson@ocf.berkeley.edu

Healthy Mothers, Healthy Babies Coalition
121 N Washington St
Suite 300
Alexandria, VA 22314
Phone: (703) 836-6110
Fax: (703) 836-3470
Web Address: www.hmhb.org

International Childbirth Education Association
PO Box 20048
Minneapolis, MI 55420
Phone: (612) 854-8660
Fax: (612) 854-8772
Web Address: www.icea.org

La Leche League
1400 N Meacham Rd
Schaumburg, IL 60173-4048
Phone: 800-LALECHE
Fax: (847) 519-0035
Web Address: www.laleche
  league.org

March of Dimes
1275 Mamaroneck Ave
White Plains, NY 10605
Phone: 888-MODIMES
Fax: (914) 428-8203
Web Address: www.modimes.
  org

National Association for Continence
PO Box 8310
Spartanburg, SC 29305
Phone: 800-BLADDER

National Cancer Institute
NCI Public Inquiries Office
Building 31, Room 10A03
31 Center Drive, MSC 2580
Bethesda, MD 20892-2580
Phone: 800-422-6237
Web Address: www.nci.nih.gov

National Center for Complementary and Alternative Medicine
NCCAM Clearinghouse
PO Box 8218
Silver Spring, MD 20907-8218
Phone: 888-644-6226
Fax: (301) 495-4957
Web Address: nccam.nih.gov

National Center for Health Statistics
6525 Bellcrest Rd, Suite 1064
Hyattsville, MD 20782-2003
Phone: (301) 458-4636
Web Address: www.cdc.gov/nchs

National Coalition Against Domestic Violence
PO Box 18749
Denver, CO 80218-0749
Phone: (303) 839-1852
Fax: (303) 831-9251
Web Address: www.ncadv.org

National Coalition Against Sexual Assault
125 N Enola Dr
Enola, PA 17025
Fax: (717) 728-9781
Web Address: www.ncasa.org

National Headache Foundation
428 W St James Place
2nd Floor
Chicago, IL 60614
Phone: 888-NHF-5552
Fax: (773) 525-7357
Web Address: www.headaches.org

National Heart, Lung, and Blood Institute
NHLBI Information Center
PO Box 30105
Bethesda, MD 20824-0105
Phone: (301) 592-8573
Fax: (301) 592-8563
Web Address: www.nhlbi.nih.gov

National Institute of Mental Health
6001 Executive Blvd
Room 8184, MSC 9663
Bethesda, MD 20892
Phone: (301) 443-4513
Fax: (301) 443-4279
Web Address: www.nimh.nih.gov

National Kidney Foundation
30 E 33rd St, Suite 1100
New York, NY 10016
Phone: 800-622-9010
Fax: (212) 689-9261
Web Address: www.kidney.org

National Osteoporosis Foundation
1232 22nd St, NW
Washington, DC 20037-1292
Phone: (202) 223-2226
Fax: (202) 223-2237
Web Address: www.nof.org

National Women's Health Network
514 10th St, NW, Suite 400
Washington, DC 20004
Phone: (202) 347-1140
Fax: (202) 347-1168
Web Address: www.womens
    healthnetwork.org

National Womens Health Resource Center
120 Albany Street, Suite 820
New Brunswick, NJ 08901
Phone: (732) 828-4503
Fax: (732) 249-4671
Web Address: www.healthy
    women.org

North American Menopause Society
PO Box 94527
Cleveland, OH 44101-4527
Phone: (440) 442-7550
Fax: (440) 442-2660
Web Address: www.menopause.org

Planned Parenthood Federation ofAmerica
810 Seventh Ave
New York, NY 10019
Phone: 800-829-7732
Fax: (212) 245-1845
Web Address: www.planned
    parenthood.org

Postpartum Support International
927 N Kellogg Ave
Santa Barbara, CA 93111
Phone: (805) 967-7636
Fax: (805) 967-0608
Web Address: www.postpar
    tum.net

Resolve
1310 Broadway
Somerville, MA 02144
Phone: (617) 623-0744
Web Address: www.resolve.org

SIECUS
130 W 42nd St
Suite 350
New York, NY 10036-7802
Phone: (212) 819-9770
Fax: (212) 819-9776
Web Address: www.siecus.org

HOTLINES

ABMS Certification Hotline
800-776-CERT

Abortion Hotline
800-772-9100

AIDS Hotline (National)
800-342-AIDS (English)
800-344-7432 (Spanish)
800-243-7889 (TTY)

C-SAT National Drug Hotline
800-662-4357

CDC Immunization Information Hotline
800-232-2522 (English)
800-232-0233 (Spanish)

National Drug and Alcohol Treatment Referral Service
800-622-HELP

Consumer Nutrition Hotline (ADA)
800-366-1655

Covenant House (suicide)
800-999-9999

Domestic Violence Hotline
800-799-SAFE

Emergency Contraception Hotline
888-NOT-2-LATE

FDA National Hotline
800-532-4440

Gay and Lesbian National Hotline
888-843-4564

Gilda Radner Familial Ovarian Cancer Registry
800-682-7426

International Association for Medical Assistance to Travelers
(716) 754-4883

National Abortion Federation
202-667-5881

National Cancer Institute's Cancer Information Service
800-4-CANCER

National Center for Victims of Crime INFOLINK Services
800-FYI-CALL

National Substance Abuse Hotline
800-DRUG-HELP

National Women's Health Information Center
800-994-WOMAN

Planned Parenthood
800-230-7526

Pregnancy Riskline
(801) 328-2229

Pregnant Workers Rights
Dept of Labor Work & Family Clearinghouse
800-827-5335

Rape, Abuse & Incest National Network (RAINN)
800-656-HOPE

Resolve (Infertility)
(617) 623-0744

STD Hotlines
(877) HPV-5868 (HPV)
(919) 361-8488 (Herpes)
800-227-8922 (other STDs)

Teen Helpline
800-637-0701

Travel Information
CDC International Travelers'
Hotline
877-FYI-TRIP

GLOSSARY

Abruptio Placentae: A condition in which the placenta has begun to separate from the inner wall of the uterus before the baby is born.

Abstinence: Not engaging in sexual intercourse.

Acquired Immunodeficiency Syndrome (AIDS): A group of signs and symptoms, usually of severe infections, occurring in a person whose immune system has been damaged by infection with human immunodeficiency virus (HIV).

Acyclovir: A drug used as treatment against herpes; it may be effective in reducing symptoms during a first outbreak of the disease and in shortening the duration of recurrences. It may also help prevent recurrences.

Adenocarcinoma: The most common kind of cancer of the uterus. About 75% of women diagnosed with adenocarcinoma of the endometrium have Stage I disease and a 5-year survival rate of up to 90%.

Adenomyosis: A condition in which tissue similar to that which normally lines the uterus begins to grow inside the uterine wall.

Adhesion: Scarring that binds together the surfaces of tissues inside the abdomen or uterus.

Adolescence: The period between puberty (appearance of secondary sex characteristics) and adulthood (end of body growth).

Alpha-Fetoprotein (AFP): A protein produced by a growing fetus; it is present in amniotic fluid and, in smaller amounts, in the mother's blood.

Amenorrhea: The absence of menstrual periods.

Amniocentesis: A procedure in which a small amount of amniotic fluid and cells are taken from the sac surrounding the fetus and tested.

Amniotic Fluid: Water in the sac surrounding the fetus in the mother's uterus.

Amniotic Sac: Fluid-filled sac in the mother's uterus in which the fetus develops.

Analgesia: Relief of pain without total loss of sensation.

Androgen: Any steroid hormone, produced by the adrenal gland or by the ovaries, that promotes male characteristics, such as a beard and deepening voice.

Anemia: Abnormally low levels of blood or red blood cells in the bloodstream. Most cases are caused by iron deficiency, or lack of iron.

Anencephaly: A type of neural tube defect that occurs when the fetus's head and brain do not develop normally.

Anesthesia: Relief of pain by loss of sensation.

Anesthesiologist: A doctor who is specially trained to give anesthesia.

Anorexia Nervosa: An eating disorder in which distorted body image leads a person to diet excessively.

Anovulation: Failure to ovulate.

Antibiotics: Drugs that treat infections.

Antibody: A protein in the blood produced in reaction to foreign substances.

Anticonvulsants: Drugs that control or prevent seizures (as in epilepsy).

Antigen: A substance, such as an organism causing infection or a protein found on the surface of blood cells, that can induce an immune response and cause the production of an antibody.

Antiprostaglandins: Drugs that relieve menstrual cramps by preventing the formation of the chemical substances (prostaglandins) responsible for uterine contractions.

Apgar Score: A measurement of a baby's response to birth and life on its own, taken 1 and 5 minutes after birth.

Areola: The darker skin around the nipple.

Artificial Insemination: A procedure in which semen from a male donor is placed into a woman's vagina, cervix, or uterus.

Aspiration Biopsy: A procedure in which fluid or tissue within a cyst is withdrawn through a needle for study.

Atherosclerosis: Narrowing and clogging of the arteries by a buildup of plaque deposited in vessel walls; also called hardening of the arteries.

Atrophic Vaginitis: A type of vaginitis that is linked with estrogen deficiency and can occur in breastfeeding and menopause.

Aura: A sensation, such as flashing lights, experienced just before the onset of certain disorders such as migraine attacks or epileptic seizures.

Auscultation: A method of listening to the fetal heartbeat during labor, either with a special stethoscope or the use of a Doppler ultrasound device.

Autoinoculation: Transfer of germs from a part of one's own body to another part.

Autopsy: An exam performed on a deceased person in an attempt to find the cause of death.

Ayurveda: A system of medicine from India that treats illness through lifestyle changes and natural therapies in the belief that all disease begins with a problem or stress in the person's awareness.

Bacterial Vaginosis: A type of vaginal infection caused by the overgrowth of a number of organisms that are normally found in the vagina.

Barrier Methods: Means of contraception that prevent sperm from entering the female reproductive system, including male condom (a thin rubber sheath covering the penis), female condom (a plastic pouch that lines the vagina, held in place by a closed inner ring at the cervix and an open outer ring at the opening of the vagina), diaphragm (a molded cup fitted over the cervix), cervical cap (a small rubber cup that fits over the cervix and stays in place by suction), and spermicidal creams, jellies, foams, and suppositories (chemicals that inactivate sperm).

Bartholin Glands: Small organs that are located just under the skin at the entrance to the vagina and produce some of the lubrication during sexual excitement.

Benign: Noncancerous growth usually confined to one part of the body.

Biofeedback: A technique in which an attempt is made to control body functions that are thought to be out of one's control—such as heartbeat or blood pressure—by using a special device to monitor the function and signal changes to it.

Biofield Therapeutics: A treatment system in which a practitioner lays hands on or near a person's body to improve general health or to treat a specific problem. The healing force is believed to come from a supernatural force, such as God or the cosmos.

Biophysical Profile: An assessment by ultrasound of fetal breathing, fetal body movement, fetal muscle tone, and the amount of amniotic fluid. May include fetal heart rate.

Biopsy: A minor surgical procedure to remove a small piece of tissue that is then examined under a microscope in a laboratory.

Bisexual: Being attracted to members of both sexes.

Bladder: A muscular organ in which urine is stored.

Blood Count: A test to detect anemia and infection.

Bone Loss: The gradual loss of calcium and protein from bone, making it brittle and susceptible to fracture.

Braxton Hicks Contractions: False labor pains.

Breakthrough Bleeding: Vaginal bleeding at a time other than the menstrual period; it sometimes occurs while taking birth control pills.

Breast Implants: Sacs filled with saline or silicone gel that are placed in the chest or breast area.

Breech Presentation: A situation in which a fetus's buttocks or feet would be born first.

Bronchitis: A lung disease that causes persistent coughing and shortness of breath.

Bulimia: An eating disorder in which a person binges on food and then forces vomiting or abuses laxatives.

CA 125: A substance in the blood that may increase at the presence of a cancerous tumor.

Carotid Artery: The chief blood vessel that carries blood to the head and neck.

Calcium: A mineral stored in bone that gives it hardness.

Calorie: A unit of heat used to express the fuel or energy value of food.

Candidiasis: Also called yeast infection or moniliasis, a type of vaginitis caused by the overgrowth of Candida (a fungus normally found in the vagina).

Cardiovascular Disease: Disease of the heart and blood vessels.

Carrier (infections): A person who is infected with the organism of a disease without showing symptoms and can transmit the disease to another person.

Carrier (genetics): A person who shows no signs of a particular disorder but could pass the gene on to his or her children.

Catheter: A tube used to drain fluid or urine from the body.

Cephalopelvic Disproportion: A condition in which a baby is too large to pass safely through the mother's pelvis during delivery.

Cervical Intraepithelial Neoplasia (CIN): Another term for dysplasia; a noncancerous condition that occurs when normal cells on the surface of the cervix are replaced by a layer of abnormal cells. CIN is graded as 1 (mild dysplasia), 2 (moderate dysplasia), or 3 (severe dysplasia).

Cervicitis: Inflammation of the cervix.

Cervix: The lower, narrow end of the uterus, which protrudes into the vagina.

Cesarean Birth: Delivery of a baby through an incision made in the mother's abdomen and uterus.

Chancre: An infectious sore caused by syphilis and appearing at the place of infection.

Chiropractic: A therapy based on the belief that disease is a result of a problem with nerves or the nervous system and the best treatment is manipulation of the spinal column.

Chlamydial Infection: A sexually transmitted disease that can cause pelvic inflammatory disease, infertility, and problems during pregnancy.

Chloasma: The darkening of areas of skin on the face during pregnancy.

Cholesterol: A natural substance that serves as a building block for cells and hormones and helps to carry fat through the blood vessels for use or storage in other parts of the body.

Chorioamnionitis: Inflammation of the membrane surrounding the fetus.

Choriocarcinoma: A cancer of the placenta.

Chorionic Villi: Microscopic, fingerlike projections that make up the placenta.

Chorionic Villus Sampling (CVS): A procedure in which a small sample of cells is taken from the placenta and tested.

Chromosomes: Structures that are located inside each cell in the body and contain the genes that determine a person's physical makeup.

Chronic Pelvic Pain: Persistent pain in the pelvic region that has lasted for at least 6 months.

Cirrhosis: A disease caused by loss of liver cells, which are replaced by scar tissue that impairs liver function.

Classical (High Vertical) Incision: An incision used for cesarean delivery, made up and down in the upper area of the uterus.

Clindamycin: An antibiotic used to treat, among other kinds of infections, certain types of vaginitis.

Clitoris: An organ that is located near the opening to the vagina and is a source of female sexual excitement.

Collaborative Practice: A type of practice where care is given by a team of professionals.

Colonized: Having bacteria in your body that could cause illness, but having no symptoms of the disease.

Colonoscopy: An exam of the entire colon using a small, lighted instrument.

Colostrum: A fluid secreted in the breasts at the beginning of milk production.

Colposcope: A special magnifying instrument used to examine the cervix, vagina, and vulva.

Colposcopy: Viewing of the cervix, vulva, or vagina under magnification with an instrument called a colposcope.

Compact Bone: A type of bone that is nearly solid.

Condyloma: Another name for the genital warts caused by human papillomavirus.

Cone Biopsy: Surgical removal of cone-shaped wedges of cervical tissue.

Congenital Disorder: A condition that is present at birth.

Conization: A procedure in which a cone-shaped wedge of tissue is removed from the cervix.

Contraception: Prevention of pregnancy.

Contraceptive Implants: Soft plastic tubes placed under the skin that slowly release a hormone to prevent pregnancy.

Contraceptive Injection: A shot given every 3 months that contains a hormone to prevent pregnancy.

Contraction Stress Test: A test in which mild contractions of the mother's uterus are induced and the fetus's heart rate in response to the contractions is recorded using an electronic fetal monitor.

Copayment: The amount you pay each time you use a health care service.

Coronary Artery Disease: A disease in which the arteries that supply blood to the heart are narrowed by the buildup of cholesterol and other deposits in the walls of the arteries.

Corpus Luteum: The remains of the egg follicle after ovulation.

Corticosteroids: Hormones given to mature fetal lungs, for arthritis, or other medical conditions.

Cryotherapy: A freezing technique used to destroy diseased tissue; also known as "cold cautery."

Culdocentesis: A test that determines the presence of blood or pus in a space behind the uterus.

Curettage: A procedure in which a sample of the endometrium is removed with a small, spoon-shaped instrument.

Cystectomy: Surgical removal of a cyst.

Cystitis: An infection of the bladder.

Cystocele: Bulging of the bladder into the vagina.

Cystoscopy: A test in which the inside of the urethra and bladder are examined.

Cystourethrocele: Bulging of the bladder neck into the vagina.

Cystourethrography: A test to determine whether urine is passing normally through the urinary tract.

Depression: A treatable medical disorder characterized by loss of interest in things you used to enjoy and feeling sad for periods of at least 2 weeks.

Diabetes: A condition in which the levels of glucose (sugar) in the blood are too high.

Diagnostic Surgery: An operation performed to discover a problem or to confirm a doctor's belief about what might be wrong.

Diastolic Blood Pressure: The force of the blood in the arteries when the heart is relaxed; the lower blood pressure reading.

Digestive System: A system in the body made up of the stomach, bowels, liver, gallbladder, and pancreas. Breaks down food and removes waste from the body.

Dilation: Stretching of the walls of the cervix so that the opening of the cervix is widened.

Dilation and Curettage (D&C): A procedure in which the cervix is opened and tissue is gently scraped or suctioned from the inside of the uterus.

Discordant: A large difference in the size of fetuses in a multiple pregnancy.

Diuretics: Drugs given to increase the production of urine.

Diverticulum: An abnormal pouch or sac in an internal organ or structure.

Doppler: A form of ultrasound that reflects motion—such as the fetal heartbeat—in the form of audible signals.

Down Syndrome: A genetic disorder caused by the presence of an extra chromosome and characterized by mental retardation, abnormal features of the face, and medical problems such as heart defects.

Dysmenorrhea: Discomfort and pain during the menstrual period.

Dyspareunia: Pain during or after intercourse.

Dysplasia: A noncancerous condition that occurs when normal cells on the surface of the cervix are replaced by a layer of abnormal cells. Dysplasia is classified as mild, moderate, or severe.

Dysuria: Pain during urination.

Early Menopause: Menopause that occurs because the ovaries have been removed during an operation or have stopped functioning at an early age.

Eclampsia: Seizures occurring in pregnancy and linked to high blood pressure.

Ectopic Pregnancy: A pregnancy in which the fertilized egg begins to grow in a place other than inside the uterus, usually in the fallopian tubes.

Edema: Swelling caused by fluid retention.

Egg: The female reproductive cell produced in and released from the ovaries; also called the ovum.

Electrical Excision: The removal of abnormal growths (of the cervix, vagina, vulva) using a thin wire loop and electric energy.

Electrocardiogram (EKG): A procedure in which the heartbeat is monitored and the results recorded as a graph.

Electrocautery: A procedure in which an instrument works with electric current to destroy tissue.

Electrode: A small wire that is attached to the scalp of the fetus to monitor the heart rate.

Electronic Fetal Monitoring: A method in which electronic instruments are used to record the heartbeat of the fetus and contractions of the mother's uterus.

Electrosurgery: A procedure used to destroy or remove diseased tissue with an electric current.

Embryo: The developing fertilized egg of early pregnancy.

Emphysema: A lung disease in which the elasticity of the lungs is destroyed.

Endometrial Biopsy: A test in which a small amount of the tissue lining the uterus is removed and examined under a microscope.

Endometriosis: A condition in which tissue similar to that normally lining the uterus is found outside of the uterus, usually on the ovaries, fallopian tubes, and other pelvic structures.

Endometrium: The lining of the uterus.

Enema: A liquid injected into the rectum to empty the intestines.

Enterocele: Bulging of the intestine into the upper part of the vagina.

Epidural Block: Anesthesia that numbs the lower half of the body.

Episiotomy: A surgical incision made into the perineum (the region between the vagina and the anus) to widen the vaginal opening for delivery.

Epithelial Ovarian Cancer: The most common kind of ovarian cancer; it accounts for about 90% of all cases of the disease.

Erection: A lengthening and hardening of the penis.

Estrogen: A female hormone produced in the ovaries that stimulates the growth of the lining of the uterus.

Estrogen Replacement Therapy: Treatment in which estrogen is taken to relieve the symptoms caused by the lack of estrogen produced by the body.

External Version: A technique, performed late in pregnancy, in which the doctor manually attempts to move a baby in the breech position into the normal, head-down position.

Fallopian Tubes: Tubes through which an egg travels from the ovary to the uterus.

Fascia: Tissue that supports the organs and muscles of the body.

Fecal Occult Blood Test: A test of a stool sample for blood, which could be a sign of cancer of the colon or rectum.

Fertilization: Joining of the egg and sperm.

Fetal Alcohol Syndrome: A pattern of physical, mental, and behavioral problems in the baby that are thought to be due to alcohol abuse by the mother during pregnancy.

Fetal Blood Sampling: A procedure in which a sample of blood is taken from the umbilical cord and tested.

Fetal Distress: A sign that the fetus may be having problems before delivery.

Fetal Monitoring: A procedure in which instruments are used to record the heartbeat of the fetus and contractions of the mother's uterus during labor.

Fetoscope: A stethoscope designed for listening to the fetal heartbeat.

Fetus: A baby growing in the woman's uterus.

Fibrocystic Changes: Formation of benign cysts and lumps of various sizes in the breast.

Fibroids: Benign (noncancerous) growths that form on the inside of the uterus, on its outer surface, or within the uterine wall itself.

Fine Needle Aspiration: A procedure in which a needle and syringe are used to withdraw a small amount of tissue. The tissue sample then is examined under a microscope to look for cancer cells.

Fistula: An abnormal opening or passage between two internal organs.

Follicle: The saclike structure that forms inside an ovary when an egg is produced.

Follicle-Stimulating Hormone (FSH): A hormone produced by the pituitary gland that helps an egg to mature and be released.

Forceps: Special instruments placed around the baby's head to help guide it out of the birth canal during delivery.

Foreskin: A layer of skin covering the end of the penis.

Fragile X: A genetic disease of the X chromosome that is the most common inherited cause of mental retardation.

Fraternal Twins: Twins that have developed from two fertilized eggs; they are not genetically identical, and each has its own placenta and amniotic sac.

Functional Cyst: A benign cyst that forms on an ovary and usually resolves on its own without treatment.

Gamete Intrafallopian Transfer (GIFT): A treatment for infertility in which eggs are removed from a woman's ovary, mixed with the man's sperm, and placed in a fallopian tube to achieve a pregnancy.

Gay: A term commonly used to mean homosexual.

Gene: A DNA "blueprint" that codes for specific traits, such as hair and eye color.

General Anesthesia: The use of drugs that produce a sleeplike state to prevent pain during surgery.

Genital Herpes: A sexually transmitted disease caused by a virus that produces painful, highly infectious sores on or around the sex organs.

Genitals: The sexual or reproductive organs.

Gestation: Pregnancy; the period from conception until birth.

Gestational Diabetes: Diabetes that arises during pregnancy; it results from the effects of hormones and usually subsides after delivery.

Glans: The head of the penis.

Glucose: A sugar that is present in the blood and is the body's main source of fuel.

Goiter: An enlarged thyroid gland that causes a lump in the neck.

Gonadotropin-Releasing Hormone (GnRH) Agonists: Medical therapy used to block the effects of certain hormones.

Gonorrhea: A sexually transmitted disease that may lead to pelvic inflammatory disease, infertility, and arthritis.

Gynecology: The branch of medicine that involves care of the female reproductive system and breasts.

Hepatitis: Inflammation of the liver.

Hepatitis B Immune Globulin: A substance given to provide temporary protection against infection with hepatitis B virus.

Hepatitis B Virus (HBV): A virus that attacks and damages the liver, causing inflammation, cirrhosis, and chronic hepatitis that can lead to cancer.

Heterosexual: Being attracted to members of the opposite sex.

High-Risk Pregnancy: A pregnancy with complications that need special medical attention.

Hirsutism: Excessive hair on the face, abdomen, and chest caused by high levels of the male hormone androgen.

Homeopathy: A system of medical treatment that uses very small amounts of remedies that in massive doses would cause symptoms like those of the disease being treated.

Homosexual: Being attracted to members of the same sex.

Hormone Replacement Therapy: Treatment in which estrogen, and often progestin, is taken to relieve the symptoms caused by the low levels of hormones produced by the body.

Hormones: Substances produced by the body to control the functions of various organs.

Hot Flashes: Sensations of heat in the skin that occur when estrogen levels are low; also called hot flushes.

Human Chorionic Gonadotropin (hCG): A hormone produced during pregnancy; its detection is the basis for most pregnancy tests.

Human Immunodeficiency Virus (HIV): A virus that attacks certain cells of the body's immune system and causes acquired immunodeficiency syndrome (AIDS).

Human Papillomavirus (HPV): The common name for a group of related viruses, some of which cause genital warts and are linked to cervical changes and cervical cancer.

Hydramnios: A condition in which there is an excess amount of amniotic fluid in the sac surrounding the fetus.

Hymen: A membrane at the entrance of the vaginal opening.

Hyperactivity: Excessive or abnormally increased activity, especially in children.

Hyperemesis Gravidarum: Severe nausea and vomiting during pregnancy that can lead to loss of weight and body fluids.

Hyperthermia: Very high body temperature.

Hyperthyroidism: A condition in which the thyroid gland makes too much thyroid hormone.

Hypnotherapy: Treatment based on using hypnosis (a created sleeplike condition in which a person responds to suggestions made by the person who hypnotized them).

Hypothyroidism: A condition in which the thyroid gland makes too little thyroid hormone.

Hysterectomy: Removal of the uterus.

Hysterosalpingography: A special X-ray procedure in which a small amount of fluid is injected into the uterus and fallopian tubes to detect abnormal changes in their size and shape or to determine whether the tubes are blocked.

Hysteroscopy: A surgical procedure in which a slender, light-transmitting telescope, the hysteroscope, is used to view the inside of the uterus or perform surgery.

Identical Twins: Twins that have developed from a single fertilized egg; they are usually genetically identical and may or may not share the same placenta and amniotic sac.

Immune System: The body's natural defense system against foreign substances and invading organisms, such as bacteria that cause disease.

Impotence: The inability in a male to achieve an erection or to sustain it until ejaculation or until intercourse takes place.

Incompetent Cervix: A cervix that begins to dilate or open earlier than it should in pregnancy.

Incontinence: Inability to control bodily functions such as urination.

Induced Abortion: The planned termination of a pregnancy before the fetus can survive outside the uterus.

Infertility: A condition in which a couple has been unable to get pregnant after 12 months without the use of any form of birth control.

Inflammation: Pain, swelling, redness, and irritation of tissues in the body.

Informed Consent: The process by which a patient gains an understanding of what will be involved in receiving a medical treatment or procedure, including why it is being done, its risks, and other alternatives, before agreeing to treatment.

Insulin: A hormone that lowers the levels of glucose (sugar) in the blood.

Intrauterine Device (IUD): A small device that is inserted and left inside the uterus to prevent pregnancy.

Intravenous Pyelography: A test performed to find defects or abnormal structures in the urinary tract.

Invasive: A term used to describe cancer that has invaded and can destroy surrounding healthy tissues.

In Vitro Fertilization: A procedure in which an egg is removed from a woman's ovary, fertilized in a dish in a laboratory with the man's sperm, and then reintroduced into the woman's uterus to achieve a pregnancy.

Jaundice: A buildup of bilirubin that causes a yellowish appearance.

Kegel Exercises: Pelvic muscle exercises that assist in bladder and bowel control.

Kick Count: A record kept during late pregnancy of the number of times a fetus moves over a certain period.

Kidneys: Two organs that cleanse the blood, removing liquid wastes.

Labia: Folds of skin on either side of the vulva.

Labia Majora: The outer folds of tissue, or lips, of the vulva.

Labia Minora: The inner folds of tissue, or lips, of the vulva.

Lactation: Production of breast milk.

Lactose Intolerant: Being unable to digest dairy products.

Laminaria: Slender rods (natural and synthetic) inserted into the opening of the cervix to dilate it.

Laparoscopy: A surgical procedure in which a slender, light-transmitting instrument, the laparoscope, is used to view the pelvic organs or perform surgery.

Laparotomy: A surgical procedure in which an incision is made in the abdomen.

Laser: A small, intense beam of light used as a surgical tool.

Laxative: An agent that is used to empty the bowels.

Lecithin/Sphingomyelin (L/S) Ratio: Measurement of substances in the amniotic fluid to determine whether the fetus's lungs are mature enough to survive outside the uterus.

Leiomyomas: Benign (not cancerous) tumors made of muscle tissue that grow in the uterus and may cause pain or bleeding; commonly called fibroids.

Lesbian: A woman who is attracted to other women.

Leukorrhea: A heavy vaginal discharge.

Libido: The desire for, or interest in, sex; sex drive.

Linea Nigra: A line running from the navel to pubic hair that darkens during pregnancy.

Lipoprotein: Substances that transport cholesterol to and from the liver throughout the blood.

Local Anesthesia: The use of drugs that prevent pain in a part of the body.

Lochia: Vaginal discharge that occurs after delivery.

Loop Electrosurgical Excision Procedure (LEEP): A surgical procedure that uses an electrified loop of wire to remove abnormal tissue from the cervix.

Low Birth Weight: Weighing less than 5½ pounds at birth.

Low Vertical Incision: An incision used on the uterus for cesarean delivery, made up and down in the lower, thinner area of the uterus.

Lumpectomy: Surgical removal of a breast lump; also called biopsy.

Luteinizing Hormone (LH): A hormone produced by the pituitary glands that helps an egg to mature and be released.

Lymph: A nearly colorless fluid that bathes body cells and moves through a system of lymph vessels and nodes in the body.

Lymph Nodes: Small glands that filter the flow of lymph (a nearly colorless fluid that bathes body cells) through the body.

Macrosomia: A condition in which a fetus grows very large; this problem is often found in babies of diabetic mothers.

Malignant: Cancerous; tending to become progressively worse and, eventually, to spread to other parts of the body.

Mammogram: An X-ray of the breast, used to detect breast cancer.

Massage: The kneading or rubbing of parts of the body to help circulation or relax muscles.

Mastectomy: Surgical removal of part or all of the breast.

Masturbation: Self-stimulation of the genitals, usually resulting in orgasm.

Meconium: A greenish substance that builds up in the bowels of a growing fetus and is normally discharged shortly after birth.

Menarche: The time in a young woman's life when menstrual periods begin.

Meningitis: Inflammation of the membranes of the brain or spinal cord.

Menopause: The process in a woman's life when ovaries stop functioning and menstruation stops.

Menstruation: The discharge of blood and tissue from the uterus that occurs when an egg is not fertilized.

Metabolism: The physical and chemical processes in the body that maintain life.

Metastasize: Spreading of cancer to other parts of the body.

Metronidazole: An antibiotic used to treat some vaginal and abdominal infections.

Minilaparotomy: A small abdominal incision used for a sterilization procedure in which the fallopian tubes are closed off.

Miscarriage: The spontaneous loss of a pregnancy before the fetus can survive outside the uterus.

Molar Pregnancy: Growth of abnormal placental tissue in the uterus. Also called gestational trophoblastic disease (GTD).

Mons Veneris: The fleshy part of the female genital area that lies directly over the joint of the pubic bone.

Multiple Pregnancy: A pregnancy in which there are two or more fetuses.

Myomectomy: Surgical removal of uterine fibroids only, leaving the uterus in place.

Naturopathy: A system of treatment that relies on natural remedies—such as sunlight, diet, and massage—to treat the sick.

Needle Aspiration: A procedure in which a small amount of fluid or tissue is withdrawn through a needle for study.

Nephrons: Parts of the kidney that remove waste products from the blood, recover some substances to be used again by the body, and eliminate what is left as urine.

Neural Tube Defect (NTD): A birth defect that results from improper development of the brain, spinal cord, or their coverings.

Nicotine: An addictive drug contained in tobacco.

Nocturia: The need to urinate frequently during the night.

Nonstress Test: A test in which fetal movements felt by the mother or noted by the doctor are recorded, along with changes in the fetal heart rate, using an electronic fetal monitor.

Nutrients: Nourishing substances supplied through food, such as vitamins and minerals.

Obstetrician–Gynecologist: A physician with special skills, training, and education in women's health.

Oral Contraceptives: Birth control pills containing hormones that prevent ovulation and thus pregnancy.

Orgasm: The climax of sexual excitement.

Osteopathy: A system of medicine based on the theory that problems in the musculoskeletal system affect other body parts, which cause disorders that can be treated with various manipulation techniques along with conventional therapies.

Osteoporosis: A condition in which the bones become so fragile that they break more easily.

Ovaries: Two glands, located on either side of the uterus, which contain the eggs released at ovulation and that produce hormones.

Ovulation: The release of an egg from one of the ovaries.

Oxytocin: A drug used to help bring on contractions.

Papillomavirus: A sexually transmitted virus that causes small growths, called condylomas or genital warts, on or around the genitals.

Pap Test: A test in which cells are taken from the cervix and vagina and examined under a microscope.

Paracervical Block: The injection of a local anesthetic into the tissues around the cervix.

Pelvic Exam: A manual internal and external examination of a woman's reproductive organs.

Pelvic Inflammatory Disease: An infection of the uterus, fallopian tubes, and nearby pelvic structures.

Penis: An external male sex organ that can become engorged with blood to increase its size and fullness.

Perforation: An injury to the wall of the uterus; it can be caused by an intrauterine device or by an instrument used in a D&C.

Perineal Laceration: Tear in the tissues between the vaginal and rectal openings.

Perineum: The area between the vagina and the rectum.

Periodic Abstinence: Prevention of pregnancy by avoiding sexual intercourse during and close to the time of ovulation.

Peritoneum: The membrane that lines the abdominal cavity and surrounds the internal organs.

Pessary: A device inserted into the vagina to support sagging organs.

Pica: The urge to eat nonfood items.

Pituitary Gland: A gland located near the brain that controls growth and other changes in the body.

Placenta: Tissue that provides nourishment to and takes away waste from the fetus.

Placenta Previa: A condition in which the placenta lies very low in the uterus, so that the opening of the uterus is partially or completely covered.

Podophyllin: A liquid drug that is used to treat genital warts.

Polycystic Ovary Syndrome (PCOS): A condition in which increased androgen causes multiple small cysts to persist on the ovaries.

Polyps: Benign (noncancerous) growths that develop from membrane tissue, such as that lining the inside of the uterus.

Postcoital Test: A test performed in infertile couples in which the woman's cervical mucus is examined after sexual intercourse to assess the ability of the man's sperm to penetrate and move into the cervical mucus.

Postpartum Blues: Feelings of sadness, fear, anger, or anxiety occurring about 3 days after childbirth and usually fading within 1–2 weeks.

Postpartum Depression: Intense feelings of sadness, anxiety, or despair after childbirth that interfere with a new mother's ability to function and that do not go away after 2 weeks.

Postpartum Sterilization: An operation that prevents a woman from becoming pregnant, performed immediately after the birth of her last child.

Postterm Pregnancy: A pregnancy that extends beyond 42 weeks.

Preeclampsia: A condition of pregnancy in which there is high blood pressure, swelling due to fluid retention, and abnormal kidney function.

Pregnancy-Induced Hypertension: High blood pressure that occurs during the second half of pregnancy and disappears soon after the baby is born.

Premature Rupture of Membranes: A condition in which the membranes that hold the amniotic fluid rupture before labor.

Premenstrual Syndrome (PMS): A term used to describe a group of physical and behavioral changes that some women experience before their menstrual periods every month.

Preterm: Born before 37 weeks of pregnancy.

Prenatal Care: A program of care for a pregnant woman before the birth of her baby.

Preinvasive: Abnormal cells that have not invaded other tissues.

Prodrome: A symptom that precedes the onset of a disease.

Progesterone: A female hormone that is produced in the ovaries and makes the lining of the uterus grow. When the level of progesterone decreases, menstruation occurs.

Progestin: A synthetic form of progesterone that is similar to the hormone produced naturally by the body.

Prostaglandins: Chemicals that are made by the body that have many effects, including causing the muscle of the uterus to contract, usually causing cramps.

Prostate Gland: A male gland that produces most of the fluid for ejaculation.

Puberty: The stage of life when the reproductive organs become functional and secondary sex characteristics develop.

Pubic Area: The external genital area.

Pudendal Block: An injection given in the vagina that relieves pain during childbirth.

Pyelonephritis: An infection of the kidney.

Quickening: The mother's first feeling of movement of the fetus.

Radiation Therapy: Treatment by exposing the affected area to high-energy radiation.

Real-Time: A type of ultrasound that uses still pictures to show movement, somewhat like a motion picture.

Rectocele: Bulging of the rectum into the vaginal wall.

Recurrent Infections: Infections that occur more than once, usually within a short time, although they may be spread out over several months.

Reflux: Backing up of urine in the urinary tract.

Regional Anesthesia: The use of drugs to block sensation in certain areas of the body.

Remodeling: A renewal process by which some bone cells add and others remove small amounts of bone.

Repeated Miscarriage: Consecutive loss of three or more pregnancies before 20 weeks of pregnancy.

Resectoscope: A slender telescope with an electrical wire loop or roller-ball tip used to remove or destroy tissue inside the uterus.

Resorption: A type of bone loss that increases its rate after menopause.

Respiratory Distress Syndrome (RDS): A condition of some babies in which the lungs are not mature.

Retracted Nipple: A nipple that has pulled inward.

Rh Immunoglobulin (RhIg): A substance given to prevent an Rh-negative person's antibody response to Rh-positive blood cells.

Salpingitis: Inflammation of the fallopian tube.

Salpingo-Oophorectomy: Removal of the ovary and fallopian tube.

Scan: A visual display of ultrasound echoes.

Screening Test: A test that looks for possible signs of disease in people who do not have symptoms.

Scrotum: The external genital sac in the male that contains the testes.

Sedative: An agent or drug that eases nervousness or tension.

Seminal Vesicles: A pair of pouchlike glands on each side of the male's bladder that secrete semen.

Sexual Abuse: Sex acts that are forced on one person by another.

Sexual Intercourse: The act of the penis of the male entering the vagina of the female (also called "having sex" or "making love").

Sexually Transmitted Disease: A disease that is spread by sexual contact, including chlamydial infection, gonorrhea, genital warts, herpes, syphilis, and infection with human immunodeficiency virus (HIV, the cause of acquired immunodeficiency syndrome [AIDS]).

Shock: A condition of very low blood pressure in response to bleeding or infection.

Sigmoidoscopy: A test in which a slender device is inserted into the rectum and lower colon to look for cancer. All women should have a sigmoidoscopy every 3–5 years beginning at age 50 years.

Smegma: A whitish, cheesy substance normally built up and shed from under the male foreskin.

Sonogram: A picture obtained by ultrasound.

Speculum: An instrument used to spread the walls of the vagina so that the cervix can be seen.

Sperm: A male cell that is produced in the testes and can fertilize a female egg cell.

Spina Bifida: A neural tube defect that results from incomplete closure of the fetal spine.

Spinal Block: A form of anesthesia that numbs the lower half of the body.

Spongy Bone: A type of bone that is not solid but is filled with holes, like a sponge.

Spontaneous Abortion: Miscarriage, or loss of a pregnancy before the fetus can survive outside the uterus.

Squamous Intraepithelial Lesion (SIL): Term used in Pap test reports that includes dysplasia, cervical intraepithelial neoplasia (CIN), and changes caused by human papillomavirus (a noncancerous condition that occurs when normal cells on the surface of the cervix are replaced by a layer of abnormal cells). SIL is classified as low grade or high grade.

Stage: Stage refers to the size of a tumor and the extent (if any) to which the disease has spread.

Stillbirth: Delivery of a baby that shows no sign of life.

Stroke: A sudden interruption of blood flow to all or part of the brain, caused by blockage or bursting of a blood vessel in the brain and often resulting in loss of consciousness and temporary or permanent paralysis.

Sudden Infant Death Syndrome (SIDS): The sudden death of any infant or young child that is unexpected and in which the cause of death is unknown.

Surrogate Motherhood: An arrangement in which a fertile woman agrees to conceive and carry a pregnancy for an infertile woman.

Syphilis: A sexually transmitted disease that is caused by an organism called *Treponema pallidum;* it may cause major health problems or death in its later stages.

Systemic Analgesia: The use of drugs that provide pain relief over the entire body without causing loss of consciousness.

Systolic Blood Pressure: The force of the blood in the arteries when the heart is contracting; the higher blood pressure reading.

Tachycardia: Rapid heartbeat.

Tai Chi: A Chinese system of exercises designed for meditation and development of self-discipline and a sense of well-being.

Target Heart Rate: The level of heartbeat that gives you the best workout—about 60–80% of your maximum heart rate, which is usually 220 minus your age.

Teratogens: Agents that can cause birth defects when a woman is exposed to them during pregnancy.

Testes: Two male organs that produce the sperm and male sex hormones.

Thermography: A technique in which a heat-sensitive device is used to detect breast lumps.

Thyroid-Stimulating Hormone (TSH): A hormone made by the pituitary gland that encourages the thyroid gland to make more thyroid hormone.

Torsion: Twisting of a bodily organ or growth.

Toxoplasmosis: An infection caused by *Toxoplasma gondii,* an organism that may be found in raw and rare meat, garden soil, and cat feces and can be harmful to the fetus.

Transducer: A device that emits sound waves and translates the echoes into electrical signals.

Transfusion: Direct injection of whole blood or plasma into the bloodstream.

Transvaginal Ultrasound: A type of ultrasound in which a transducer specially designed to be placed in the vagina is used.

Transverse Incision: An incision used for cesarean delivery, made horizontally across the lower, thinner area of the uterus.

Trichomoniasis: A type of vaginal infection caused by a one-celled organism that is usually transmitted through sex.

Trimester: Any of the three 3-month periods into which pregnancy is divided.

Tubal Occlusion: Blockage of the fallopian tubes.

Tubal Sterilization: A method of female sterilization in which the fallopian tubes are closed by tying, banding, clipping, or sealing with electric current.

Tumor: Growth or lump made up of cells.

Twin–Twin Transfusion (TTS): A condition of identical twin fetuses when the blood passes from one twin to the other through a shared placenta.

Ultrasound: A test in which sound waves are used to examine internal structures. During pregnancy, it can be used to examine the fetus.

Umbilical Cord: A cordlike structure containing blood vessels that connects the fetus to the placenta.

Ureters: A pair of tubes, each leading from one of the kidneys to the bladder.

Urethra: A short, narrow tube that conveys urine from the bladder out of the body.

Urethritis: Infection of the urethra.

Urethrocele: Protrusion of the urethra into the vagina.

Urgency: A sudden, strong desire to urinate, even though the bladder may not be full.

Urinalysis: A test in which a sample of urine is analyzed.

Urinary Frequency: Urinating at short intervals, usually defined as more than every 2 hours or more than 7 times a day.

Urine: A liquid that is excreted by the body and is made up of wastes, water, and salt removed from the blood.

Uterine Prolapse: Falling of the uterus into the vagina.

Uterus: A muscular organ located in the female pelvis that contains and nourishes the developing fetus during pregnancy.

Vacuum Extraction: The use of a special instrument attached to the baby's head to help guide it out of the birth canal during delivery.

Vagina: A passageway surrounded by muscles leading from the uterus to the outside of the body, also known as the birth canal.

Vaginal Prolapse: Bulging of the top of the vagina into the lower vagina or outside the opening of the vagina.

Vaginismus: Involuntary spasm of the pubic muscles and lower vagina that makes penetration by the penis difficult, painful, or impossible.

Vanishing Twin: Loss of a twin in the first 3 months of pregnancy.

Varicocele: Varicose veins in the scrotum.

Vas Deferens: A small tube that carries sperm from a male testis to the prostate gland.

Vasectomy: A method of male sterilization in which a portion of the vas deferens is removed.

Veins: Blood vessels that carry blood from various parts of the body back to the heart.

Venereal Disease: Another term for sexually transmitted disease (STD)—a disease that is transmitted by sexual contact.

Vernix: The greasy, whitish coating of a newborn.

Vertex Presentation: A normal position assumed by a fetus in which the head is positioned down ready to be born first.

Vestibule: The space within the labia minora into which the vagina and urethra open.

Viable: Able to live outside the uterus; usually referring to a fetus.

Voiding: Passage of urine out of the body; urination.

Vulva: The lips of external female genital area.

Vestibulitis: Inflammation of an area near the opening of the vagina, the vestibule.

Wet Dream: When a male ejaculates during an erotic dream.

X-Ray Pelvimetry: A type of X-ray showing the size of both the mother's pelvis and the baby's head.

Zygote Intrafallopian Transfer (ZIFT): A procedure in which a zygote (a fertilized egg that has not divided) is placed in a fallopian tube to achieve a pregnancy.

INDEX

Note: Italicized letters *f* and *t* following page numbers indicate figures and tables, respectively.

F

FACOG. *See* Fellows
Fallopian tube(s), 8
  blockage of, 305, 306
  in ectopic pregnancy, 228–229,
    229*f*
  infection of. *See* Pelvic inflamma-
    tory disease
  in ovulation, 12*f*
  removal during hysterectomy, 303,
    327
  in tubal sterilization, 465–468
Falls, prevention of, 25, 34, 368
False labor, 322, 322*t*, 426
Family history
  in first prenatal visit, 422
  and pregnancy planning, 402
FASTER. *See* First and Second
    Trimester Evaluation of Risk
    (FASTER) study
Fat, 65
  body, 65, 81–82
  and cholesterol, 179–180, 183
  in diet, 65, 179–180, 183
  needs during pregnancy, 362*t*
  and nutrition, 65
  saturated, 65, 183
  unsaturated, 65, 183
  and weight, 81–82
Fathers, feelings with miscarriage,
    345
FDA. *See* U.S. Food and Drug
    Administration
Fecal incontinence. *See* Bowel con-
    trol, problems with
Female reproductive system, 8
Feminine hygiene products. *See*
    Menstrual hygiene products
Fertility awareness. *See* Natural family
    planning
Fertility drugs, 315, 350. *See also*
    Infertility
Fertilization, 14, 112, 113*f*, 312
Fetal alcohol syndrome, 103–104,
    136, 218
Fetal fibronectin test, 428
Fetal heart rate, 248
Fetal monitoring, 245–249
  auscultation, 246
  electronic, 209, 246–247, 248,
    249
  external, 247, 247*f*
  internal, 247, 247*f*
  risks of, 248
  types of, 246–247
Fiber, in diet, 147, 195*t*
Fibroadenomas, 151
Fibrocystic breast changes, 151,
    249–251
  detection of, 250
  versus premenstrual syndrome, 419
  relief of symptoms, 251
Fibroids (uterine). *See* Uterine
    fibroids

First and Second Trimester
    Evaluation of Risk (FASTER)
    study, 5
Fistulas, 474
Flunitrazepam, 432
Folic acid, 66–67, 361
  antiepileptic drugs and, 437, 438
  food sources of, 362, 362*t*
  functions of, 362*t*
  supplements, 67, 251–252,
    361–363, 404–405
Follicle-stimulating hormone (FSH),
    10
Food Guide Pyramid, 63–64, 64*f*
Food labels, 62, 63, 183
Foods, triggering headache, 265. *See
    also* Nutrition
Footling breech, 160
Forceps, 252
Fractures, 365. *See also* Hip fractures
Frank breech presentation, 160, 162
Fraternal twins, 350, 351*f*
FSH. *See* Follicle-stimulating hor-
    mone
Functional ovarian cysts, 371, 372

G

Gallbladder disease, 83
Gamete intrafallopian transfer
    (GIFT), 112
Gas, 252–253
Gastrointestinal disorders, and pelvic
    pain, 380, 383
Gastrointestinal reflux disease
    (GERD), 270
Gateways, 514
General anesthesia, 110
Generic drugs, 61
Genetic counseling, 256–257, 346,
    402
Genetic disorders, 253–258. *See also*
    Birth defects
  and genetic counseling, 256–257,
    402
  risk factors for, 255, 256
  testing for, 257–258
  types and causes of, 254–255
Genetic testing, 257–258
  for cancer risk, 368
  types of, 257–258
Genetics, 5, 253–254, 257
Genital herpes. *See* Herpes
Genital warts, 168, 301, 446, 504.
    See also Human papillomavirus
    (HPV) infection
  and pregnancy, 449*t*, 450
  treatment of, 301, 504
  and vulvar intraepithelial neoplasia,
    505
GERD. *See* Gastrointestinal reflux
    disease
Germ cell tumors, 368
Gestational diabetes, 201, 205, 209,
    210

Gestational trophoblastic disease
    (GTD), 348. *See also* Molar
    pregnancy
GIFT. *See* Gamete intrafallopian
    transfer
Glue sniffing, during pregnancy, 220
GnRH. *See* Gonadotropin-releasing
    hormone
GnRH agonists
  for endometriosis, 240
  for uterine fibroids, 492
Goiter, 462
Gonadotropin-releasing hormone
    (GnRH), 10
Gonorrhea, 258–261, 445–446
  and chlamydia, 174, 258
  diagnosis of, 260
  health risks of, 259–260
  incidence of, 258
  infection rate, 446
  and pelvic inflammatory disease,
    259, 376, 379, 446
  and pregnancy, 259–260, 448,
    449*t*
  prevention of, 261
  risk factors for, 260
  symptoms of, 259, 445–446, 449*t*
  treatment of, 261
Graves' disease, 463
Great American Smokeout, 79
Grief, at death of baby/miscarriage,
    345
Group B streptococcus (GBS), 261,
    262
  colonization with, 262
  effects on baby, 262
  infection during pregnancy,
    261–263
  risk factors for, 263
  testing for, 262–263
  treatment for infection, 263
GTD. *See* Gestational trophoblastic
    disease
Gum (nicotine replacement product),
    78
Guns, 34
Gynecologic oncology, 3
Gynecology. *See* Obstetrics and gyne-
    cology

H

Hair growth. *See* Hirsutism
Hashimoto's disease (thyroiditis),
    462
Hazardous substance exposure, and
    pregnancy, 136, 406–407
HBIG. *See* Hepatitis B immune glob-
    ulin
hCG. *See* Human chorionic
    gonadotropin
HDL. *See* High-density lipoprotein
Headache, 263–266
  doctor's questions about, 266
  prevention and control of, 264